Color Atlas of Hemoglobin Disorders

A Compendium Based on Proficiency Testing

Hemoglobinopathy Atlas Subcommittee
of the
Hematology and Clinical Microscopy
Resource Committee

James D. Hoyer, MD
Chairman and Editor

Steven H. Kroft, MD
Co-Editor

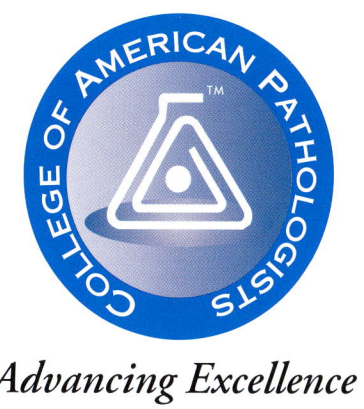

Advancing Excellence

Copyright 2003 College of American Pathologists (CAP). All rights reserved. None of the contents of this publication may be reproduced, stored in a retrieval system, or transmitted in any form or by any means (electronic, mechanical, photocopying, recording, or otherwise) without prior written permission from the publisher.

The inclusion of a product name or service in a CAP publication should not be construed as an endorsement of such product or service, nor is a failure to include the name of a product or service to be construed as disapproval.

Library of Congress Control Number: 2003106194
ISBN: 0-930304-80-2

Printed in U.S.A.

College of American Pathologists
325 Waukegan Road
Northfield, Illinois 60093-2750
800-323-4040
www.cap.org

Color Atlas of Hemoglobin Disorders

A Compendium Based on Proficiency Testing

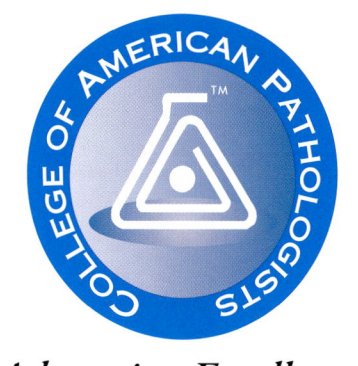

Advancing Excellence

Co-Editors
James D. Hoyer, MD
Steven H. Kroft, MD

Hemoglobinopathy Atlas Subcommittee
Virgil F. Fairbanks, MD
James D. Hoyer, MD
Steven H. Kroft, MD
Linda M. Sandhaus, MD

Illustrations, Design, and Layout
Eric F. Glassy, MD

Table of Contents

Preface vii
Acknowledgements viii

Section I: Introduction

Introduction: Methods used in the evaluation of hemoglobinopathies 3

Section II: Case Studies

Case 1:	Normal adult	11
Case 2:	Iron deficiency	15
	A Closer Look At…Alpha-Thalassemia	18
Case 3:	β-Thalassemia trait	21
	A Closer Look At…Beta-Thalassemia	24
Case 4:	HPFH trait	29
Case 5:	δβ-Thalassemia trait	33
Case 6:	Homozygous β⁺-thalassemia	37
Case 7:	Hb S trait	41
Case 8:	Hb C trait	45
Case 9:	Hb E trait	49
Case 10:	Hb Lepore trait	53
Case 11:	Hb D-Los Angeles trait	57
Case 12:	Hb O-Arab trait	61
Case 13:	Hb G-Philadelphia trait	65
Case 14:	Homozygous Hb E	69
	A Closer Look At…Hb E-Associated Disorders	72
Case 15:	Homozygous Hb C	75
Case 16:	Homozygous Hb S	79
Case 17:	Hb S/C disease	85
Case 18:	Hb S/β⁺-thalassemia	89
Case 19:	Hb S/G-Philadelphia	93
Case 20:	Hb S/Hb Korle-Bu	97
Case 21:	Hb S/Hb E	101
Case 22:	Hb S/HPFH	105
Case 23:	HPFH trait/β-Thalassemia trait and HPFH trait/Hb C trait	109

Case 24:	Hb G-Coushatta trait	113
Case 25:	Hb J-Baltimore trait	119
Case 26:	Hb I trait	121
Case 27:	Hb S/Hb N-Baltimore	127
Case 28:	Hb S/Hb Hope	131
Case 29:	Hb C/β^+-thalassemia	135
Case 30:	Hb C/β^0-thalassemia	139
Case 31:	Homozygous Hb A_2'	143
Case 32	β-Thalassemia trait with Hb A_2' trait	147
Case 33	Hb S trait/Hb A_2' trait/α-thalassemia-2 trait	151
Case 34:	Hb E trait/α-thalassemia trait	155
Case 35:	Hb Q-Thailand trait/α-thalassemia-2 trait	159
Case 36:	Hb Hasharon trait	161
Case 37:	Hb Köln trait	167
Case 38:	Hb Zürich trait	173
Case 39:	Hb Malmö trait	177
Case 40:	Hb Andrew-Minneapolis trait	183
Case 41:	Hb British Columbia trait	187
Case 42:	Hb Kempsey trait	191
Case 43:	Hb S/C disease after transfusion	195
Case 44:	Hb M-Saskatoon trait	199
Case 45:	Hb Russ/Hb Raleigh	207

Section III: Dry Lab Challenges

DL-1:	Hb H disease	215
DL-2:	Hb G-Philadelphia trait/α-thalassemia-2 trait	219
DL-3:	Hb F-Texas-I trait	223
DL-4:	Hb AE-Bart's disease	229
DL-5:	Hb S/β°-thalassemia in a neonate	233
DL-6:	Hb S/C/G-Philadelphia in a neonate	237
DL-7:	Hb E trait/α-thalassemia trait in a neonate	241
DL-8:	Hb S/O-Arab in a neonate	245
DL-9:	Hb S/C-Harlem	249
DL-10:	Hb Q-Thailand/Hb H disease	253
DL-11:	Homozygous Hb S with high Hb F levels	257
DL-12:	Hb H/Hb Constant Spring	261
DL-13:	Homozygous Hb S/Hb G-Philadelphia	265
DL-14:	Laboratory artifacts	269
DL-15:	Hb S/Hb J-Baltimore	273
DL-16:	Hb C/G-Philadelphia	277
DL-17:	Hb Bart's hydrops fetalis	281
DL-18:	Hb E/β°-thalassemia	285
DL-19:	β-Thalassemia trait	289
DL-20:	Hb S/Hb A_2'	293
DL-21:	Hb S/Hb K-Woolwich	297
DL-22:	Hb Q-Thailand/Hb E	301
DL-23:	Homozygous β°-thalassemia and Homozygous HPFH	305
DL-24:	Hb S/D-Los Angeles	309

Section IV: Appendix

A:	General references pertaining to hemoglobinopathies and thalassemias	314
B:	Listing of cases used in the CAP Hemoglobinopathy Survey by year	315

Index 320

Preface

The College of American Pathologists' (CAP) Hemoglobinopathy Survey began in 1986 as an outgrowth of the Electrophoresis-Chromatography Survey. For most of its existence, the Survey has consisted of three separate mailings per year with three wet specimens per mailing. Participants are asked to quantitate Hb A_2 and perform a sickle solubility test on each specimen. On the first specimen of each mailing, Hb F quantitation is also required. Identification of any hemoglobin variants that are present is also requested; the completeness of identification is dependent upon the level of complexity of the participating laboratory. Also included in two mailings per year are exercises, which have been termed "Dry Lab Challenges." These cases are usually those in which a sufficient volume of blood could not be obtained to distribute to all participants, or where a specimen could otherwise not be obtained. Rather than an actual specimen, a series of diagrams that illustrate the electrophoretic findings of the case are included.

The first part of this atlas represents a compilation of the wet cases that have been included in the College of American Pathologists Hemoglobinopathy Survey since its inception. In almost all cases, the illustrations that are included are electrophoresis gels of the actual specimens included in the Survey, as run in Dr. Hoyer's and Dr. Fairbank's laboratory at the Mayo Clinic.

The cases are set up as a series of learning exercises. On the first page is the case history and the alkaline and acid electrophoresis gels. Alkaline and acid electrophoresis were chosen, as this is the method still employed by the majority of laboratories. However, examples of both high performance liquid chromatography and isoelectric focusing are also included in the discussion of the majority of these cases. After reviewing the case history and electrophoresis gels, the identification of the case and Survey participant performance is found on the second page. The discussion of the case and references follow. Most of these discussions are modified from those that originally appeared in the Survey summary for that sample. The cases are set up in increasing order of complexity and represent a very comprehensive list of hemoglobin disorders that may be encountered by laboratories. For reference purposes, a listing of the individual cases is included in the table of contents, although it is hoped that readers will first use the book as a series of unknowns.

The second section of this atlas represents a compilation of almost all of the Dry Lab Challenges that have been included in the Hemoglobinopathy Survey over the years. In the original survey set, the participants were asked a series of questions pertaining to this case. However, for the purposes of this atlas, these Dry Lab Challenges have been modified to resemble the format of the wet cases included in the atlas. Some of the illustrations for the Dry Lab Challenges have been modified to make the format of all cases standard. The Dry Lab Challenges are generally in the order that they appeared in the Hemoglobinopathy Survey.

Acknowledgements

The *Color Atlas of Hemoglobin Disorders* represents the culmination of a multi-year effort. There are many individuals we wish to acknowledge, without whose support and input this atlas would not have been possible.

Virgil F. Fairbanks, MD, first proposed the concept of this atlas as the *Color Atlas of Hematology* was being developed. Many individuals had remarked to him about the usefulness of the discussions in the Hemoglobinopathy Survey, and that it might be beneficial to compile them. Joanne Cornbleet, MD, Chair of the Hematology and Clinical Microscopy Resource Committee (HCMRC) from 1993 to 1996, was instrumental in encouraging the initial phases of development of this project. Katherine Galagan, MD, recent chair of the HCMRC, was very helpful in pushing the project to its final completion.

There are many past and present CAP staff members who were also instrumental in this project. They include Jill Kachin, Stacy Junge, Krista Curcio, and Caryn Tursky. Many HCMRC members, both past and present, also gave many helpful comments.

Patrick C.J. Ward, MD, deserves special acknowledgement as the photographer for the majority of the photomicrographs in this atlas. LoAnn Peterson, MD, also supplied photomicrographs of some of the cases.

James D. Hoyer, MD, would like to thank Sara Brackett and Ruth Hutchinson for the countless hours of secretarial support they provided for this project. Ayrika Gunn was indispensable in assisting with the layout of the atlas. Dr. Hoyer would also like to thank the staff of the Metabolic Hematology Laboratory at the Mayo Clinic, especially the supervisor, Regina Scheidt, for their extra efforts in assisting with many of the illustrations found in this atlas. Finally, he would like to thank his wife, Kathy, and his daughters, Emily and Alison, for their support and patience for the hard work that the completion of this atlas required.

Steven H. Kroft, MD, would like to thank his wife, Laura, for putting up with him, and his sons, Max and Charlie, for being generally okay with the concept that Daddy has to go to work every day.

Dr. Hoyer
Dr. Kroft

Section I: Introduction

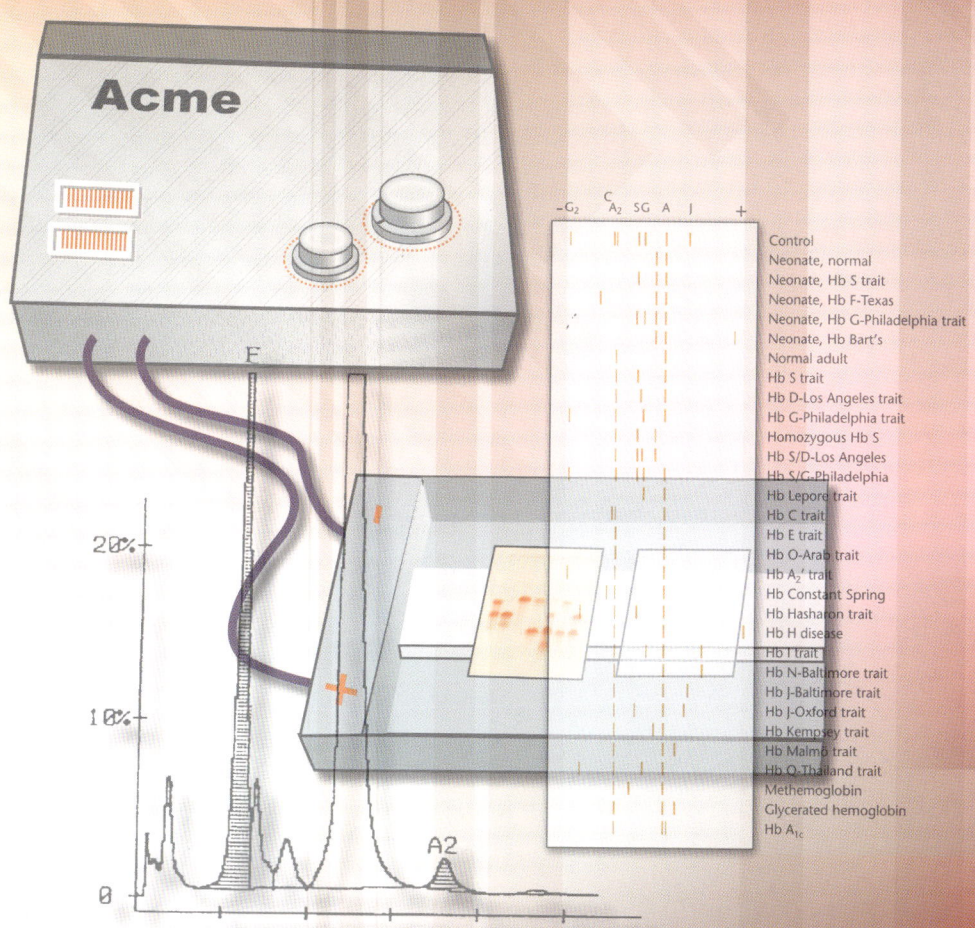

Introduction

Methods Used in the Evaluation of Hemoglobinopathies

This chapter outlines methods used by laboratories in the evaluation of hemoglobin disorders. It is important to stress that in conjunction with any of these methods, evaluation of the peripheral blood smear, as well as correlation with the results of a complete blood count (CBC), are very important. Many of the clinically significant hemoglobin disorders show characteristic peripheral blood findings. These are illustrated by photomicrographs throughout this atlas.

Solubility Test for Sickling Hemoglobins

Although a simple test, this test is still useful for confirmation of the presence of hemoglobin (Hb) S. A lysate of red blood cells is placed in a high phosphate buffer solution. Dithionate (sodium hydrosulfite) is added to the solution, which lowers the oxygen tension of the solution. Hb S, if present, will form a cloudy solution as it precipitates in this environment. This test only confirms the presence of Hb S in the solution and cannot differentiate Hb S trait from homozygous Hb S or Hb S in combination with another hemoglobin variant (such as Hb S/Hb C). Furthermore, any doubly substituted hemoglobin variant which contains the Hb S mutation (such as Hb C-Harlem) will also produce a positive sickling solubility test. False-negative results can be obtained if the percentage of Hb S is below 15-20%, such as in a sickle cell patient after a large number of transfusions, or in an infant. False-positive tests can also be obtained if nucleated red blood cells are present in the peripheral blood or the patient has marked hypergammaglobulinemia (such as in multiple myeloma). Many manufacturers have produced kits using a variation on this principle.

Alkaline Electrophoresis

This electrophoretic method is the initial method most commonly utilized by the majority of laboratories in the United States. Electrophoresis is typically carried out at a pH of 8.6 using cellulose acetate or agar as the support medium. At this pH, the overall hemoglobin molecule is negatively charged and, when placed in an electric field, will move towards the positive terminal (anode). This procedure is based on the fact that, if an amino acid substitution alters the overall charge of the molecule, then the mobility of the variant hemoglobin will be different from that of Hb A. Figure 1 illustrates this principle. Although this method is extremely useful, it has limitations in that many hemoglobin variants will migrate in the same position. For example, Hbs S, D, G, and Lepore all migrate in the same position (S position). Hbs C, E, and O-Arab all migrate in the A_2 position.

Acid Electrophoresis

This method complements alkaline electrophoresis as it gives further information on many hemoglobin variants. This electrophoretic method is run at a pH of 6.2, typically using a citrate buffer. Agar is usually used as the support medium. Agar contains agarose and the negatively charged sulfate polysaccharide agaropectin. In an agar gel, agarose is polymerized to form an immobile matrix; agaropectin does not polymerize and can bind reversibly with a small number of amino acids of hemoglobin that are on the external surfaces, in the heme pockets, or at the 2,3-DPG binding sites of the globin chains. The hemoglobin-agaropectin complex migrates electrophoretically through the immobile agarose matrix towards the anode, whereas noncomplexed hemoglobin is carried towards the cathode by electroendosmotic flow of the citrate buffer. This method is very useful in the confirmation of Hb S and the separations of Hb C from Hb E and Hb O-Arab. Unfortunately, many variants, which have their substitution within the hemoglobin molecule, show no altered mobility from Hb A with this method. This method is also illustrated in Figure 1.

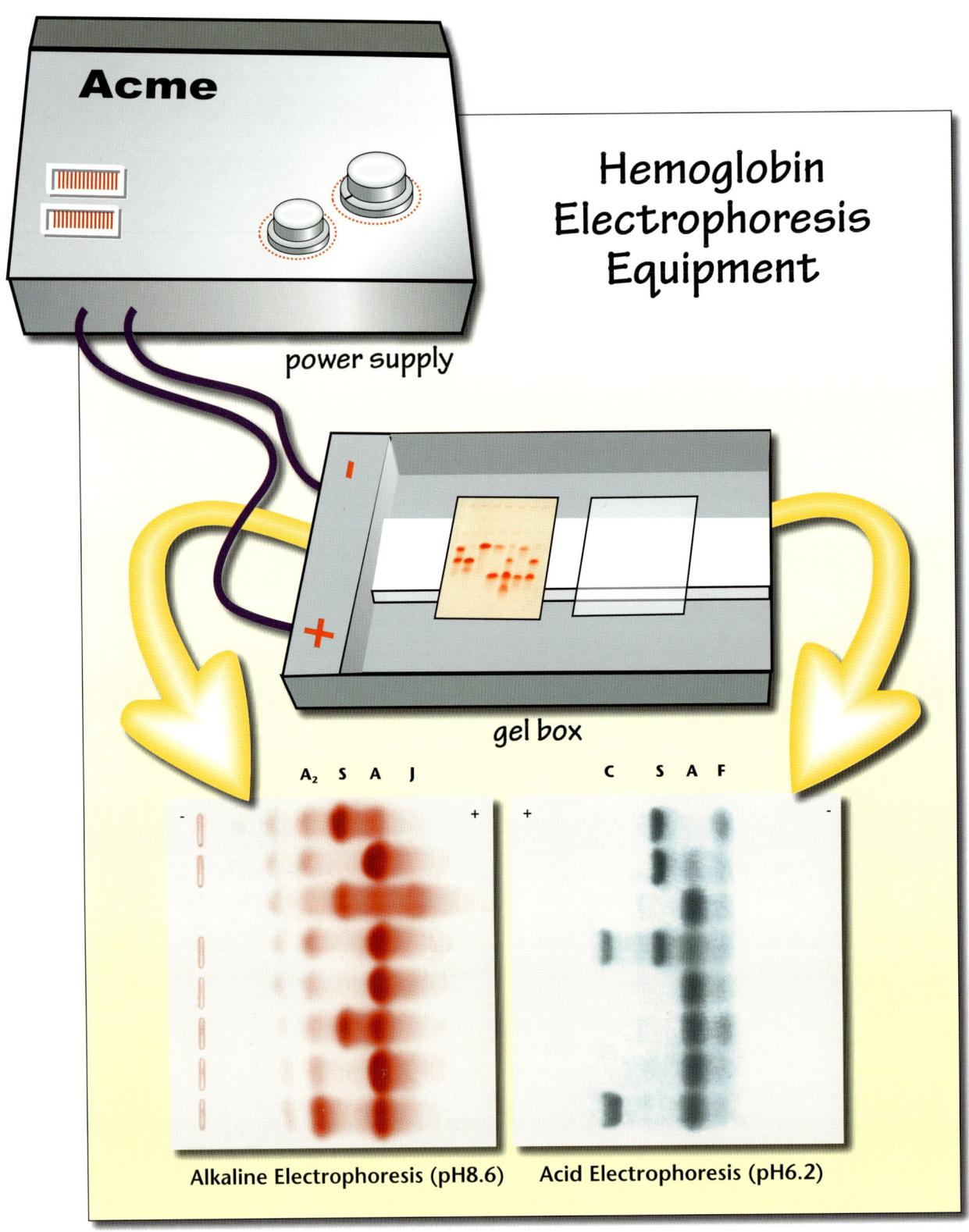

Figure 1
Examples of many hemoglobin variants and their migration patterns on isoelectric focusing.

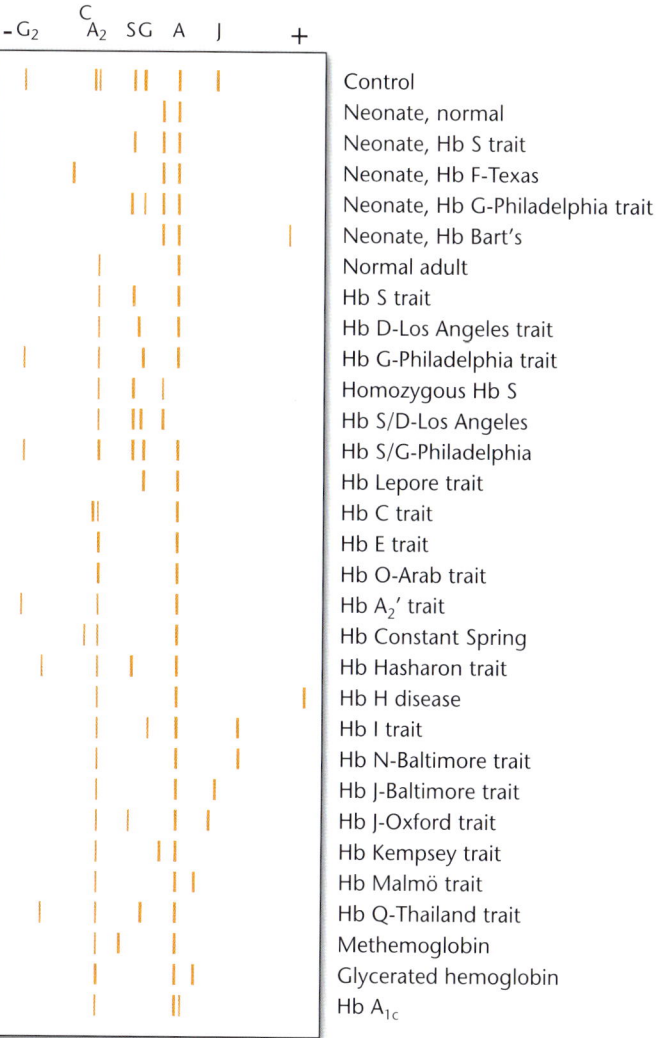

Figure 2
Examples of many hemoglobin variants and their migration patterns on isoelectric focusing.

Isoelectric Focusing (IEF)

This electrophoretic method utilizes carrier ampholytes, small proteins that are able to carry both current and pH. These compounds have molecular weights of 300-1000 daltons and are used in mixtures of 50-100 individual compounds. The ampholytes are incorporated into the support medium (usually agarose). When a current is applied to the support medium, these ampholytes will gradually establish a pH gradient throughout the gel (for example, a pH range of 6-8 for hemoglobin analysis). High voltages must be used because the carrier ampholytes are present in high concentrations. When samples are placed on the gel, they will travel to their isoelectric point (the point at which they carry a net zero charge), where migration stops. Isoelectric focusing offers several advantages. Due to minor differences in isoelectric points of various hemoglobin variants, IEF gives better separation of hemoglobin variants that show similar mobilities on alkaline electrophoresis. For example, Hbs S, D-Los Angeles, and G-Philadelphia all show identical mobilities on alkaline electrophoresis, whereas these can be differentiated on IEF. The bands present are much sharper than those seen on alkaline electrophoresis. Some hemoglobin variants, such as Hb Malmö, show separation from Hb A, which is not seen on alkaline electrophoresis. Additionally, minor bands (such as Hb H, Bart's, and δ chain variants) are easily seen. Unlike alkaline electrophoresis and other electrophoretic methods, there is no danger of running the gel too long. Therefore, fast variants, such as Hb I or Hb H, will not be overlooked. A disadvantage of IEF is that minor bands (due to glycosylated hemoglobins) and aging bands (methemoglobin, glycerated hemoglobin) are also seen and may cause confusion in interpretation. Examples of several hemoglobin variants are illustrated in Figure 2.

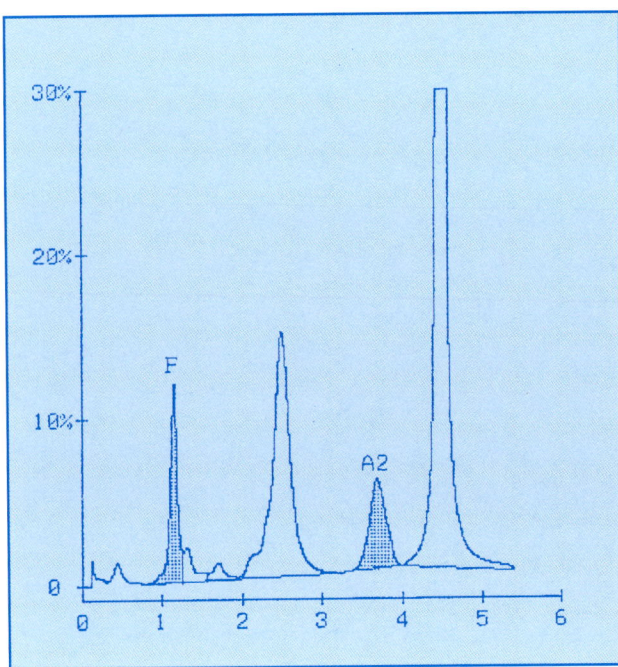

Figure 3
An example of a patient with Hb S/β^+-thalassemia by weak cation exchange HPLC. There is a peak at 2.5 minutes, corresponding to Hb A. The Hb A_2 peak at 3.68 minutes is elevated (6.4%). The majority of the hemoglobin present is Hb S, which has a retention time of 4.48 minutes. There is also a slight increase in Hb F, which has a retention time of 1.15 minutes.

High Performance Liquid Chromatography (HPLC)

This method has been available for many years but has been used primarily by research laboratories. However, in the past decade, HPLC instruments have become available that are compact, user-friendly and dedicated to the detection of hemoglobins and their variants. Run lengths have been shortened from greater than 20 minutes to 6-7 minutes. These instruments are FDA approved for the measurements of Hbs A_2 and F but also give useful information for other hemoglobin variants that may be present.

These instruments generally utilize a weak cation exchange column. As the ionic strength of the eluting solution is increased, hemoglobin variants will come off of the column at a particular retention time. Amino acid substitutions that are present in the hemoglobin variant will alter the retention time relative to Hb A. There is some correlation between the retention times obtained by HPLC and the pattern seen on alkaline electrophoresis. Amino acid substitutions that give the hemoglobin molecule an overall more negative charge at alkaline pH will run faster than Hb A. Similarly, these same substitutions usually result in a shorter retention time than Hb A on the HPLC column. Conversely, those amino acid substitutions that would result in a more positively charged molecule on alkaline electrophoresis will run slower than Hb A and usually result in a longer retention time than Hb A on HPLC. This method also has the advantage that Hb C does not co-elute with Hb A_2, and so Hb A_2 can be measured in the presence of Hb C. Hb E, however, still co-elutes with Hb A_2 by this method. An example of an HPLC chromatogram is given in Figure 3.

Globin Chain Electrophoresis

A hemoglobin lysate is treated with a mixture of hydrochloric acid (HCl) and acetone, and the heme group is removed by repeated washing of the precipitated globin with acetone. The globin chains are dissociated into monomers by urea and then are separated on the basis of charge differences by electrophoresis on two cellulose acetate membranes that contain 8 M urea buffer: one at alkaline pH and the other at acid pH. Mercaptoethanol is incorporated into these solutions because it protects the globin chains from oxidative denaturation. The alpha (α) and beta (β) globin chains are clearly separated by this method. Furthermore, any hemoglobin variants present often show altered mobility of the affected chains compared to their normal chains. Globin chain electrophoresis is run at both alkaline and acid pH because some hemoglobin variants show slight differences in mobility at the two pHs. This method often gives additional information on hemoglobin variants that have similar mobilities by other methods. In confusing cases, this method may be useful to document the presence of both an α and a β chain variant. Illustrations of globin chain electrophoresis are used in selected cases in this *Atlas*. Examples of different hemoglobin variants on globin chain electrophoresis are shown in Figure 4.

Amino Acid/DNA Sequencing

These procedures are undertaken by very few laboratories due to the expertise required and the expense of performing these tests. These tests are important for confirmation of previously undetected or extremely rare variants. This is particularly true of clinically important variants (unstable hemoglobins, high or low oxygen affinity hemoglobins, and M-hemoglobins), many of which do not separate from Hb A because of a neutral charge substitution. Examples of these are Hbs

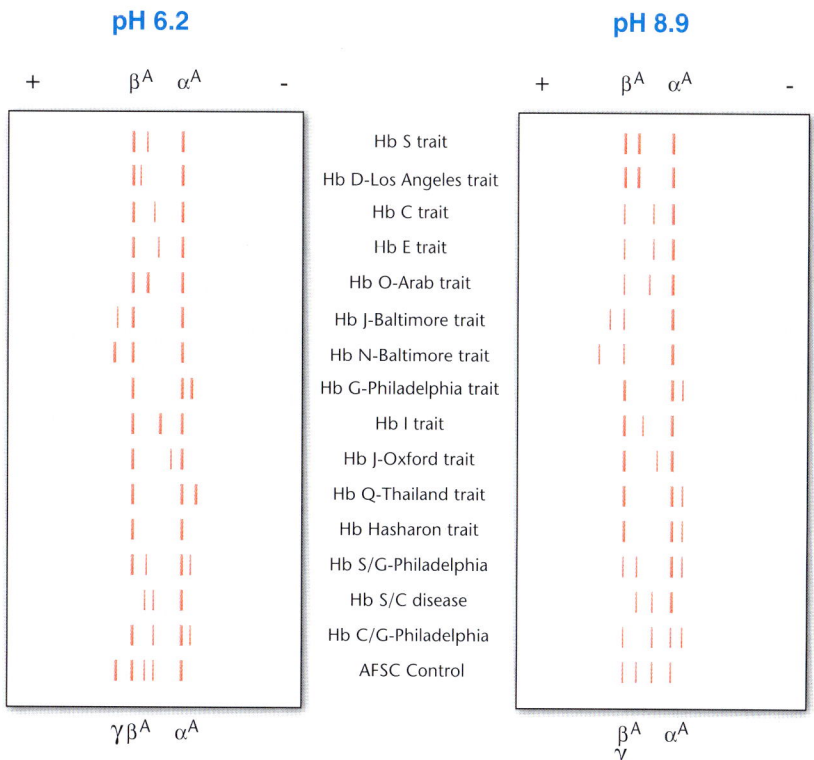

Figure 4
Examples of many hemoglobin variants on both acid (pH 6.2) and alkaline (pH 8.9) globin chain electrophoresis.

Bethesda, Hammersmith, and Little Rock.

Amino acid sequencing is usually preceded by reverse phase HPLC analysis of the hemoglobin molecule after trypsin digestion. Trypsin digestion breaks the intact globin chains into smaller protein sequences (tryptic peptides). One looks for a tryptic peptide with an altered retention time compared to its normal counterpart. Isolation of an abnormal tryptic peptide is useful because then only that portion of the protein needs to be sequenced.

DNA sequencing usually involves polymerase chain reaction (PCR) amplification of one, two, or three exons (coding regions) of each globin chain. This is followed by a second sequencing reaction to determine the nucleotide sequence of the segment that has been amplified. Three sets of primers will amplify the three exons of the β chain. The nucleotide sequences of the two α globin genes are very similar; however, sets of PCR primers have been developed that will sequentially amplify one or the other of the α chain genes.

The nucleotide substitution causing the alteration in the amino acid sequence is usually easily identified. DNA sequencing may also be of value in showing the nucleotide substitution of many types of β-thalassemia mutations.

Capillary Electrophoresis (CE)

As the name implies, electrophoresis is performed in a capillary tube. Much higher voltages (and hence shorter run times) can be used as the high surface-to-volume ratios in the capillary tube allow for good dissipation of the heat that is generated. There are several variations of CE, such as capillary zone electrophoresis and capillary isoelectric focusing. These methods are at least semi-automated, use a very small sample size, and offer the potential of more precise separation of different hemoglobin variants.

References

Bartlett RC. Rapid cellulose acetate electrophoresis, II: qualitative and quantitative hemoglobin fractionation. *Clin Chem.* 1963;9:325-329.

Beuzard Y, Galacteros F, Braconnier F, et al. Isoelectric focusing of human hemoglobins. *Prog Clin Biol Res.* 1981;60:177-195.

Black J. Isoelectric focusing in agarose gel for detection and identification of hemoglobin variants. *Hemoglobin.* 1984;8:117-127.

Briere RO, Golias T, Batsakis JG. Rapid qualitative and quantitative hemoglobin fractionation: cellulose acetate electrophoresis. *Am J Clin Pathol.* 1965;44:695-701.

Greenberg MS, Harvey HA, Morgan C. A simple and inexpensive screening test for sickle hemoglobin. *N Engl J Med.* 1972;286:1143-1144.

Huisman THJ. Separation of hemoglobins and hemoglobin chain by high-performance liquid chromatography. *J Chromatog.* 1987;418:277-304.

Koepke JA, Thomas JF, Schmidt RM. Identification of human hemoglobins by use of isoelectric focusing in gel. *Clin Chem.* 1975;21:1953-1955.

Milner PF, Gooden HM, General RT. Rapid citrate agar electrophoresis in routine screening for hemoglobinopathies using a simple hemolysate. *Am J Clin Pathol.* 1975;64:58-64.

Ou CN, Rognerud CL. Rapid analysis of hemoglobin variants by cation-exchange HPLC. *Clin Chem.* 1993;39:820-824.

Schmidt RM. Laboratory diagnosis of hemoglobinopathies. *JAMA.* 1973;225:1276-1280.

Schmidt RM, Wilson SM. Standardization in detection of abnormal hemoglobins: solubility tests for hemoglobin S. *JAMA.* 1973;225:1225-1230.

Schneider RG. Differentiation of electrophoretically similar hemoglobins such as S, D, G and P; or A_2, C, E and O by electrophoresis of globin chains. *Clin Chem.* 1974;20:1111-1115.

Schneider RG, Barwick RC. Measuring relative electrophoretic mobilities of mutant hemoglobins and globin chains. *Hemoglobin.* 1978;2:417-435.

Section II: Case Studies

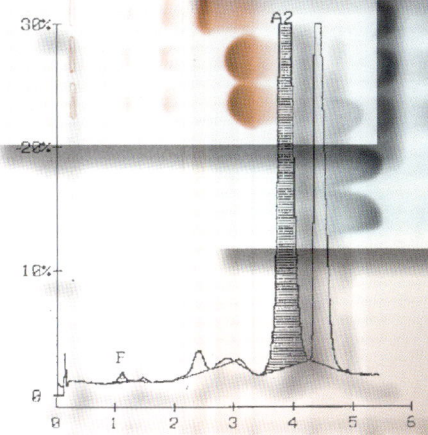

HISTORY
The patient is an asymptomatic 33 year-old African-American male who was told that he has sickle cell anemia when he was younger. No abnormalities noted on the physical examination.

BLOOD COUNT DATA
RBC .... 4.94 x 10^{12}/L
Hb .... 14.8 g/dL
MCV .... 89.0 fL
WBC .... 10.2 x 10^9/L
Plt .... 196 x 10^9/L

PERIPHERAL BLOOD SMEAR
No abnormalities.

Case 1

HISTORY
The patient is a 33-year-old asymptomatic woman of Cuban ancestry. No abnormalities were noted on the physical examination.

BLOOD COUNT DATA
RBC .... 4.8 x 10^{12}/L
Hb .... 13.3 g/dL
MCV .... 83.0 fL
WBC .... 5.8 x 10^9/L
Plt .... 289 x 10^9/L

PERIPHERAL BLOOD SMEAR
No abnormalities noted.

Alkaline Electrophoresis (pH 8.6)   Acid Electrophoresis (pH 6.2)

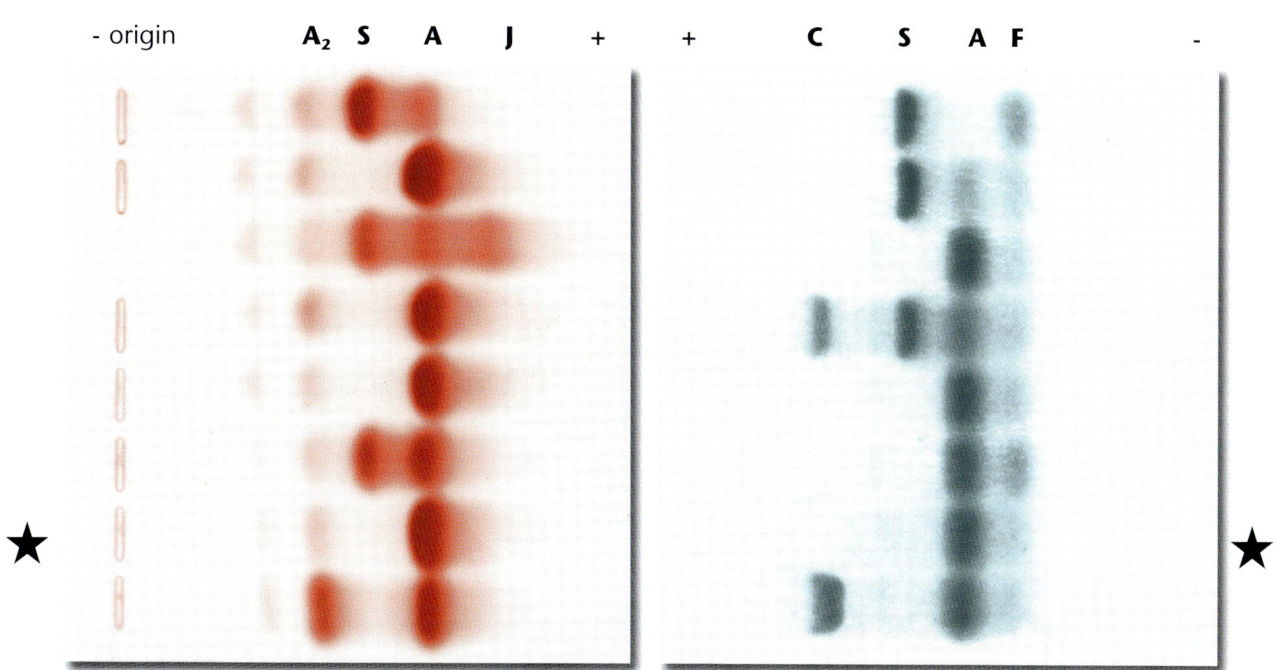

Case 1 Discussion

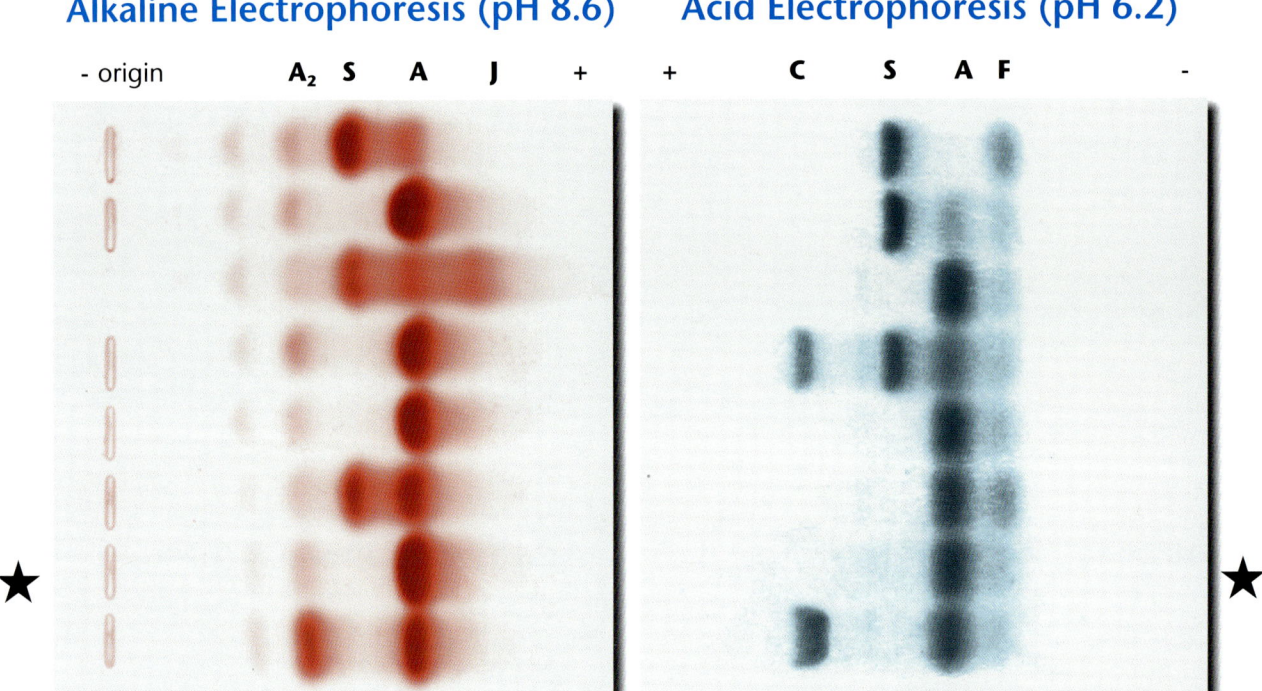

Interpretation
On alkaline electrophoresis, there is a band in the A position and a minor band in the A_2 position. No other abnormal bands are present. On acid electrophoresis, there is a band in the A position.

Diagnosis
Normal adult.

Performance
Normal specimens have been used numerous times in the survey. Typically, >95% of laboratories correctly identify a normal specimen.

Discussion

This sample is included to illustrate the pattern seen on a normal specimen. On alkaline electrophoresis, there is a major band in the A position and a minor band in the A_2 position. There is also a minor band seen cathodal to the A_2 position, which represents carbonic anhydrase. On acid electrophoresis, a normal specimen shows a band in the A position and a small band in the F position. This band likely represents a small amount of glycated hemoglobin. Hb A_2 runs with Hb A.

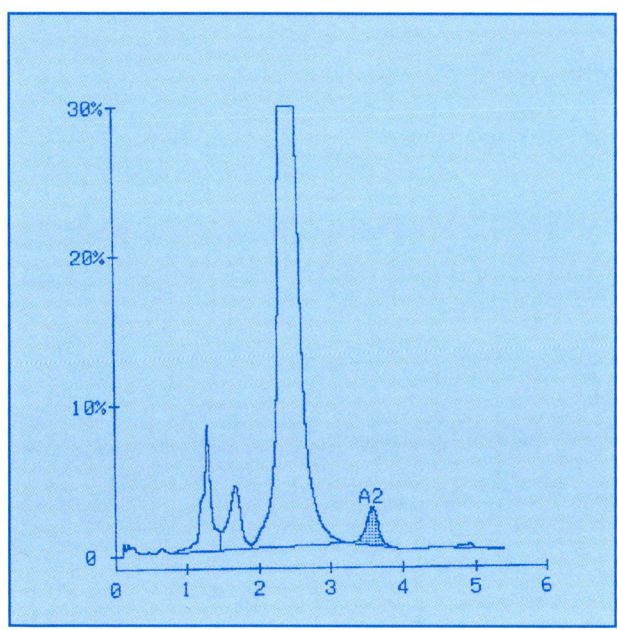

Figure 1.1
An example of a normal patient by high performance liquid chromatography. The large peak is the normal Hb A, which has a retention time of approximately 2.5 minutes. The Hb A_2 peak has a retention time of 3.3-3.9 minutes. There are two small peaks that elute before Hb A (called the P2 and P3 peaks on this instrument). These peaks usually contain glycated hemoglobin (such as Hb A_{1c}).

Case 2

HISTORY
The patient is a 26-year-old male of Southeast Asian origin who was evaluated for anemia. The physical exam was normal.

BLOOD COUNT DATA
RBC.................................4.1 x 10^{12}/L
Hb...................................10.0 g/dL
MCV ....74 fL
WBC ....9.7 x 10^9/L
Plt...................................234 x 10^9/L

PERIPHERAL BLOOD SMEAR
Microcytosis, hypochromia, scattered elliptocytes, and mild eosinophilia.

OTHER LABORATORY TESTS
Serum iron was 86.0 µg/dL, TIBC was 277 µg/dL, and serum ferritin was 5 µg/L.

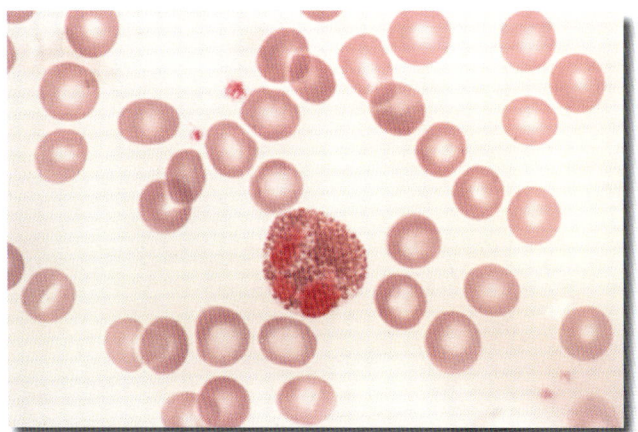

Alkaline Electrophoresis (pH 8.6)

- origin A_2 S   A   +

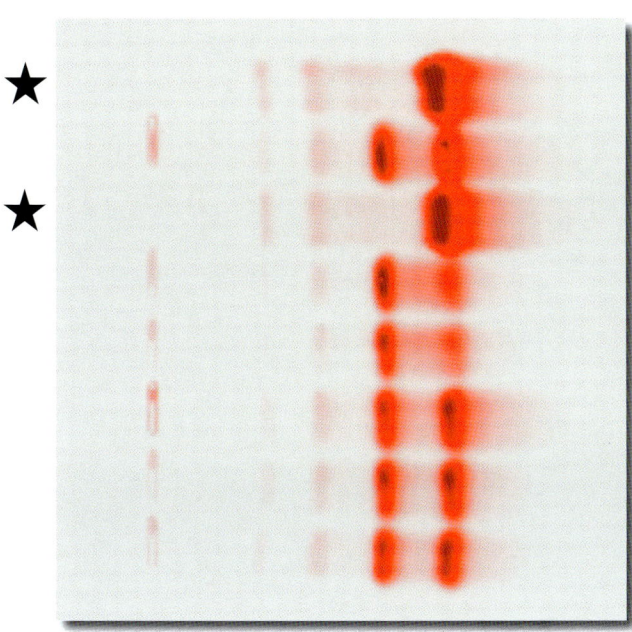

Acid Electrophoresis (pH 6.2)

+   C   S   A F   -

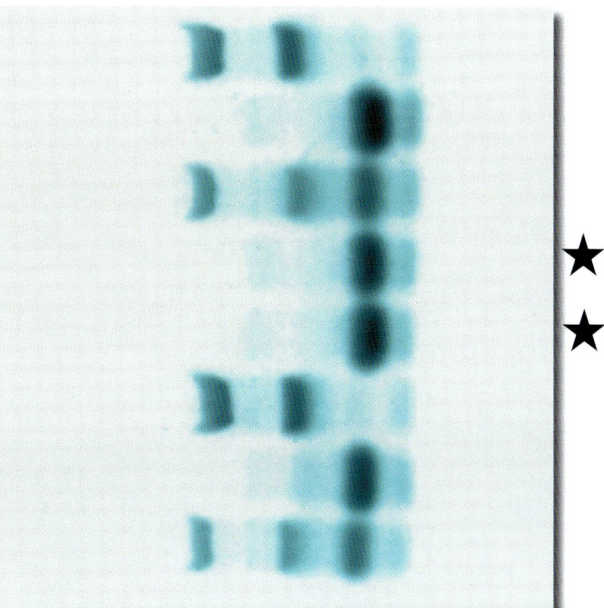

Case Studies

Case 2 Discussion

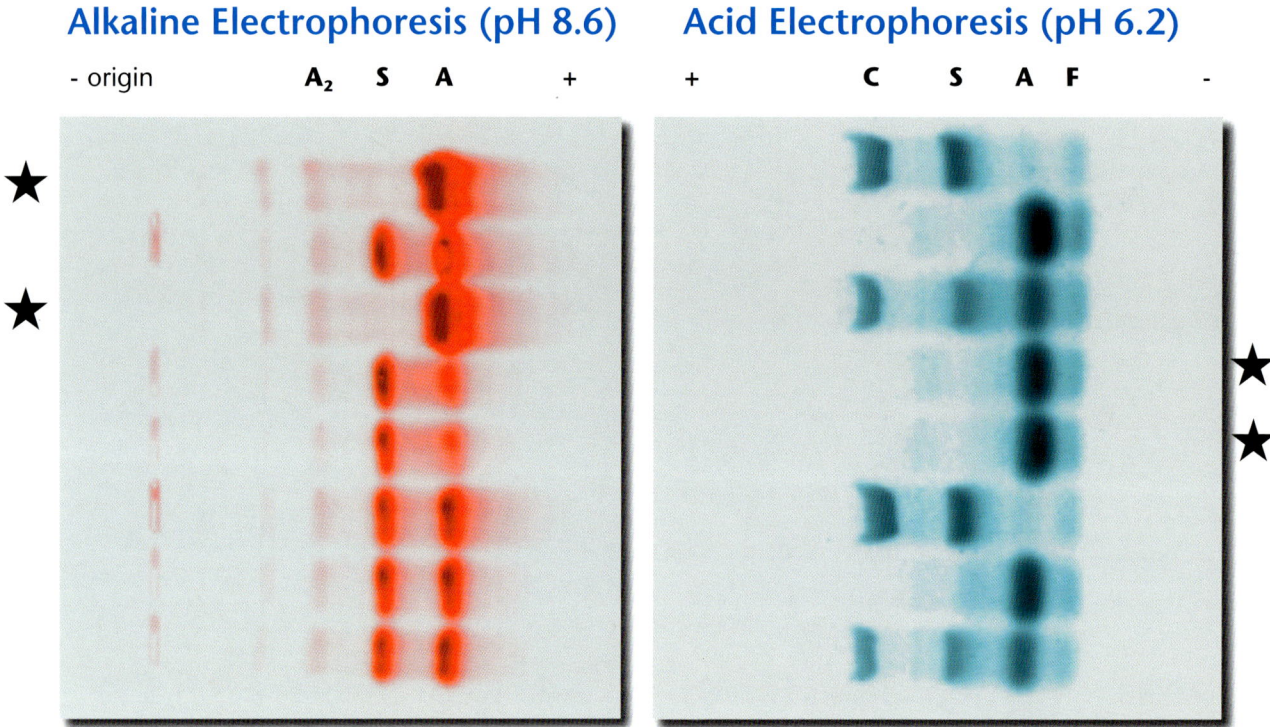

Interpretation
Alkaline and acid electrophoresis show a single dominant band in the A position and a normal appearing Hb A$_2$ band. Hb A$_2$ quantification revealed 2.5% Hb A$_2$.

Diagnosis
Iron deficiency anemia.

Performance
Iron deficiency anemia in a Southeast Asian patient has been used once previously in the survey. Interpretation was not required.

Discussion

The differential diagnosis in a Southeast Asian patient with a mild microcytic anemia includes the following in descending order of probability: α-thalassemia, Hb E, iron deficiency, and β-thalassemia. The low serum ferritin in this case is diagnostic of iron deficiency. It was subsequently determined that the iron deficiency was a result of chronic blood loss associated with hookworm infection, thus explaining the mild eosinophilia. However, differential diagnostic considerations in this case bear mentioning. Hb E disease is easily excluded in this case based on the absence of a major band in the C/E/O/A$_2$ position on alkaline electrophoresis. Heterozygous β-thalassemia (β-thalassemia minor) typically produces an elevation in Hb A$_2$, a finding that was absent in this case. However, it is important to point out that Hb A$_2$ may be in the normal range in this condition when there is concomitant iron deficiency. Thus, a re-evaluation of this patient's hemoglobin and MCV following iron repletion, and possibly a repeat Hb A$_2$ determination, would be necessary to completely rule out β-thalassemia in this patient. Finally, mild forms of α-thalassemia produce no electrophoretic abnormalities in adult patients, as discussed in *A Closer Look At...Alpha-Thalassemia* (page 18), and re-evaluation after iron repletion would be necessary to rule out this possibility as well. This particular patient's hematologic abnormalities completely resolved with iron therapy.

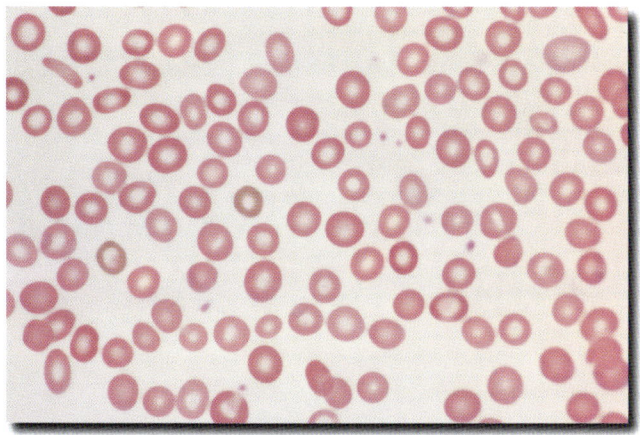 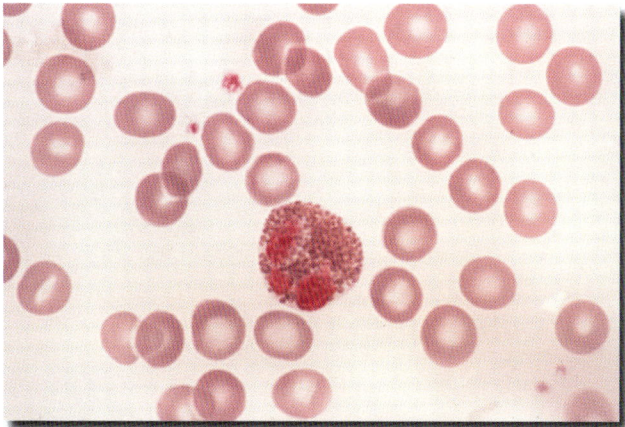

Figure 2.1 (Wright-Giemsa, 160x and 400x)
The peripheral blood smear in a patient with iron deficiency anemia. The red blood cells are hyochromic and microcytic.
Central pallor is mild and there is no coarse basophilic stippling. The leukocyte is an eosinophil.

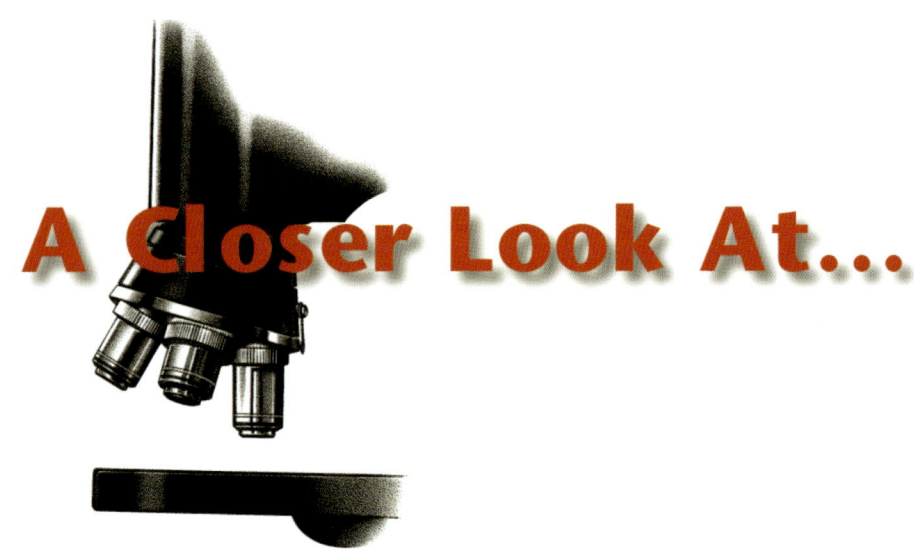

A Closer Look At...

Alpha-Thalassemia

The α globin gene cluster on chromosome 16 contains two functioning α globin genes (designated α1 and α2), as well as the embryonic ζ gene and four pseudogenes. Thus, normal individuals possess four α genes [designated (αα/αα)], with the α2 genes contributing 1.5 to 3 times more to the production of a globin chains than the α1 genes. The α-thalassemias result primarily from large deletions in the α cluster, with rare non-deletional variants. Two general haplotypes are recognized for α-thalassemia: the α-thalassemia-1 haplotype (also known α^0), in which both α genes are deleted in one α cluster [designated (--)]; and the α-thalassemia-2 haplotype (also known as α^+), in which there is a single α gene deletion in the α cluster [designated (-α)]. These two forms of mutation exist at different frequencies in different patient populations, and this becomes important from the standpoint of genetic counseling (see below). Specifically, α-thalassemia-2 trait (-α/αα) is present in 28% of African Americans, whereas the α-thalassemia-1 haplotype is virtually nonexistent in this population. In Southeast Asian, Mediterranean, and Middle Eastern populations, both types of mutation are relatively common. The α-thalassemia-1 (α^0) haplotype primarily results from a variety of deletions which abrogate both α genes on a single chromosome 16. The α-thalassemia-2 haplotype (α^+) results most commonly from a 3.7 kB deletion, which spans the 5' end of the α1 gene, the 3' end of the α2 gene, and intervening intronic sequences. This haplotype [designated (-$\alpha^{3.7}$), also known as the "rightward" deletion] results in a fusion α gene, with the net effect of deleting a single α gene on that chromosome. This mutation has a worldwide distribution. The second major mutation producing the α-thalassemia-2 haplotype is a 4.2 kB deletion [designated (-$\alpha^{4.2}$), also known as the "leftward" deletion] which spans and deletes only the α2 gene. This mutation is seen in Southeast Asia and Saudi Arabia but is rare in Mediterranean and black populations.

The pathophysiology of the anemia in the thalassemic disorders relates to the imbalance between the production of the α and β globin chains. When α chains are under-produced in the α-thalassemias, the excess β chains tetramerize to form Hb H. These tetramers are soluble but unstable, and thus denature and precipitate as the circulating red cells age. This leads to decreased deformability and ultimate removal by the spleen.

The clinical consequences of the α-thalassemias depend on how many α genes are deleted. The one-gene deletion [heterozygous α-thalassemia-2, (-α/αα)] is clinically and hematologically silent. The 2-gene deletions, known as α-thalassemia minor or trait [heterozygous α-thal-1 (--/αα) or homozygous α-thal-2 (-α/-α)] produce a mild, asymptomatic, microcytic anemia similar to β-thalassemia minor (Figure 2.1). (See also Case 3.) Three-gene deletions [compound heterozygous state for α-thalassemia-1 and α-thalassemia-2 (-α/--) or co-inheritance of α-thalassemia-1 and hemoglobin Constant Spring (--/$\alpha^{CS}\alpha$)] produce a moderately severe, chronic hemolytic anemia (similar to β-thalassemia intermedia) that does not require regular transfusion support. Finally, the complete absence of α genes, and thus α globin chains, produces a severe non-immune hydrops fetalis and is essentially incompatible with life (although rarely an infant may be rescued with intrauterine transfusions). The two clinically significant α-thalassemia syndromes are extremely rare in the African-American population because they both involve α-thalassemia-1 mutations. The α-thalassemias are summarized in Table 2.1 and Figure 2.2.

In regard to laboratory diagnosis, the silent carrier state is undetectable with routine laboratory studies but may be suspected from family studies. However, the common 3.7 and 4.2 kB deletions may be easily detected with Southern blot analysis. Alpha-thalassemia minor/trait is a diagnosis of exclusion in routine practice, as it produces no electrophoretic abnormalities in adult patients. However, it may be detected at birth, as there will be a small amount of fast-moving Hb Bart's (γ tetramers) present. In addition, it may be confirmed with molecular analysis of the α gene cluster. Hemoglobin H disease is diagnosed by the presence of 20-40% Hb Bart's at birth or 5-40% fast-moving Hb H (β tetramers) in adult patients. A very small, slow moving Hb Constant Spring band may be detected as well. In addition, supravital staining with brilliant cresyl blue will produce numerous pale blue Hb H inclusions in patient red cells. Finally, 4-gene deletion hydrops fetalis is characterized electrophoretically by a predominance of Hb Bart's with smaller amounts of Hb H and Hb Portland (an embryonic hemoglobin that normally is absent by the twelfth week of gestation).

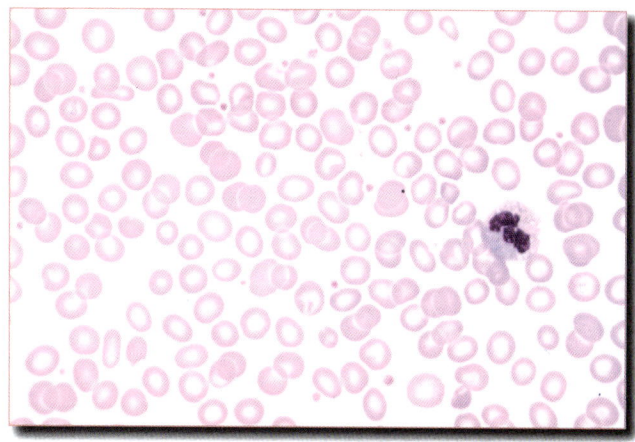

Figure 2.1 (Wright-Giemsa, 200x)
The peripheral blood smear from a patient with alpha-thalassemia due to a two alpha gene deletion. The red blood cells are mildly microcytic with slight anisopoikilocytosis.

Table 2.1 Summary of α-Thalassemias

Subtype	α Genes Deleted	Genotype	Associated Disorder	Clinical Effect
Normal	0	$\alpha\alpha/\alpha\alpha$	None	None
Heterozygous α-thal-2	1	$-\alpha/\alpha\alpha$	Silent Carrier	Asympotmatic
Homozygous α-thal-2	2	$-\alpha/-\alpha$	Thalassemia minor	Microcytosis +/- mild anemia
Heterozygous α-thal-1	2	$--/\alpha\alpha$	Thalassemia minor	Microcytosis +/- mild anemia
α-thal-1/α-thal-2	3	$--/-\alpha$	Hemoglobin H disease	Chronic hemolytic anemia
Homozygous α-thal-1	4	$--/--$	Bart's hydrops fetalis	Lethal

Figure 2.2 Alpha-Thalassemia Mutations

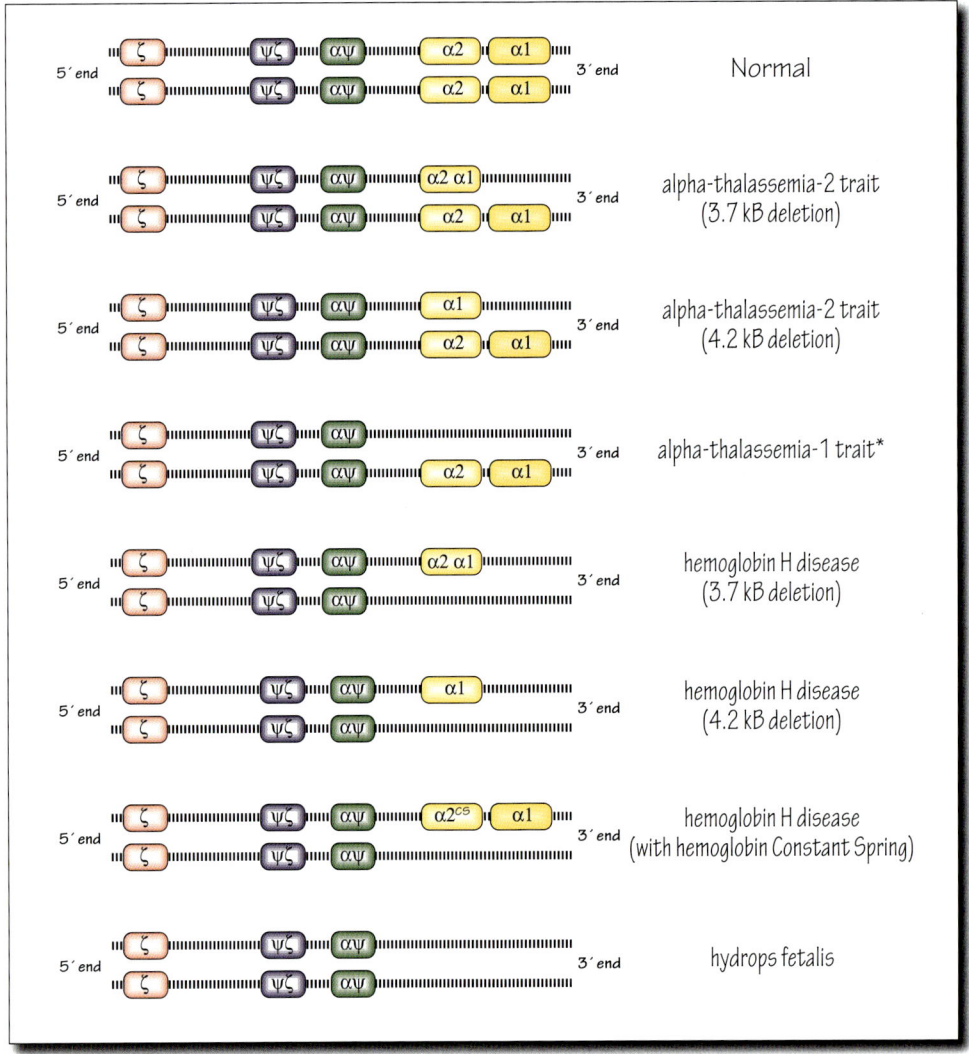

*some α-thalassemia-1 mutations involve one or more of the pseudogenes and the ζ genes

References

Higgs DR, Bowden DK. Clinical and laboratory features of α-thalassemia syndromes. In: Steinberg MH, Forget BL, Higgs DR, Nagel RL, eds. *Disorders of Hemoglobin: Genetics, Pathophysiology, and Clinical Management.* Cambridge, England: Cambridge University Press. 2001:431-469.

Liebhaber SA. Alpha thalassemia. *Hemoglobin.* 1989; 13:685-731.

Lukens JN. The thalassemias and related disorders: quantitative disorders of hemoglobin synthesis. In: Lee GR, Foerster J, Lukens J, et al, eds. *Wintrobe's Clinical Hematology.* Baltimore, MD: Williams and Wilkins; 1999:1405-1448.

Weatherall DJ. The thalassemias. In: Beutler E, Lichtman MA, Coller BS, Kipps TJ, Seligsohn U, eds. *Williams Hematology.* 6th ed. New York, NY: McGraw-Hill; 2001:547-580.

Weatherall DJ, Clegg JB. The α-thalassemias and their interaction with hemoglobin variants. In: *The Thalassemia Syndromes.* 4th ed. Oxford, England: Blackwell Science, Ltd; 2001:484-525.

Case 3

HISTORY
The patient is an asymptomatic 29-year-old African-American male. The physical examination showed no abnormalities.

BLOOD COUNT DATA
RBC .... 6.6×10^{12}/L
Hb .... 14.1 g/dL
MCV .... 64 fL
WBC .... 5.8×10^9/L
Plt .... 253×10^9/L

PERIPHERAL BLOOD SMEAR
The red blood cells show microcytosis, hypochromia, targets, basophilic stippling.

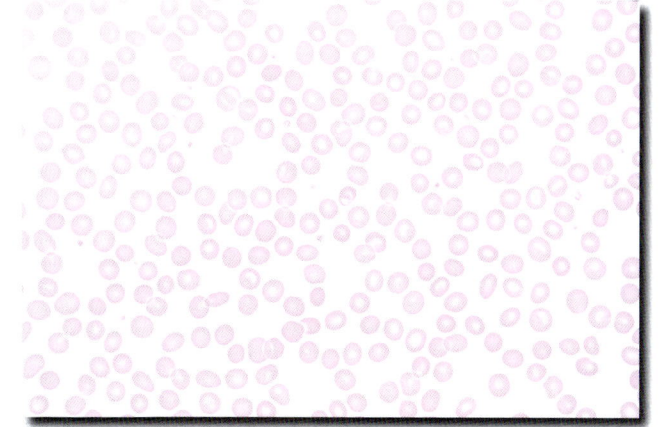

Alkaline Electrophoresis (pH 8.6)

- origin   A₂   S   A   +

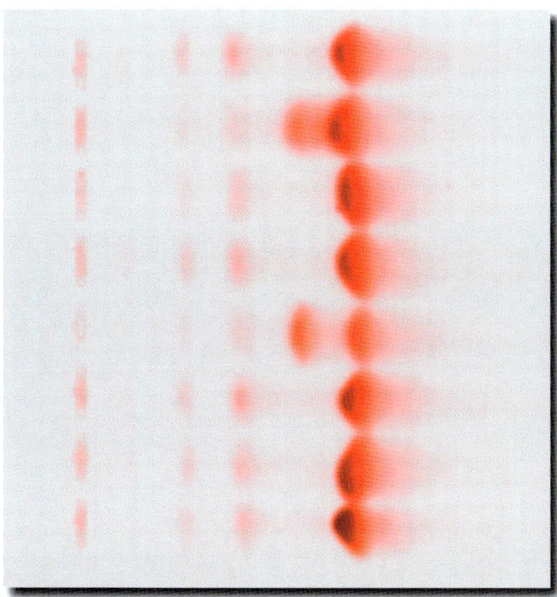

Acid Electrophoresis (pH 6.2)

\+   C   S   A   F   -

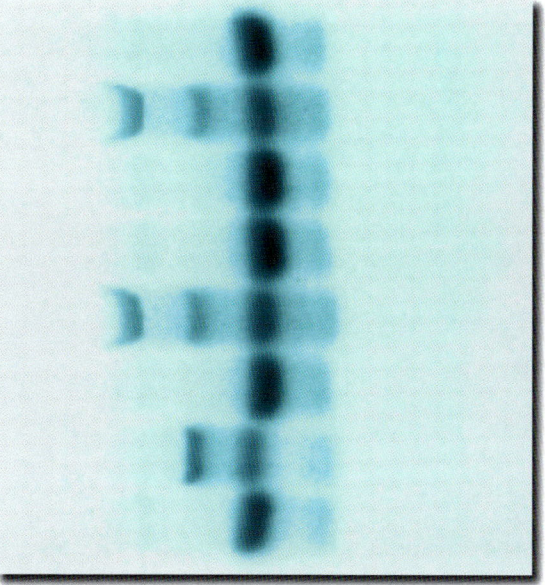

Case Studies

Case 3 Discussion

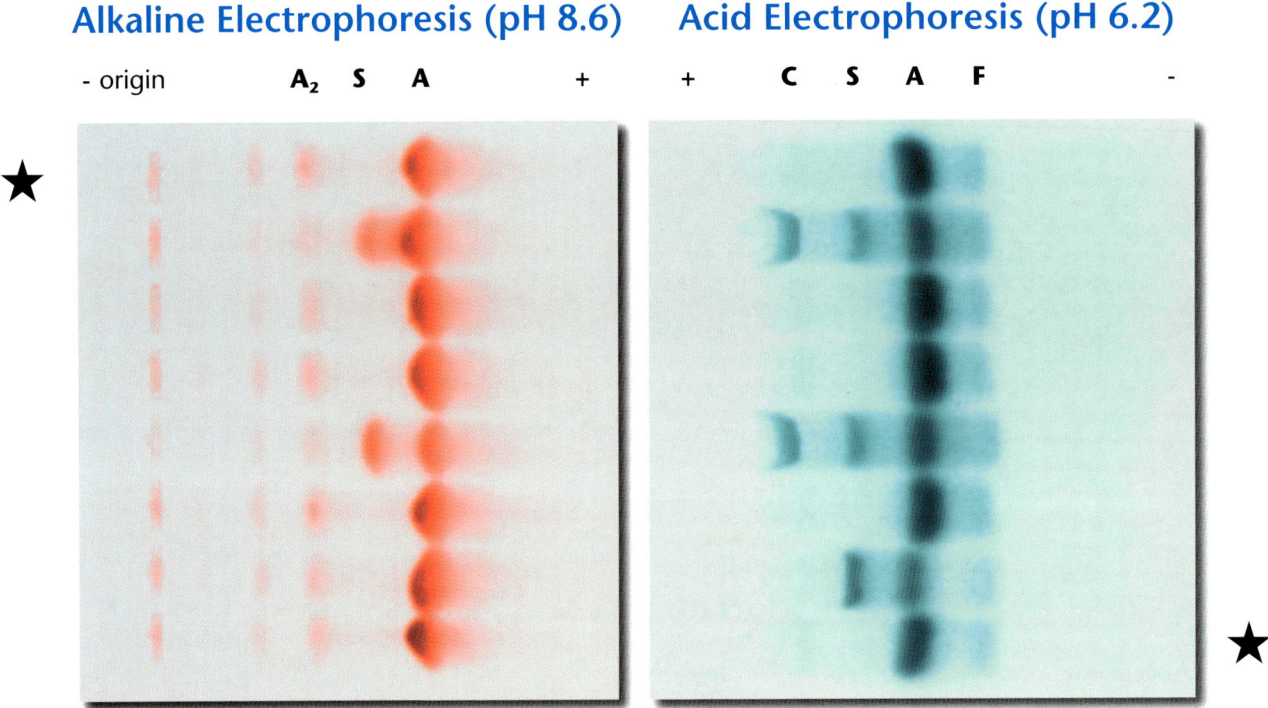

Interpretation

On alkaline electrophoresis, there are no abnormal bands seen. However, the Hb A_2 band is slightly more prominent than usual, and quantitative methods for Hb A_2 revealed an elevated Hb A_2. There are no abnormal bands seen on acid electrophoresis.

Diagnosis

Beta-thalassemia trait.

Performance

Beta-thalassemia trait has been included in the survey seven times, with correct identification generally ranging from 89-96%. In one specimen (1999 HG-05), a correct identification of beta-thalassemia trait was made by 31.6% of laboratories. However, this was a challenging case in which the Hb A_2 level was only slightly elevated (3.9-4.1%).

Discussion

In contrast with the α-thalassemias, which are predominantly due to deletions of the α globin genes (see *A Closer Look At...Alpha-Thalassemia,* page 18), β-thalassemias are due mostly to point mutations in the DNA code for the β globin chain. A wide variety of mutations result in β thalassemia (see *A Closer Look At...Beta-Thalassemia,* page 24). These may be broadly divided into those that completely abrogate β chain production by the affected allele ($β^0$) and those that reduce but don't completely eliminate β chain production ($β^+$). Inheritance of one β-thalassemia gene results in the disorder known as β-thalassemia trait (or minor). Inheritance of two β-thalassemia alleles results in more severe disease, either β-thalassemia major (Cooley's anemia) or β-thalassemia intermedia (see Case 6, page 37). An exception to these rules is a rare form of autosomal dominant β-thalassemia that results in a moderately severe anemia despite being present in the heterozygous state (see case DL-19, page 289). The severity of the β-thalassemias is inversely related to the amount of residual β globin chain production left. β-thalassemia has a wide distribution in the Mediterranean region, Middle East, India, Pakistan, and Southeast Asia.

β-thalassemia minor (trait) is an asymptomatic condition characterized by mild or no anemia (Hb>10 g/dL), microcytosis with MCVs ranging from 50-70 fL, and normal or elevated red cell counts. The last feature is a consequence of a decrease in cell size out of proportion to the decrease in hemoglobin concentration. Morphologic features include red blood cells with mild hypochromia, and little anisocytosis. Target cells are usually present and may be numerous. In some cases, basophilic stippling is present

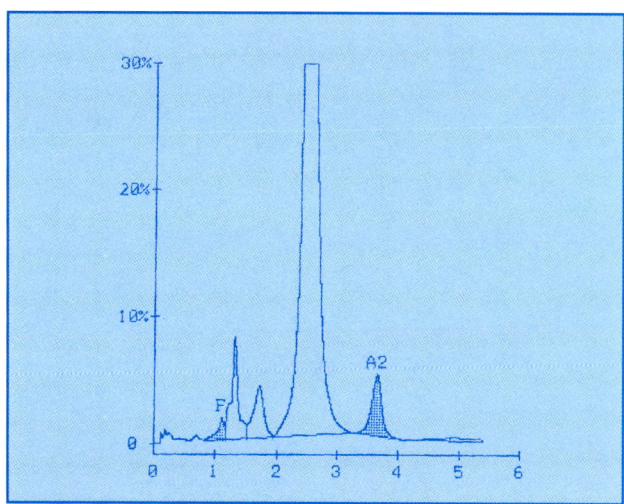

Figure 3.2
An example of beta-thalassemia trait by HPLC. There is an increase in the A_2 peak which measures approximately 5%. There is also a small amount of Hb F present.

(Figure 3.1).

The importance of diagnosing β-thalassemia minor is largely to prevent unnecessary lab testing (iron studies at every doctor visit) or treatment (unnecessary chronic iron supplementation). The hallmark of this disorder is an elevation in Hb A_2 (>3.5%) (Figure 3.2), which in the context of appropriate laboratory findings is pathognomonic for β-thalassemia minor. Hemoglobin electrophoresis typically demonstrates a more prominent Hb A_2 band than normal, but precise quantification requires other methodology, most commonly microcolumn chromatography or HPLC. It should be emphasized that Hb A_2 almost never represents more than 10% of total hemoglobin. When

continued page 26

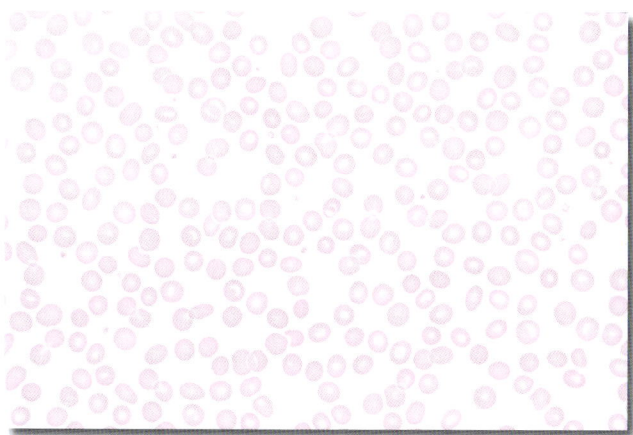

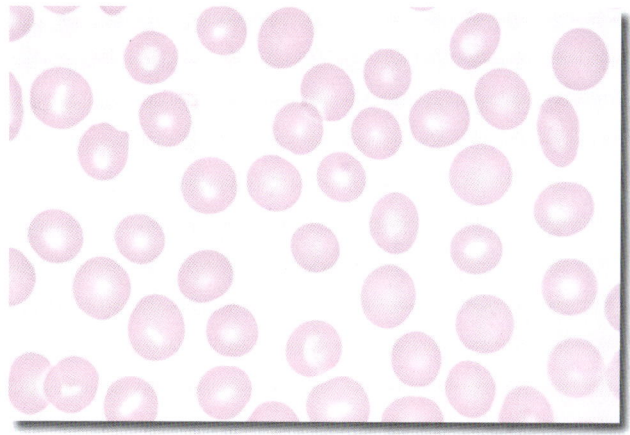

Figure 3.1 (Wright-Giemsa, 160x and 400x)
The peripheral blood smear in a patient with beta-thalassemia trait. The red blood cells are microcytic with only slight anisocytosis. Occasional target cells are present.

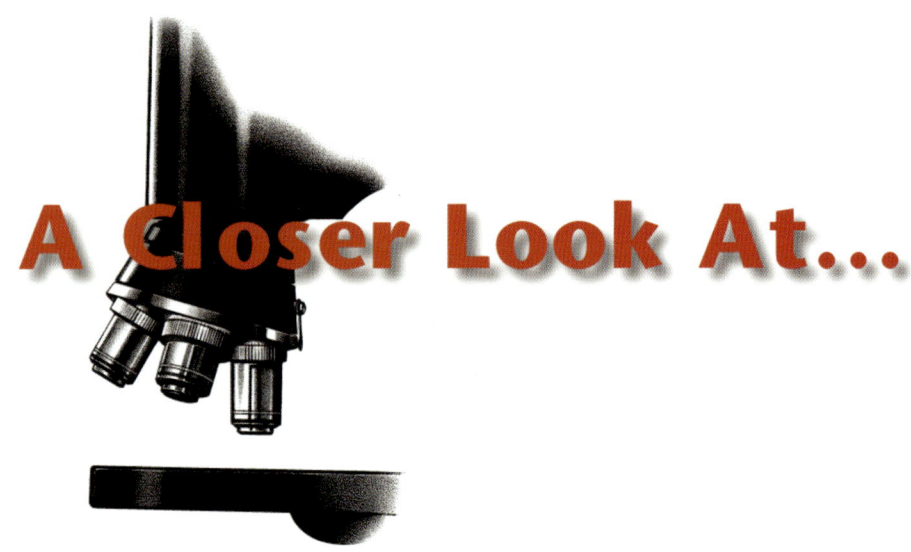

Beta-Thalassemia

The β cluster on chromosome 11 consists of one β gene, a δ gene, a pseudo-β gene, two γ genes (G and A), and the embryonic ε gene. More than 170 mutations that cause β-thalassemia have now been characterized. Some of these are summarized in the following tables (Tables 3.1 and 3.2) and illustration (Figure 3.3). A few of these mutations are in the exons of the β globin chain. For example, nucleotide substitutions at amino acid codons 17 and 39, in exon 1 and exon 2, respectively, cause a change to a nonsense codon that signals termination of synthesis of the globin chain at that point. Such major change results in absence of β chains, i.e., $β^0$-thalassemia. Most of the mutations causing β-thalassemia occur within the introns, often near the splice junctions. These mutations result in abnormal processing of mRNA and are generally associated with $β^+$-thalassemia.

Some mutations are due to insertion or deletion of nucleotides; these mutations cause frameshifts, so that the remainder of the downstream mRNA cannot be read correctly. These are generally associated with $β^0$-thalassemia, whether they are located in exons or introns. Finally, mutations have been described in the promoter region of the β globin gene. These result in reduced formation of mRNA, and hence in $β^+$-thalassemia. Two nucleotide sequences in the promoter region seem to be present in the β globin genes of nearly all species and phyla; their preservation throughout evolution implies that they are particularly critical for transcription. These are the "CAT box" sequence, so named because the nucleotide sequence is CCAAT, and the "TATA box", so named because it includes ATA; in humans, the sequence is C<u>ATA</u>AAA. Eight mutations in the TATA box are known as causes of $β^+$-thalassemia.

Like the α-thalassemias, the primary cause of the anemia in the β-thalassemias is the accumulation of the normally produced globin chain (in this case the α chains). However, in contrast to the β chains, α chains do not form soluble tetramers. Instead, the α chains precipitate in the erythroblasts, resulting in intramedullary cell death. The red cells that are produced have a shortened life span. Therefore, the anemia in the β-thalassemias is characterized by components of both ineffective erythropoiesis and hemolysis.

Globin Gene Loci

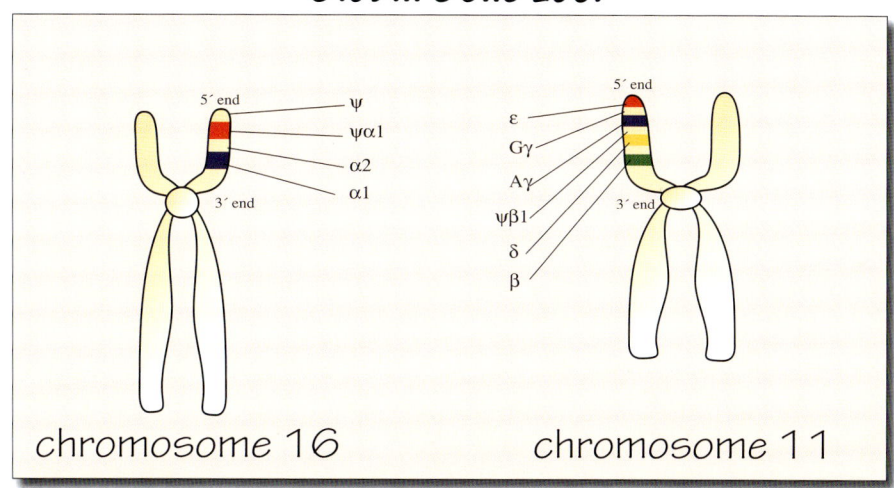

Anatomy of the Beta Globin Gene

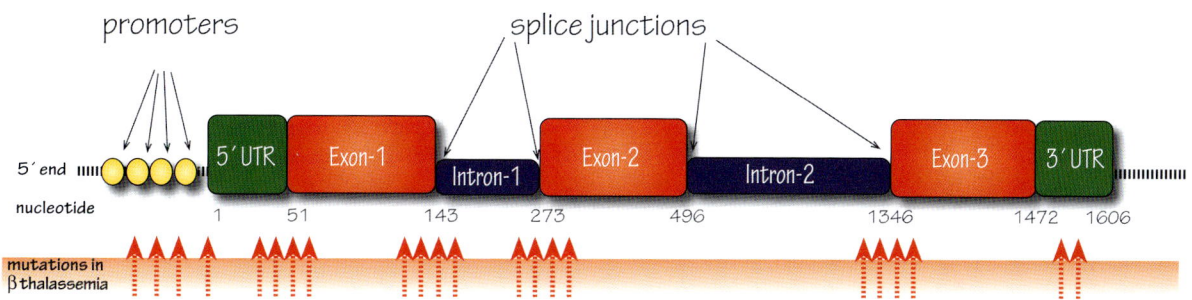

Nucleotide Number	Designation	Function
-88		transcription promoter
-87		transcription promoter
-76 to -72	CAT box (CCAAT)	transcription promoter
-32 to -26	TATA box (CATAAAA)	transcription promoter
1 to 53	5´ untranslated region	
51 to 53	Initiator codon (ATG)	starts translation
54 to 142	Exon-1	coding region for amino acids 1 to 30
143 to 272	Intron-1	exact function unknown
273 to 495	Exon-2	coding region for amino acids 31 to 104
496 to 1345	Intron-2	exact function unknown
1346 to 1471	Exon-3	coding region for amino acids 105 to 146
1472 to 1474	Stop codon (TAA)	terminates translation
1475 to 1606	3´ untranslated region	
1582 to 1587	Polyadenylation site	adds poly A tail (post transcriptional modification of mRNA)

Figure 3.3

continued from page 23

a band in the A$_2$ position does represent more than 10% of hemoglobin, there is almost certainly another abnormal hemoglobin species present (see Case 19, page 93). The differential diagnosis of β-thalassemia trait includes iron deficiency, α-thalassemia trait, and heterozygous or homozygous Hb E. Iron deficiency may be easily excluded based on serum ferritin and other iron studies, and the lack of Hb A$_2$ elevation. However, the reader should be cautioned that iron deficiency anemia and β-thalassemia minor may coexist, and in this scenario Hb A$_2$ may be in the normal range. Although Hb E migrates in the same position as Hb A$_2$ on alkaline electrophoresis, it will represent at least 25% in the heterozygous state and the large majority of the hemoglobin in the homozygous state (see *A Closer Look At…Hb E-Associated Disorders*, page 72). Finally, it should be noted that hemoglobins C, E, and O all co-elute with Hb A$_2$ in microcolumn chromatography systems, and thus this method is not useful for differential diagnosis of hemoglobins migrating in this position.

Table 3.1 Common β-Thalassemia Mutations

Population	Site	Mutation	Effect	Type
African American	-88 (promotor)	C→T	Decreased transcription	β$^+$
	-29 (promotor)	A→G	Decreased transcription	β^{++}
North African	Codon 39	C→T	Stop codon	β^0
	IVS-I nt 110	G→A	Decreased mRNA processing	β$^+$
	Codon 6	Del A	Frameshift	β^0
	IVS-I nt 1	G→A	Splice error	β^0
	IVS-I nt 6	T→C	Splice error	β$^+$
Turkey	Codon 8	+G	Frameshift	β^0
	IVS-II nt 1	G→A	Splice error	β^0
	IVS-I nt 6	T→C	Splice error	β^0
Northern Mediterranean	IVS-I nt 110	G→A	Decreased mRNA processing	β$^+$
	Codon 39	C→T	Stop codon	β^0
	IVS-I nt 1	G→A	Splice error	β^0
	IVS-1 nt 6	T→C	Splice error	β$^+$
	IVS-II nt 745	C→G	Decreased mRNA processing	β$^+$
Kurdish Jews	Codon 44	-C*	Frameshift	β^0
India	IVS-1 nt 5	G→C	Splice error	β$^+$
	Codon 41/42	-TTCT	Frameshift	β^0
	Codon 8/9	+G	Frameshift	β^0
	IVS-I nt 1	G→A	Splice error	β^0
	-619 bp	Large deletion	Defective mRNA	β^0
Thailand and S. China	Codon 41/42	-TTCT	Frameshift	β^0
	Codon 17	A→T	Stop codon	β^0
	IVS-II nt 654	C→T	Splice error	β$^+$
	-28 (promotor)	A→G	Decreased transcription	β$^+$

* *Several other mutations unique to this ethnic group.*

Abbreviations: IVS— intervening sequence   nt— nucleotide

Table 3.2 Some Mutations That Cause β-Thalassemia

5'	Nucleotide Number	Position	Type of Mutation	Effect	Type of β-Thalassemia	Frequency and Ethinic Group
Promotor Region	-88 -87 -29 -28	Promotor Promotor Promotor "TATA box"	C→T C→G A→G A→C	Error in transcription	All β⁺	Blacks, U.S. Mediterraneans (rare) US Blacks (most common) Kurdish Jews (frequency unknown)
Exon-1	70 77,78 102 125 129 132	Exon-1 Cdn 6 Exon-1 Cdn 8/9 Exon-1 Cdn 17 Exon-1 Cdn 24 Exon-1 Cdn 26 Exon-1 Cdn 27	-A +G A→T T→A G→A G→T	"frameshift" "frameshift" Termination of chain Cryptic splice junction Cryptic splice junction Cryptic splice junction	β⁰ β⁰ β⁰ β⁺ (β⁺) Hb E Hb Knossos (β⁺)	Mediterraneans, US Blacks (uncommon) India (common), Turkey (uncommon) Chinese, SE Asia (common) Blacks, U.S (uncommon) SE Asia (common) Mediterranean (uncommon)
Intron-1	143 147 148 252	IVS-I-1 IVS-I-5 IVS-I-6 IVS-I-110	G→A G→C T→C G→A	5' splice junction, false signal 5' splice junction, false signal 5' splice junction, false signal New (false) Splice junction near 3' end	β⁰ β⁺ β⁺ β⁺	Mediterranean, Iran (common) India (most common), Iran (common) Mediterranean (common) Mediterranean (most common), Iran (common)
Exon-2	298 304-307 315	Exon-2 Cdn 39 Exon-2 Cdn 41/42 Exon 2 Cdn 44	C→T -TTCT -C	Termination of chain "frameshift" "frameshift"	β⁰ β⁰ β⁰	Mediterranean (common) India, SE Asia (common) Kurdish Jews (most common)
Intron-2	496 1339	IVS-II-1 IVS-II-844	G→A C→G	5' splice site eliminated New (false) splice junction near 3' end	β⁰ β⁺	Iran (common) Mediterraneans (uncommon) Mediterraneans (rare)
Exon-3	1394	Exon-3 Cdn 121	G→T	Termination of chain	β⁰ (dominant)	Swiss, British, Dutch, Czech, Japanese

Common= 5-20% of cases of beta-thalassemia
Most Common= 40-70% of cases of beta-thalassemia

IVS= Intervening Sequence (intron)
Cdn= Codon

References

Olivieri N, Weatherall DJ. Clinical aspects of β thalassemia. In: Steinberg MH, Forget BG, Higgs DR, Nagel RL, eds. *Disorders of Hemoglobin: Genetics, Pathophysiology, and Clinical Management.* Cambridge, England: Cambridge University Press; 2001:277-341.

Weatherall DJ, Clegg JB. The β thalassemias. In: *The Thalassemia Syndromes.* 4th ed. Oxford, England: Blackwell Science, Ltd; 2001:287-356.

Case 4

HISTORY
The patient is an asymptomatic 34-year-old black male investigated because of abnormal results noted in a hemoglobinopathy screening program. The physical examination was unremarkable.

BLOOD COUNT DATA
RBC ....5.0 x 10^{12}/L
Hb................................13.0 g/dL
MCV ....81.0 fL
WBC..............................4.1 x 10^9/L
Plt.................................232 x 10^9/L

PERIPHERAL BLOOD SMEAR
No abnormalities.

Alkaline Electrophoresis (pH 8.6)   Acid Electrophoresis (pH 6.2)

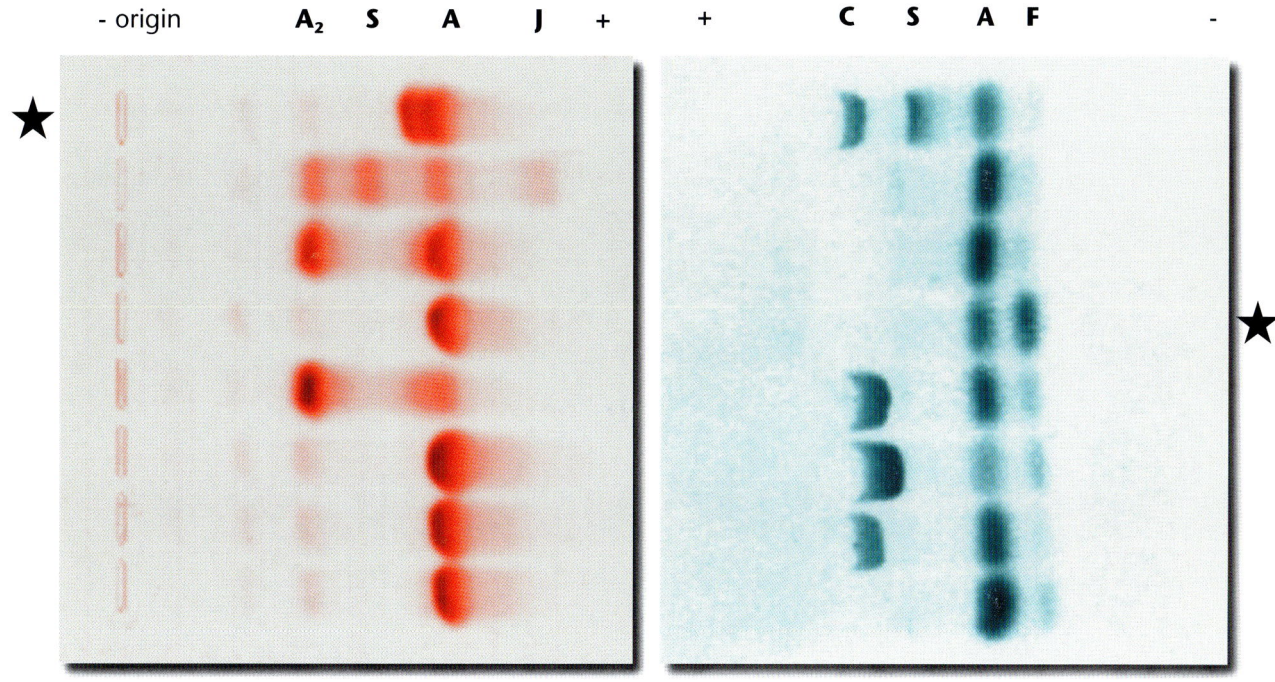

Case 4 Discussion

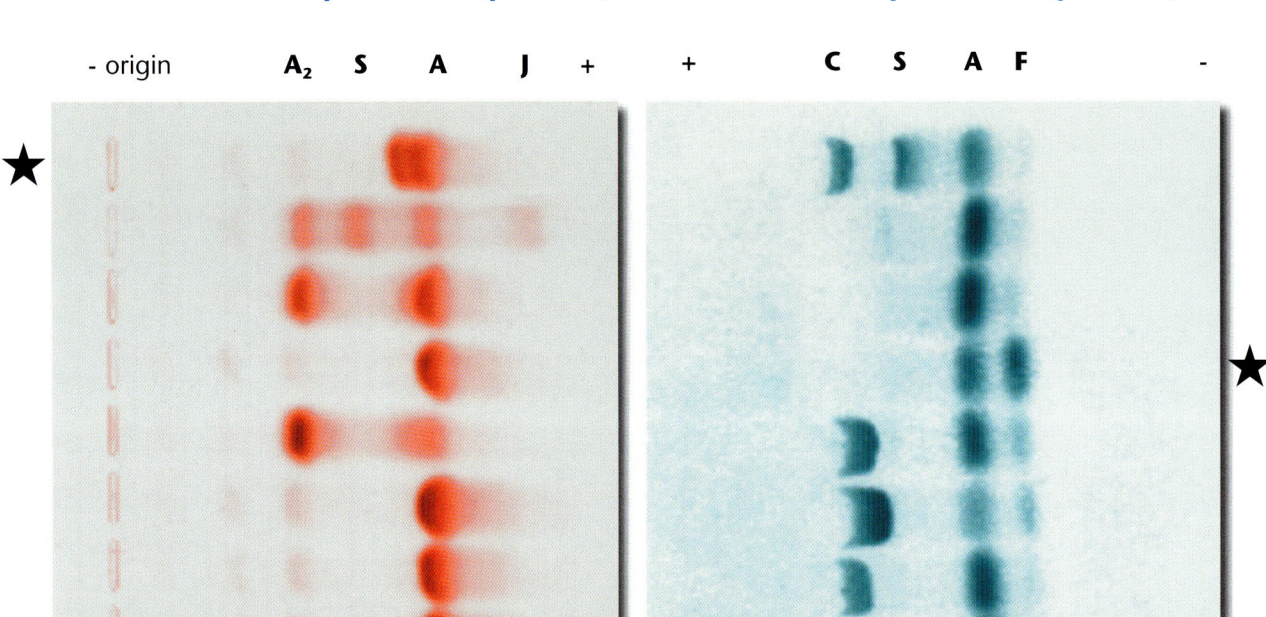

Interpretation
There are two bands seen on alkaline electrophoresis. One in the A position, one in the F position. Similarly, acid electrophoresis also shows a band in the A position and the F position. Quantitative measurement of Hb F shows an elevation of Hb F of 28%.

Diagnosis
Hereditary persistence of fetal hemoglobin (HPFH) trait.

Performance
HPFH trait has been used once as an identification, with 82.4% of laboratories giving a correct response. Patients with HPFH trait have also been used at other times for quantitative Hb F measurement.

Discussion

Hereditary persistence of fetal hemoglobin represents a heterogeneous group of disorders which, as the name implies, is characterized by elevation of Hb F into adulthood. These are found in several different ethnic groups and can be classified in several ways. At the molecular level, they can be divided into deletional and nondeletional forms. The deletional mutations involve large deletions of DNA which span both the β and δ globin genes on the affected chromosome 11. As in this case, the Hb F is elevated in the range of 25-35%. The MCV is either normal or slightly decreased, and there is no anemia. The nondeletional types of HPFH typically involve a point mutation in the promoter region of one of the γ globin genes. These mutations result in persistent expression of Hb F into adulthood (i.e., the γ globin "switch" is not turned off). The elevation of Hb F is not as high as in the deletional forms.

HPFH can also be classified by the cellular distribution of Hb F. This can be either pancellular (or homocellular), in which all of the red cells contain similar amounts of Hb F, or heterocellular, in which a small number of red cells contain a high proportion of Hb F. The deletional forms usually show a pancellular distribution of Hb F. The nondeletional forms can show either a pancellular or heterocellular distribution. Other conditions with high Hb F levels, such as β-thalassemia trait or δβ-thalassemia trait, will show a heterocellular distribution. The evaluation of the cellular distribution of Hb F has traditionally been done by the Kleihauer-Betke acid elution test. However, in recent years, a monoclonal antibody for Hb F has become available, and this cellular distribution can be evaluated by flow cytometry (see also Case 22, page 105).

Finally, HPFH can be categorized based on the types of gamma chains that are present ($^G\gamma$ versus $^A\gamma$). Because the nondeletional forms of HPFH involve a point mutation in one of the γ globin genes, measurement of the individual γ chains usually shows an abnormal $^G\gamma$ to $^A\gamma$ ratio compared to that seen in normal individuals. Table 4.1 is a summary of some of the types of HPFH. An example of homozygous HPFH is presented in one of the dry lab exercises (case DL-23, page 305).

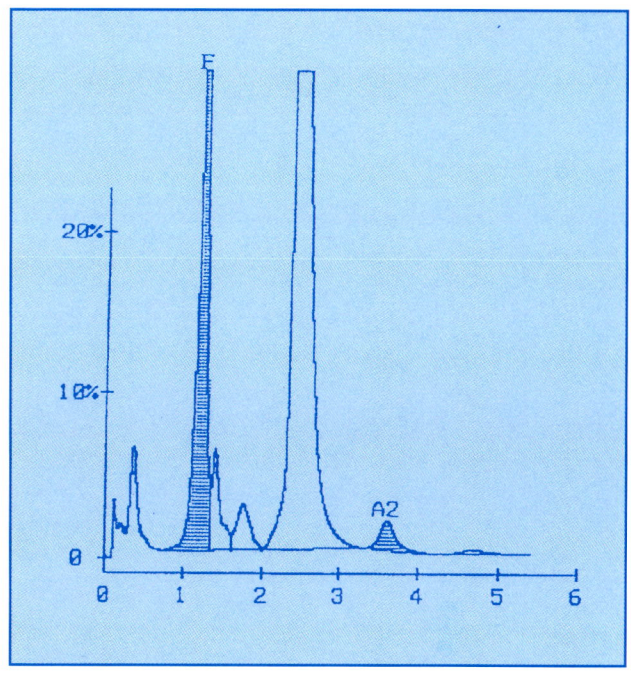

Figure 4.1
An example of HPFH trait by HPLC. There is a prominent increase in the Hb F peak which accounts for approximately 30% of the total hemoglobin.

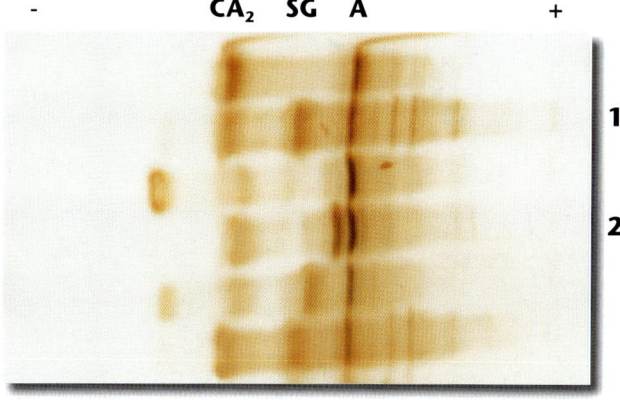

Figure 4.2
An example of a patient with HPFH trait by isoelectric focusing (lane 2). In addition to hemoglobins A and A_2, there is an increased proportion of Hb F for this patient's age. Lane 1 is a control which combines Hb C, Hb S, Hb G-Philadelphia, and Hb J-Baltimore.

Table 4.1 HPFH and Related Conditions

Type	% Hb F	$^G\gamma{:}^A\gamma$	Hb F Cellular Distribution
African [$^G\gamma^A\gamma(\delta\beta)^\circ$]			
Heterozygous	13-31	2:3	Pancellular
Homozygous	100	Variable	Pancellular
African ($^G\gamma\beta^+$)			
Heterozygous	15-20	$^G\gamma$ only	Pancellular
Swiss			
Heterozygous	1-3	Variable	Heterocellular
British			
Heterozygous	4-13	9:1	Heterocellular
Homozygous	20	9:1	Heterocellular
Georgian (U.S.)	4-7	$^G\gamma$ only	Heterocellular
Hb Kenya trait ($^G\gamma$)	5-9	$^G\gamma$ only	Pancellular
Greek ($^A\gamma$)			
Heterozygous	10-20	$^A\gamma$ only	Pancellular
$\delta\beta$-Thalassemia			
Heterozygous	5-15	$^G\gamma$ only or	Heterocellular
Homozygous	100	$^A\gamma$ only	Heterocellular
Normal neonate	50-80	3:1	Heterocellular
Normal adult	<2	2:3	Heterocellular

References

Bollekens JA, Forget BG. $\delta\beta$ thalassemia and hereditary persistence of fetal hemoglobin. *Hematol Oncol Clin North Am.* 1991;5:399-422.

Fairbanks VF. *Hemoglobinopathies and Thalassemias.* New York, NY: Brian C. Decker; 1980:24-25.

Hoyer JD, Penz CS, Fairbanks VF, et al. Flow cytometric measurement of hemoglobin F in RBCs: diagnostic usefulness in the distinction of hereditary persistence of fetal hemoglobin (HPFH) and hemoglobin S-HPFH from other conditions with elevated levels of hemoglobin F. *Am J Clin Pathol.* 2002;117:857-863.

Weatherall DJ, Clegg JB. Hereditary persistence of fetal hemoglobin. In: *The Thalassemia Syndromes.* 4th ed. Oxford: Blackwell Science, Ltd; 2001:450-484.

Wood WB. Hereditary persistence of fetal hemo-globin and $\delta\beta$ thalassemia. In: Steinberg MH, Forget BG, Higgs DR, Nagel RL. *Disorders of Hemoglobin: Genetics, Pathophysiology, and Clinical Management.* Cambridge, England: Cambridge University Press; 2001:356-388.

Case 5

HISTORY
A 30-year-old Egyptian physician was seen for mild abdominal discomfort. He is otherwise asymptomatic and has no significant past medical history. The physical examination is normal. His brother is said to have microcytic erythrocytes.

BLOOD COUNT DATA
RBC ....6.57 x 10^{12}/L
Hb ....13.7 g/dL
MCV ....63.0 fL
WBC ....8.9 x 10^9/L
Plt ....250 x 10^9/L

PERIPHERAL BLOOD SMEAR
The blood smear showed 2+ anisocytosis, 1+ elliptocytes, occasional spherocytes, and occasional basophilic stippling.

OTHER LABORATORY TESTS
The Kleihauer-Betke stain on the blood film showed a heterocellular distribution of Hb F.

Alkaline Electrophoresis (pH 8.6)

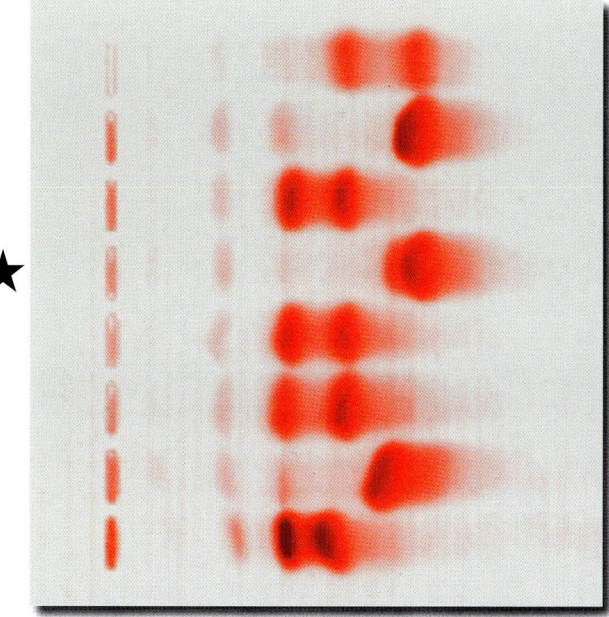

Acid Electrophoresis (pH 6.2)

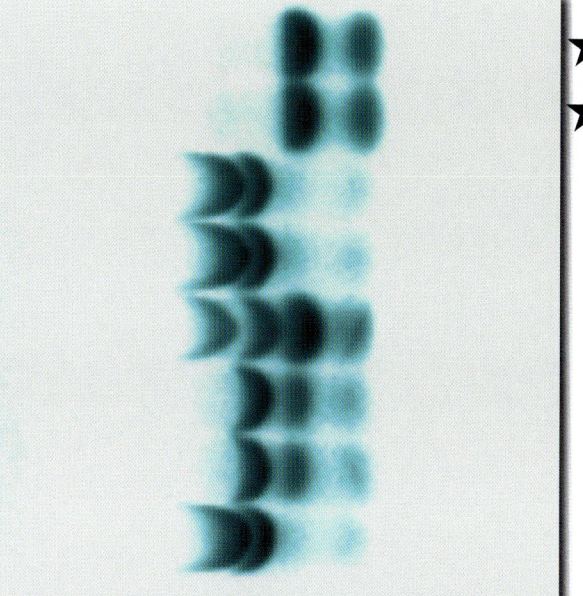

Case 5 Discussion

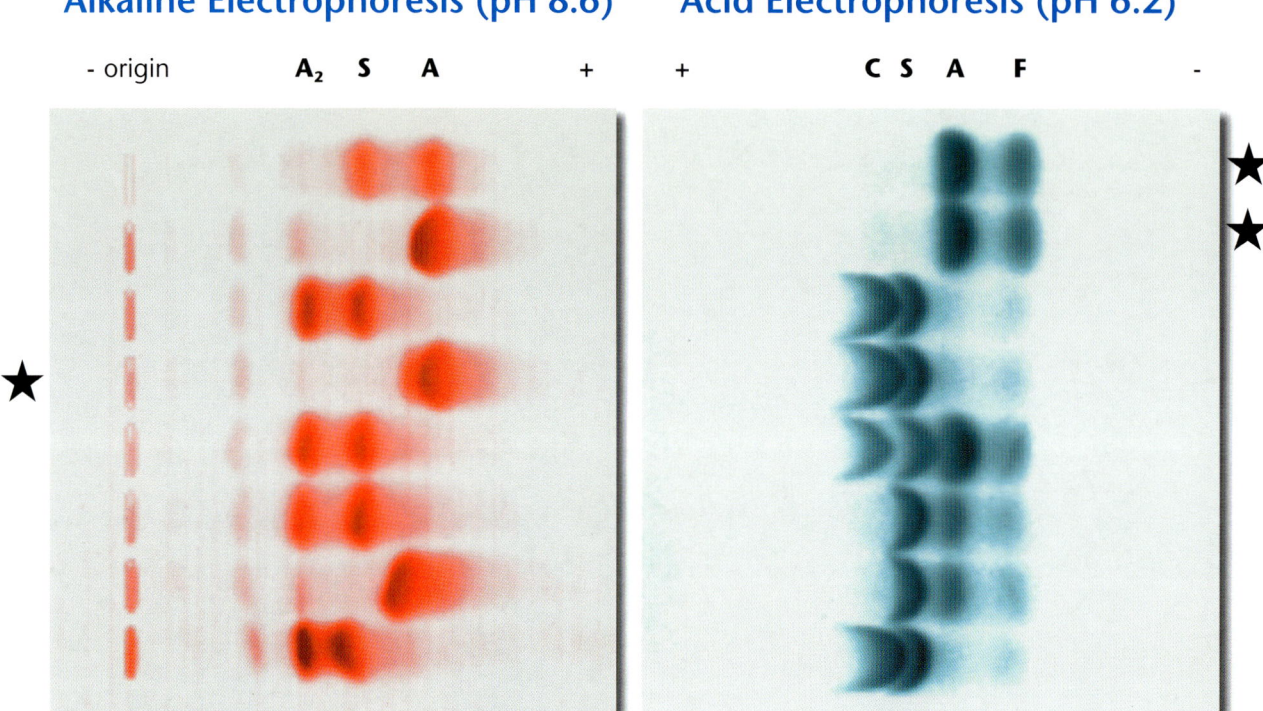

Interpretation

On both alkaline and acid electrophoresis, there is an increase in Hb F. The quantitative measurement of Hb F was 15.0%. The quantitative measurement of Hb A_2 was 1.0%.

Diagnosis

δβ-thalassemia trait.

Performance

δβ-thalassemia trait has been included twice in the survey, but identification has been required only once. The correct response was given by 75.1% of laboratories. 12.9% of laboratories incorrectly labeled this β-thalassemia trait.

Discussion

δβ-thalassemia is caused by deletions of large segments of DNA on chromosome 11 that include both the δ and β genes. Rare types of deletions also include the $^A\gamma$ gene ($^A\gamma\delta\beta^0$-thalassemia) or even show total deletion of the entire β globin gene complex ($^G\gamma^A\gamma\ \delta\beta^0$-thalassemia). δβ-thalassemia trait is approximately one-fiftieth as common as β-thalassemia trait. The most common of the δβ-thalassemia mutations is termed the Sicilian type, which involves a -13.4 kB deletion. This mutation has been found in multiple ethnic groups in Mediterranean countries (including Egypt).

The gene deletions seen in δβ-thalassemia are very similar to those seen in the deletional forms of HPFH. Like HPFH, δβ-thalassemia is characterized by persistent elevation of Hb F into adulthood. However, the increase in γ globin chains does not entirely compensate for the decreased β chains. Therefore, there is an α chain excess, and thus a β-thalassemic phenotype. Hb F in δβ-thalassemia trait is typically elevated to 5-15% of the total Hb; Hb A_2 is normal or low. The patients also show microcytosis without anemia. Analysis of the cellular distribution of Hb F (such as by the Kleihauer-Betke test or flow cytometry) shows a heterocellular distribution. Patients homozygous for this δβ mutation have been reported. These patients have 100% Hb F and clinical features of thalassemia intermedia.

References

Bunn HF, Forget BG. *Hemoglobin: Molecular, Genetic and Clinical Aspects.* Philadelphia, PA: WB Saunders Co; 1980:338.

Bollekens JA, Forget BG. δβ thalassemia and hereditary persistence of fetal hemoglobin. *Hematol Oncol Clin North Am.* 1991;5:399-422.

Gimferren E, Biaget M, Rutllant MF. Homozygous δβ thalassemia in a Spanish woman. *Acta Hematol.* 1979;61:226-229.

Huisman THJ, Carver, MFH, Baysac E. *A Syllabus of Thalassemia Mutations (1997).* Augusta, GA: Sickle Cell Anemia Foundation; 1977:211-234.

Weatherall DJ, Clegg JB. The δβ and related thalassemias. In: *The Thalassemia Syndromes.* 4th ed. Oxford, England: Blackwell Science, Ltd; 2001: 357-392.

Wood WB. Hereditary persistence of fetal hemo-globin and δβ thalassemia. In: Steinberg MH, Forget BG, Higgs DR, Nagel RL. *Disorders of Hemoglobin: Genetics, Pathophysiology, and Clinical Management.* Cambridge, England: Cambridge University Press; 2001:356-388.

Case 6

HISTORY
The patient is a 46-year-old male of English ancestry examined because of life-long anemia. Splenectomy had been performed at age 20. This was followed by minimal amelioration of the anemia. No other member of his family was similarly affected. The physical examination showed mild scleral icterus, slight hepatomegaly, and a surgical scar in the upper left abdomen.

BLOOD COUNT DATA
RBC .... 3.6 x 10^{12}/L
Hb .... 8.9 g/dL
MCV .... 71.0 fL
WBC .... 6.8 x 10^9/L
Plt .... 876 x 10^9/L

PERIPHERAL BLOOD SMEAR
Erythrocyte hypochromia and microcytosis with numerous target cells, elliptocytes, schistocytes, RBCs with basophilic stippling, numerous normoblasts, Howell-Jolly bodies, and Pappenheimer bodies.

OTHER LABORATORY TESTS
Reticulocytes 4.8%
Serum indirect bilirubin 1.9 mg/dL
Serum total bilirubin 2.5 mg/dL
Serum iron 297 µg/dL

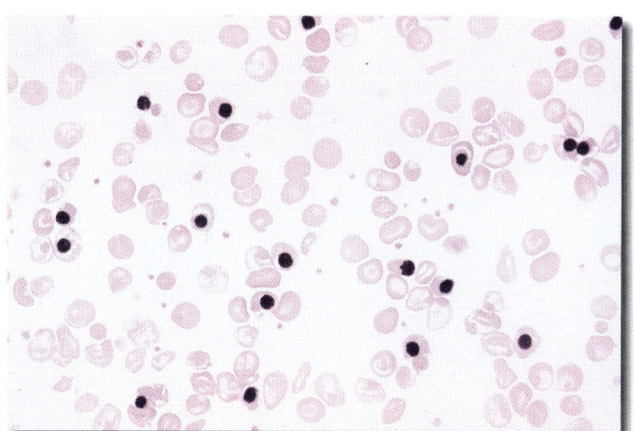

Alkaline Electrophoresis (pH 8.6)

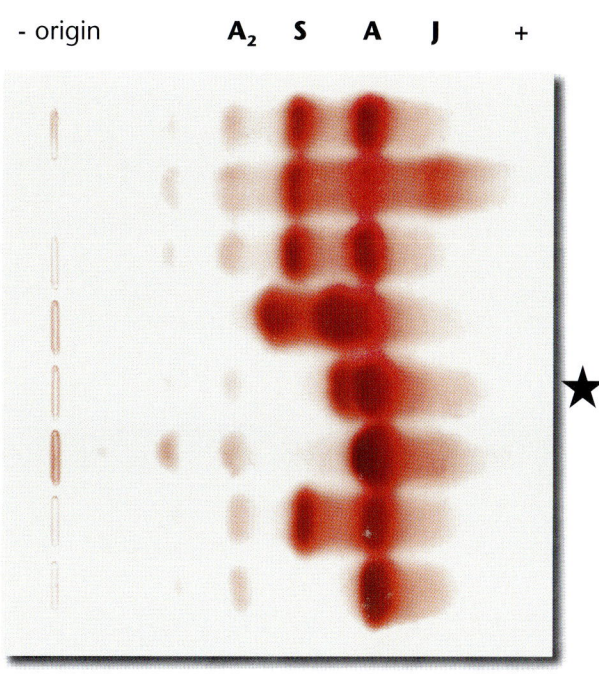

Case Studies

Case 6 Discussion

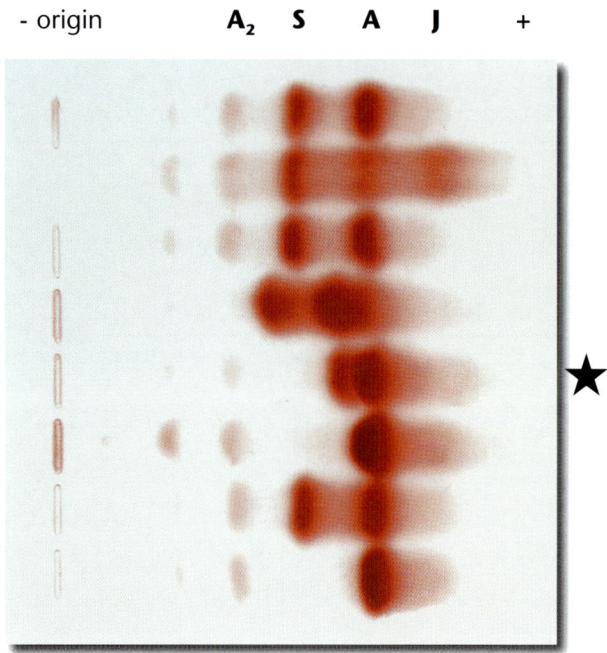

Alkaline Electrophoresis (pH 8.6)

Interpretation
On alkaline electrophoresis, there is a band in the A position and a band in the F position. Acid electrophoresis (not shown) confirms the increase in Hb F, and quantitative measurement for Hb F shows a level of 33%. Quantitative measurement of Hb A_2 was 3.1%.

Diagnosis
Homozygous β^+-thalassemia.

Performance
48.9% of laboratories correctly interpreted this case as homozygous β-thalassemia; other incorrect answers were HPFH trait (34.2%), δβ-thalassemia (22.4%), and β-thalassemia trait (11.8%).

Discussion

Because of the genetic complexity of the β-thalassemias (see *A Closer Look At...Beta-Thalassemia,* page 24), these disorders are generally classified on a clinical basis. The mild end of the spectrum (β-thalassemia minor or trait) is the heterozygous form that results in only a modest decrease in β chain production. This is an asymptomatic disorder with little or no anemia (see Case 3). On the other end of the spectrum is β-thalassemia major (Cooley's anemia), resulting from total or near-total abrogation of β chain production by both alleles. This is a profound transfusion-dependent anemia that is fatal in childhood if untreated; adequately transfused patients ultimately succumb to iron overload in early adulthood. β-thalassemia intermedia (of which this case is an example) encompasses a wide range of clinical severity between these two extremes. The distinction between β-thalassemia major and β-thalassemia intermedia rests primarily on whether a patient is transfusion-dependent or not. β-thalassemia intermedia is usually due to inheritance of two β⁺-thalassemia alleles. Both parents of the patient in this case had slight microcytosis and slight elevation of Hb A_2. Genetic analysis of the β globin genes of the parents demonstrated a guanine to adenine mutation in nucleotide 252, near the 3′ end of intron-1 of mRNA (IVS-1-110 (G→A) in both; the patient was homozygous for this abnormality. This mutation is the most common cause of β-thalassemia in Mediterranean peoples, in that it is responsible for approximately 50% of β-thalassemia in that region. This is a β⁺ mutation, and thus the patient's erythroblasts are able to produce β globin chains in sufficient quantity such that the anemia is not as severe as in β-thalassemia major.

The diagnosis of one of the severe β-thalassemias (major or intermedia) is usually straightforward. The blood smear will demonstrate marked anisopoikilocytosis, including hypochromia, target cells, elliptocytes, and fragments. Prominent erythroblastosis is also an important diagnostic feature. Other morphologic abnormalities include Howell-Jolly bodies and basophilic stippling (Figure 6.1). In a patient with severe life-long anemia, the finding of a prominent elevation in the proportion of hemoglobin F (20-40% for β-thalassemia intermedia and 60-98% for β-thalassemia major) without any abnormal hemoglobin species establishes the diagnosis. Note that Hb A_2 may or may not be elevated in patients with severe forms of β-thalassemia. The most frequent misdiagnosis on an electrophoretic basis in severe β-thalassemias is hereditary persistence of fetal hemoglobin; however, this is easily ruled out on clinical and hematologic grounds, as such patients will have normal (or elevated) hemoglobin levels, and will usually not be microcytic. The hematologic and electrophoretic findings in this case could be consistent with compound heterozygosity for δβ-thalassemia and β⁺-thalassemia, but this is unlikely.

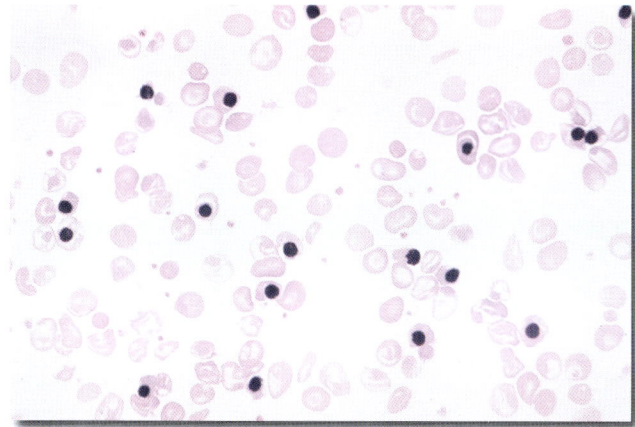
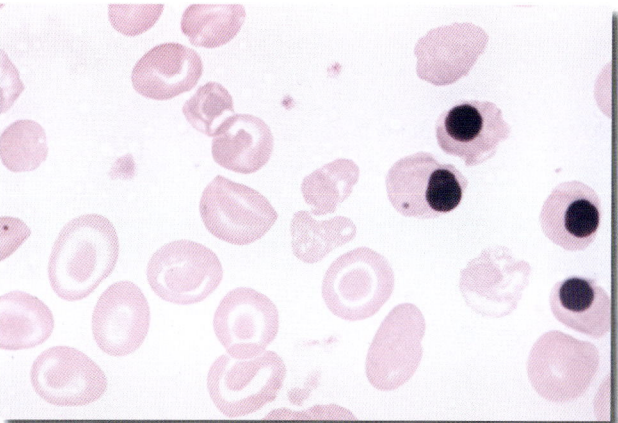

Figure 6.1 (Wright-Giemsa, 160x and 400x)
The peripheral blood appearance of a patient similar to Case 6. There is prominent anisopoikilocytosis with increased target cells and misshapen cells. There are numerous nucleated RBCs present. Some red blood cells contain Howell-Jolly bodies consistent with a previous splenectomy.

References

Antonarakis SE, Kazazian HH, Jr. Molecular basis of the thalassemia syndromes. In: *CRC Handbook Series in Clinical Laboratory Science, Section I: Hematology,* Volume IV. Boca Raton, FL: CRC Press Inc; 1986: 249-261.

Bunn HF, Forget BG. The thalassemias clinical manifestations. In: *Hemoglobin: Molecular, Genetic, and Clincal Aspects.* Philadelphia, PA: WB Saunders Co; 1986:322-380.

Bussliner M, Moschonas N, Flavell RA. β+-thalassemia: aberrant splicing results from a single point mutation in an intron. *Cell.* 1982;27:289.

Spritz RA, Jagadeesvaran P, Choudary PV, et al. Base substitution in an IVS of a β+ thalassemia human globin gene. *Proc Natl Acad Sci USA.* 1981;78: 2455-2459.

Weatherall DJ, Clegg JB. The β-thalassemias. In: *The Thalassemia Syndromes.* 4th ed. Oxford: Blackwell Science, Ltd; 2001:287-356.

Case 7

HISTORY
The patient is a 25-year-old African-American male who is asymptomatic. The physical examination is unremarkable.

BLOOD COUNT DATA
Hgb..............................14.8 g/dL
MCV ....93.1 fL
WBC ....4.6 x 10⁹/L
Plt ....279 x 10⁹/L

PERIPHERAL BLOOD SMEAR
The peripheral blood smear shows no abnormalities.

OTHER LABORATORY TESTS
The solubility test for sickling hemoglobin was positive.

Alkaline Electrophoresis (pH 8.6)

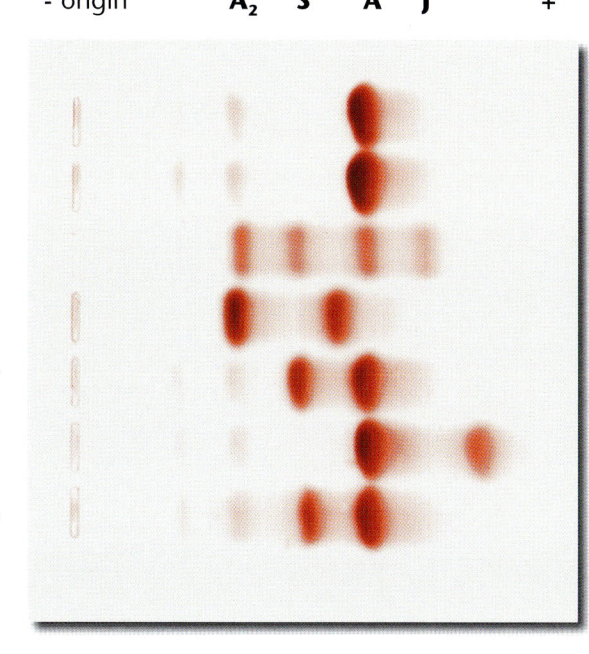

Acid Electrophoresis (pH 6.2)

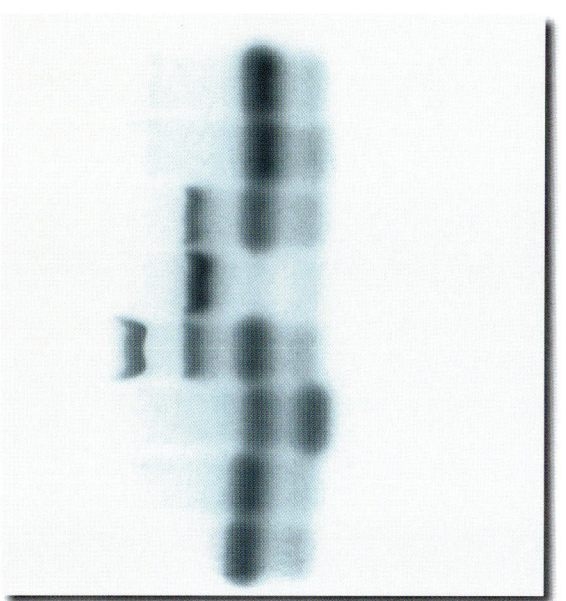

Case Studies

Case 7 Discussion

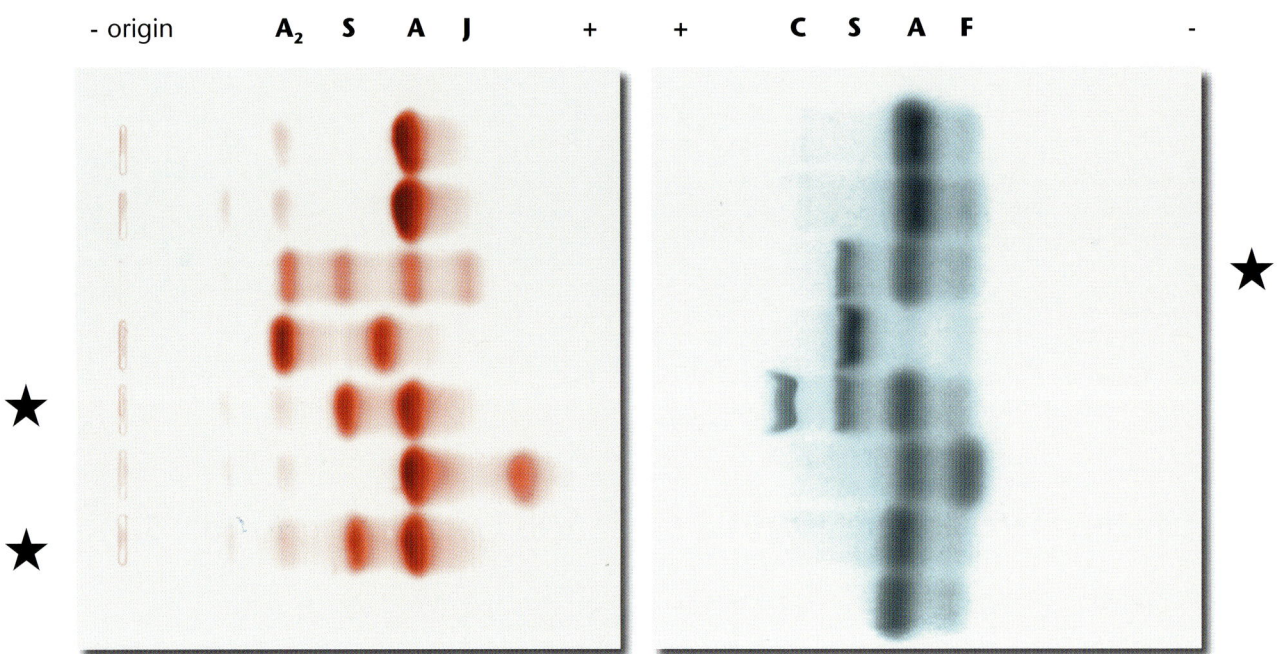

Interpretation

In addition to the bands corresponding to Hb A and Hb A_2, there is an additional band which accounts for approximately 30-35% of the total hemoglobin present. This band is in the S position on both alkaline and acid electrophoresis.

Diagnosis

Hb S trait.

Performance

Hb S trait has been used in the survey 21 times. The identification of this has been excellent, with correct responses ranging from 95–99.6%.

Discussion

Hb S results from a glutamic acid to valine mutation at the 6th amino acid position of the β chain [β6 (A3) Glu→Val]. Hb S was the first hemoglobin variant to be discovered and is the most well studied. Although sickle cell anemia, the disease entity caused by homozygous Hb S, was first described in 1910, Dr. Linus Pauling and associates in 1949 were the first to demonstrate that the disease itself was due to an abnormal hemoglobin. In 1959, Dr. Vernon Ingram demonstrated the nature of the amino acid substitution resulting in the abnormal hemoglobin. Worldwide, Hb S is found in highest frequency in Africa. Although found throughout the African continent, it is found in highest proportion in two areas in west (Nigeria and Ghana) and central (Gabon and Zaire) Africa, in which a gene frequency as high as 0.165 has been reported. There are two other notable pockets of high gene frequency: (1) the northeast corner of Saudi Arabia and Kuwait and (2) an area in east central India. The gene frequency in these two areas approaches 0.1. Hb S is also found throughout the Mediterranean littoral, and can be found in overall low frequencies in Greece, Sicily, Italy, and Turkey. The overall prevalence of Hb S trait in these areas is approximately 1%, but there are areas in which the prevalence is higher. For example, in Turkey, the prevalence is very low in the eastern, central, and northern areas of the country; but on the Mediterranean coast, it is much higher. It is highest in the Eti Turks, where in some areas the prevalence of Hb S trait approaches 35-40%. In American blacks, Hb S trait occurs in approximately 8% of individuals, with a gene frequency of 0.04. Based on haplotype analysis, it appears that the Hb S mutation has likely occurred several times in different ethnic groups (see case DL-11).

Hb S trait is usually asymptomatic. Hematologic parameters and blood smear findings are within normal limits. Hematuria is one of the few clinical manifestations of Hb S, occurring in <1% of cases. For unknown reasons, the hematuria seems most often to result from bleeding from the left kidney. The hematuria is usually mild but recurrent. It usually requires no other treatment but reassurance. Very rare sickling complications have been reported under extreme circumstances, such as flying in an unpressurized airplane, severe pneumonia, and high altitude exercise. The electrophoretic findings in this case are typical, in that the percentage of the variant obtained is approximately 35-40%. If the percentage of Hb S is <33%, one should expect a concurrent α-thalassemia or iron deficiency. Many other hemoglobin variants have a similar electrophoretic pattern as Hb S on alkaline electrophoresis. However, other simple techniques, such as a sickle solubility test or acid electrophoresis, will confirm the presence of Hb S. Examples of Hb S trait are shown on HPLC (Figure 7.1) and isoelectric focusing (Figure 7.2).

There are many other variants (both α and β) which migrate in the "S position" on cellulose acetate. Definite identification of these variants usually requires other methodology, such as isoelectric focusing and globin chain electrophoresis. The most significant of these are Hb D-Los Angeles and Hb G-Philadelphia. These variants will be presented in subsequent cases.

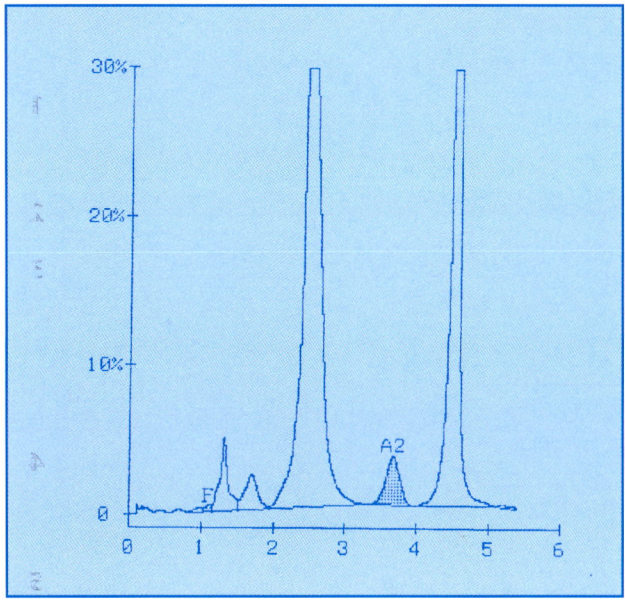

Figure 7.1

An example of Hb S trait by HPLC. There is a prominent peak, accounting for approximately 30-35% of the total hemoglobin which elutes in the S window (4.3-4.7 minutes). The Hb A_2 level appears slightly elevated (4.0-4.5%), which is typical for Hb S trait by this method but does not imply concurrent β-thalassemia trait.

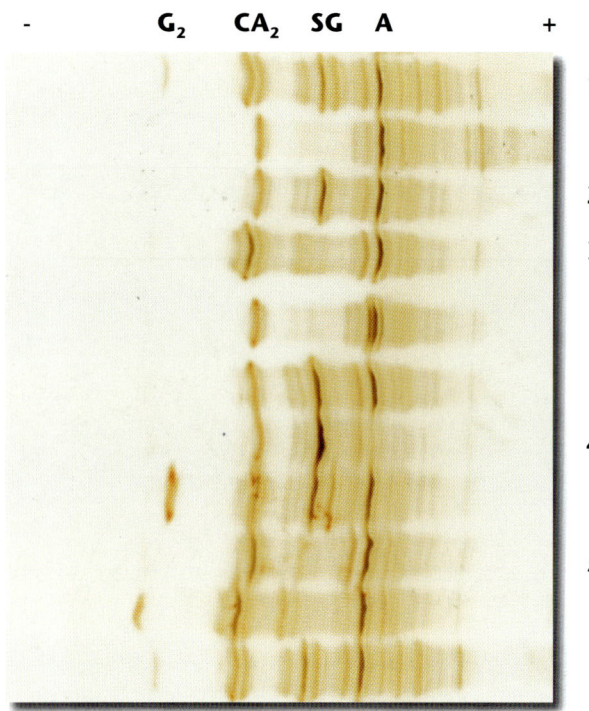

Figure 7.2
An example of Hb S trait by isoelectric focusing. 1-control, 2-Hb S trait, 3-Hb C trait, 4-Homozygous S, 5-Hb E trait.

References

Bunn HF, Forget BG. *Hemoglobin: Molecular Genetic and Clinical Aspects.* 1st ed. Philadelphia, PA: WB Saunders Co; 1986:508-510.

Fairbanks VF. *Hemoglobinopathies and Thalassemias.* New York, NY: Brian C. Decker; 1980:10-11.

Pauling S, Itano HA, Singer ST, Wells IC. Sickle cell anemia: a molecular disease. *Science.* 1949;110: 543-548.

Steinberg MH. Sickle cell trait. In: Steinberg MH, Fogret BG, Higgs DR, Nagel RC, eds. *Disorders of Hemoglobin: Genetics, Pathophysiology and Clinical Management.* Cambridge, England: Cambridge University Press; 2001:811-830.

Winter WP, ed. *Hemoglobin Variants in Human Populations.* Vols. I and II. Boca Raton, FL: CRC Press; 1986.

Case 8

HISTORY
The patient is a 27-year-old African-American male examined because his sister was found to have a sickling disorder. The physical examination showed no abnormalities.

BLOOD COUNT DATA
RBC ....5.7 x 10^{12}/L
Hgb ....14.3 g/dL
MCV ....78.0 fL
WBC ....4.7 x 10^9/L
PLT ....324 x 10^9/L

PERIPHERAL BLOOD SMEAR
The peripheral blood smear shows mild microcytosis and numerous codocytes (target cells).

OTHER LABORATORY TESTS
The solubility test for sickling hemoglobin was negative.

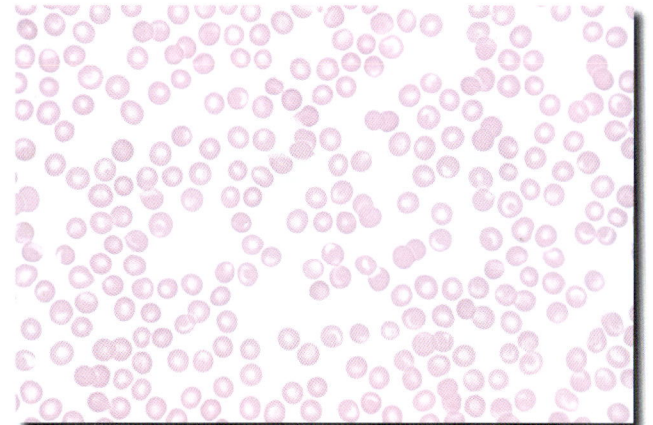

Alkaline Electrophoresis (pH 8.6)

-     origin   A₂   S   A   J   +

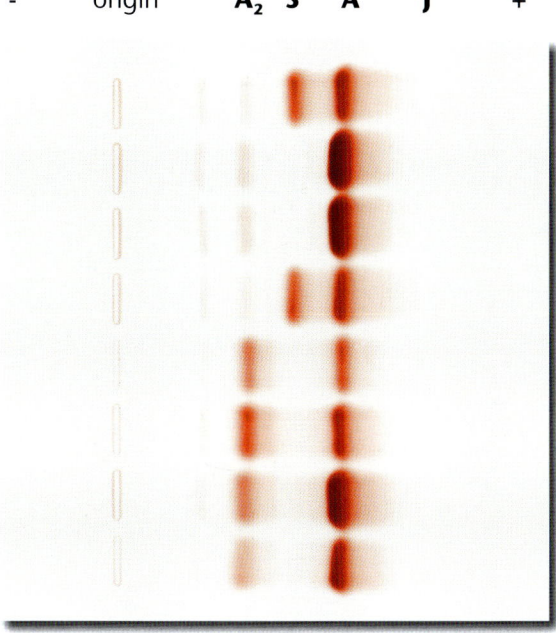

Acid Electrophoresis (pH 6.2)

+   C   S   A   F   -

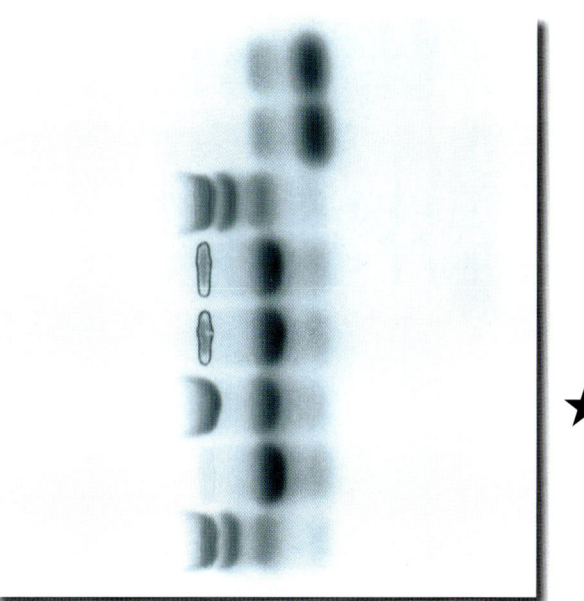

Case Studies

Case 8 Discussion

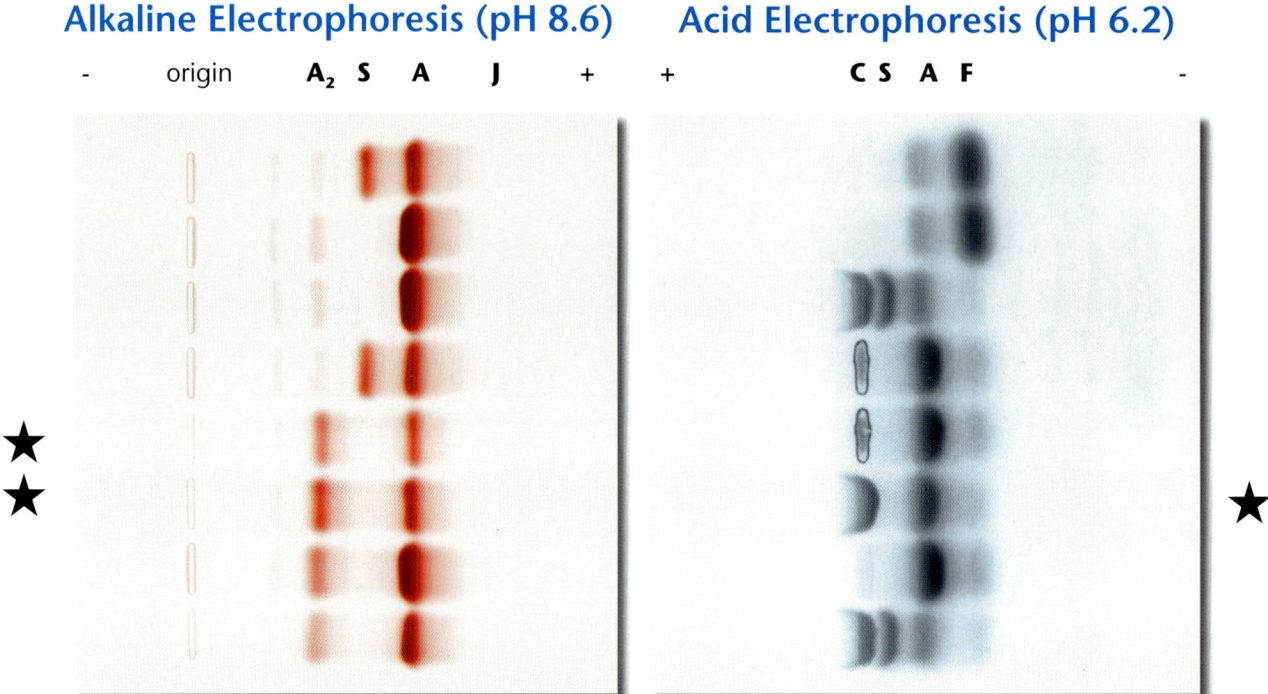

Interpretation
In addition to the band in the Hb A position, there is a major band in the Hb A_2 position which accounts for approximately 35-40% of the total hemoglobin. Acid electrophoresis reveals two bands: one in the A position and one in the C position.

Diagnosis
Hb C trait.

Performance
Hemoglobin C trait has been included in the survey six times. Identification of this variant as been excellent, with correct responses ranging from 89.9–99%.

Discussion

Hb C results from a substitution of glutamic acid by lysine at the 6th amino acid of the β chain [β 6 (A3) Glu→Lys]. Note that this is the same amino acid position involved in Hb S. Hb C trait occurs in 2-3% of African Americans. The presence of Hb C trait implies ancestry back to the western part of Africa, particularly areas of Ghana and the upper Volta region, in which the gene frequency approaches 0.15. Thus, in this area, about 25% of individuals are heterozygous for Hb C. Hb C is rarely found in other ethnic groups.

Hb C trait is characterized by target cells in the blood smear, often accompanied by a mild microcytosis (Figure 8.1). It has no other clinical or hematologic manifestations. Hb C can be seen in combination with other hemoglobin variants, in particular Hb S, as will be discussed in subsequent cases. The cause of the mild microcytosis in Hb C trait is not completely understood. This may simply be a manifestation of somewhat decreased production of Hb C itself. It does not appear to be the result of a concurrent α-thalassemia because the frequency of α-thalassemia in African Americans is insufficient to explain all cases of Hb C trait with microcytosis. Furthermore, in such cases, although there is microcytosis present, the percentage of Hb C is in the 35-40% range, which is not suggestive of concurrent α-thalassemia.

Hb E, Hb O-Arab, and Hb C-Harlem all migrate with Hb C on alkaline electrophoresis. However, none of these migrate in the C position on acid electrophoresis, making diagnosis of Hb C a straightforward task. Examples of Hb C trait on HPLC and isoelectric focusing are shown in Figures 8.2 and 8.3.

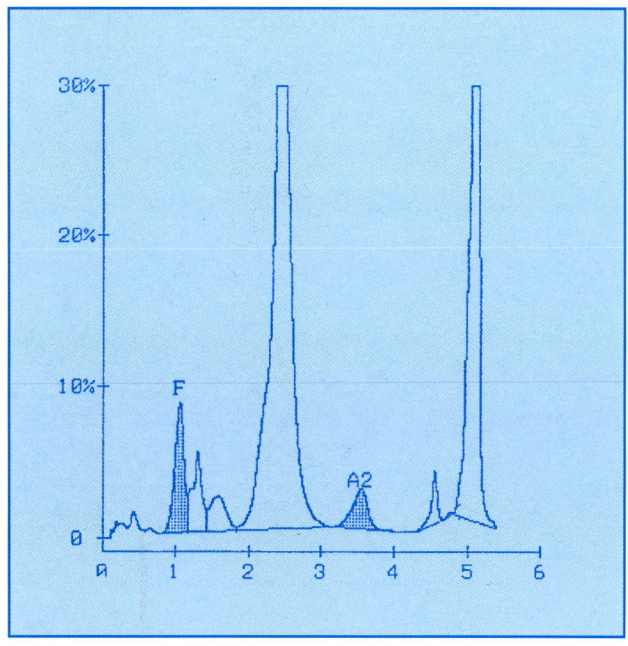

Figure 8.2
An example of Hb C trait by HPLC. There is a prominent peak in the "C window" (4.85-5.15 minutes), which accounts for approximately 35-45% of the total hemoglobin. There is also a very small peak that elutes in front of the main Hb C peak, which is felt to represent glycosylated hemoglobin C (Hb C_{1c}).

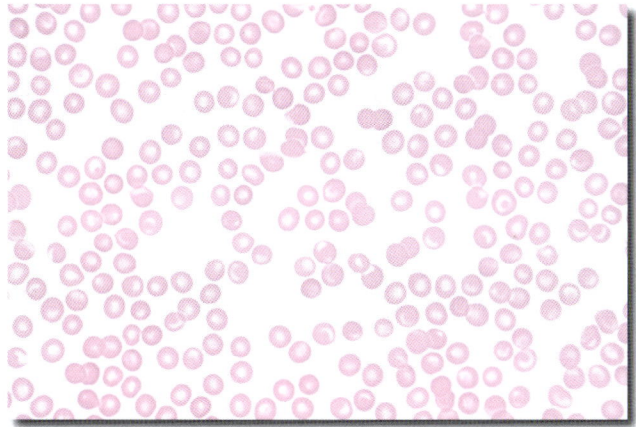
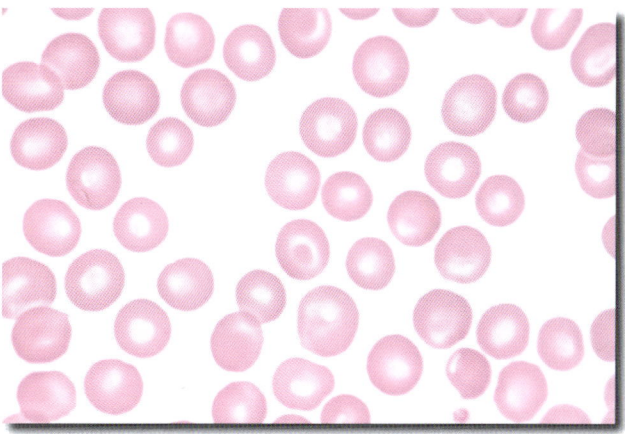

Figure 8.1 (Wright-Giemsa, 160x and 400x)
Low- and high-power views of the peripheral blood smear in a patient with Hb C trait. The red blood cells are mildly microcytic; occasional target cells are present.

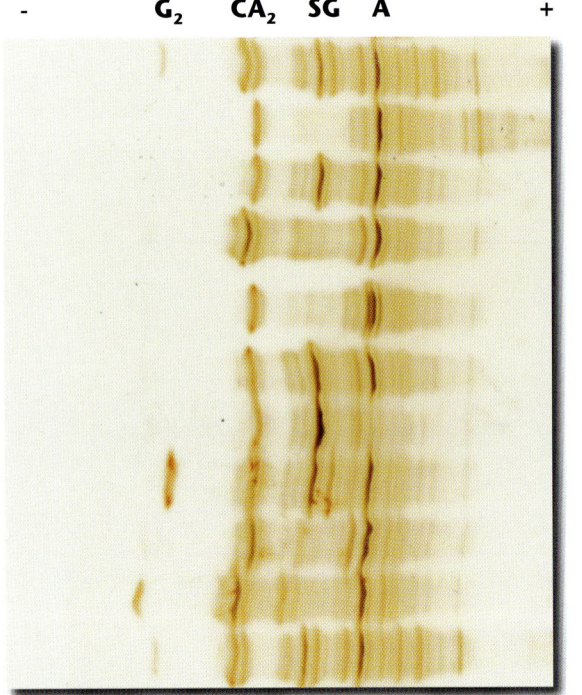

Figure 8.3
An example of Hb C trait by isoelectric focusing. 1-control, 2-Hb S trait, 3-Hb C trait, 4-Homozygous Hb S, 5-Hb E trait.

References

Bunn HF, Forget BG. *Hemoglobin: Molecular, Genetic and Clinical Aspects.* 1st ed. Philadelphia, PA: WB Saunders Co; 1986:421-425.

Fairbanks VF. *Hemoglobinopathies and Thalassemias.* New York, NY: Brian C. Decker; 1980:11-12.

Fairbanks VF. Letter-to-the-editor. *Blood.* 1980; 56: 141-142.

Itano HA, Neel JV. A new inherited abnormality of human hemoglobin. *Proc Natl Acad Sci USA.* 1950;36: 613.

Winter WP. *Hemoglobin Variants in Human Populations.* Volume II. Boca Raton, FL: CRC Press; 1986:11-28.

Case 9

HISTORY
The patient is a 25-year-old male of Asian descent who is asymptomatic. The physical examination showed no abnormalities.

BLOOD COUNT DATA
RBC .... 6.3×10^{12}/L
Hgb .... 14.9 g/dL
MCV .... 76.0 fL
WBC .... 8.9×10^9/L
Plt .... 324×10^9/L

PERIPHERAL BLOOD SMEAR
There is minimal microcytosis and occasional target cells.

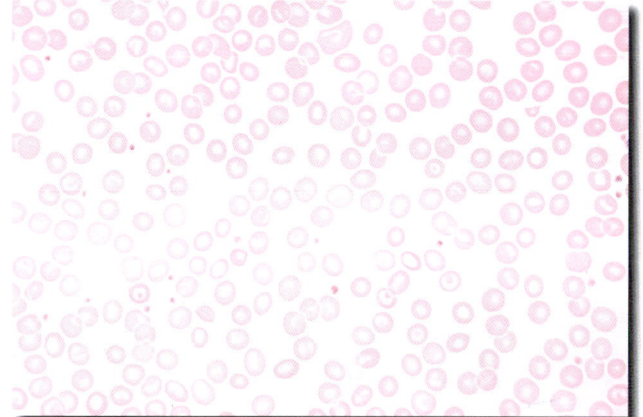

Alkaline Electrophoresis (pH 8.6)

Acid Electrophoresis (pH 6.2)

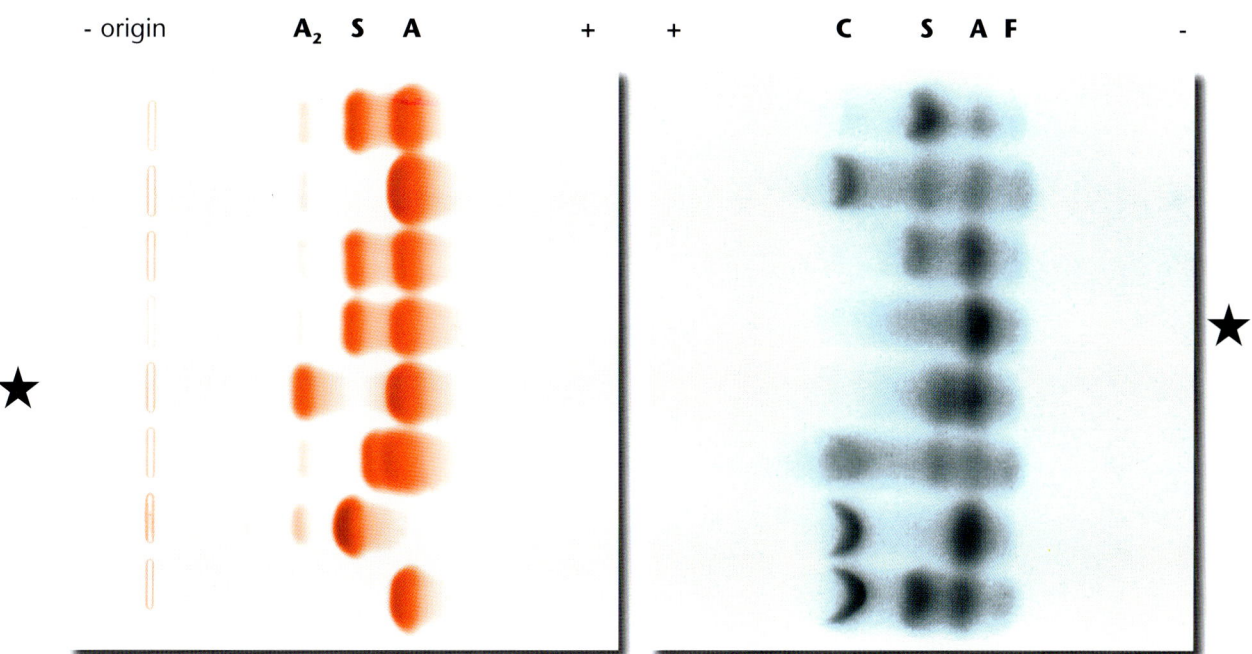

Case 9 Discussion

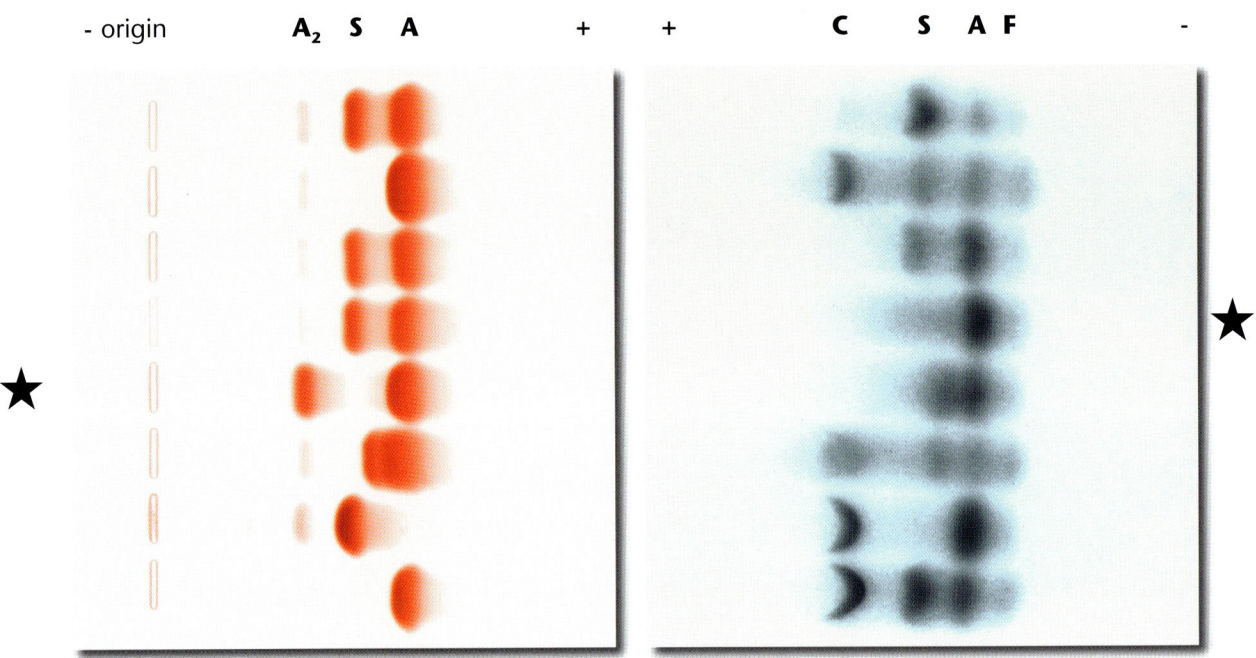

Interpretation
On alkaline electrophoresis, there are two major bands seen, one in the A position and one in the A_2 (CEO) position. On acid electrophoresis, there is only one band seen in the A position.

Diagnosis
Hb E trait.

Performance
Hb E trait has been included in the survey 4 times, with correct responses ranging from 87.4–96.3%.

Discussion

Hb E results from a substitution of lysine for glutamic acid at the 26th amino acid of the β globin chain [β26 (β8) Glu→Lys]. The 26th codon at which the nucleotide substitution of Hb E occurs is near the end of the first exon of the β globin gene. The alteration in the 26th codon from GAG (Glu) to AAG (Lys) creates a nucleotide sequence in the messenger RNA that is very similar to the splicing site that is present at the beginning of the first intron. This "donor" splice site is critical in removing the intron nucleotide sequences to form the resultant messenger RNA that is used for translation into the β globin protein. If the normal splicing sequence is used, an intact β globin protein with the Hb E mutation is produced. If the cryptic splicing site formed by the Hb E mutation is utilized, an abnormal and probably non-functional mRNA is produced. This process is similar to some types of β-thalassemia mutations, which can also involve activation of cryptic splicing sites. The end result of this alteration of the splicing process is the production of smaller amounts of functional β-globin mRNA, and thus under-production relative to normal β chains. This results in a thalassemic phenotype. Hb E is unstable by the heat and isopropanol tests but does not cause clinical signs of hemolysis.

Hb E is very common in Southeast Asia. However, within different countries and ethnic groups, there is a wide variability in its prevalence. For example, Hb E is very common in Cambodia, Laos, and Thailand. At the junction of these three countries, the prevalence of Hb E trait reaches 50-60% (the so-called "Hb E triangle"). Conversely, Hb E is uncommon in persons of ethnic Chinese or Vietnamese origin. Hb E is also found on the Indian subcontinent, particularly in Bengalese from Bangladesh or West Bengal and in the Indian state of Assam. Hb E is also rarely seen in Europeans and African Americans.

Hb E trait does not cause anemia but is associated with a mildly thalassemic picture, including mild microcytosis and target cells on the peripheral blood smear (Figure 9.1). The percentage of Hb E in the trait form is usually 30-35% of the total hemoglobin, which is lower than that seen with Hb S trait or Hb C trait. With concurrent α-thalassemia, the percentage of Hb E is <30% (see *A Closer Look At...Hb E-Associated Disorders*, page 72). On alkaline electrophoresis, Hb E co-migrates with Hb C, Hb O-Arab, and Hb C-Harlem. However, while Hb E migrates with Hb A on acid electrophoresis, the other three abnormal hemoglobins separate from Hb A. Examples of Hb E trait by HPLC and isoelectric focusing are shown in Figures 9.2 and 9.3.

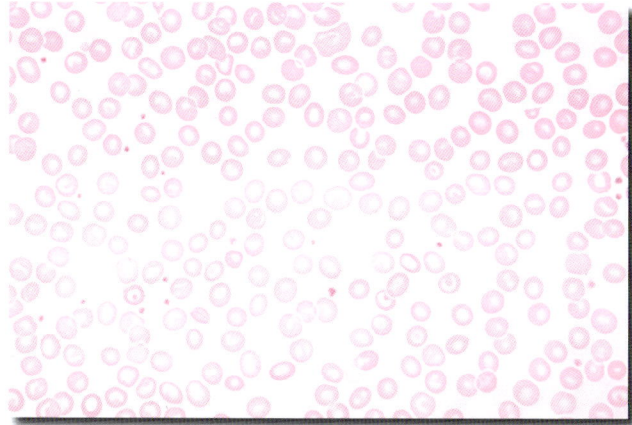 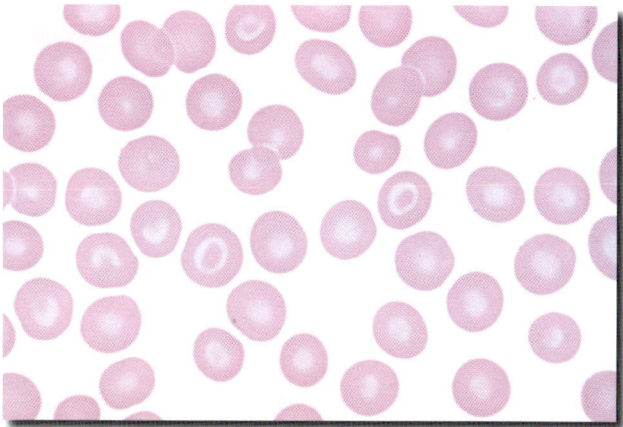

Figure 9.1 (Wright-Giemsa, 160x and 400x)
Low- and high-power views of the peripheral blood smear in a patient with Hb E trait. The red blood cells are mildly microcytic with slight anisocytosis and occasional target cells.

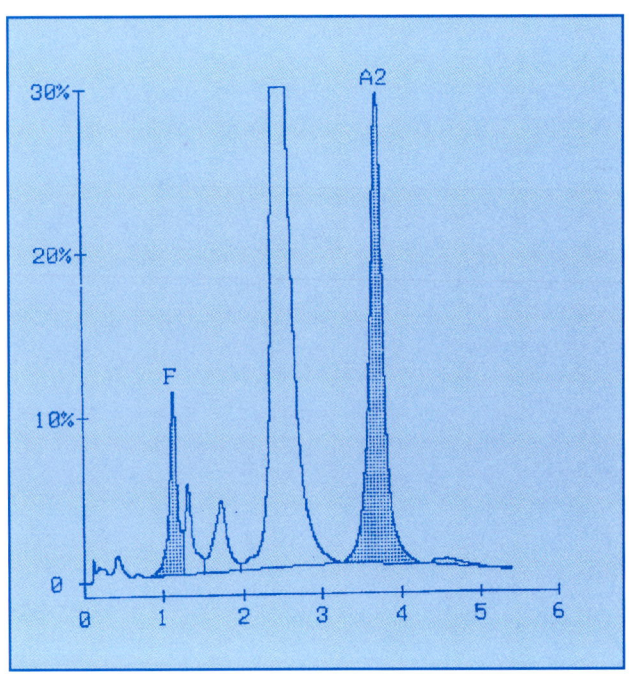

Figure 9.2
An example of Hb E trait by HPLC. There is a prominent peak in the A_2 position, which accounts for 30-35% of the total hemoglobin. The mild increase in Hb F is due to the young age of this patient.

References

Chernoff AI, Minnich V, Chongchareonsuk S. Hemoglobin E, a hereditary abnormality of human hemoglobin. *Science.* 1954;120:605-606.

Fairbanks VF, Gilchrist GS, Brimhall B, et al. Hemoglobin E trait reexamined: a cause of microcytosis and erythrocytosis. *Blood.* 1979;53:109-115.

Itano HA, Bergren WR, Monzon CM, Fairbanks VF, Burgert EO Jr, et al. Hematologic genetic disorders among Southeast Asian refugees. *Am J Hematol.* 1985;19:27-36.

Sturgeon P. Identification of a fourth abnormal human hemoglobin. *J Am Chem Soc.* 1954;75:2278.

Thompson MW, McInnes RR, Willard HF. *Genetics in Medicine.* 5th ed. Philadelphia, PA: WB Saunders Co; 1991:266-269.

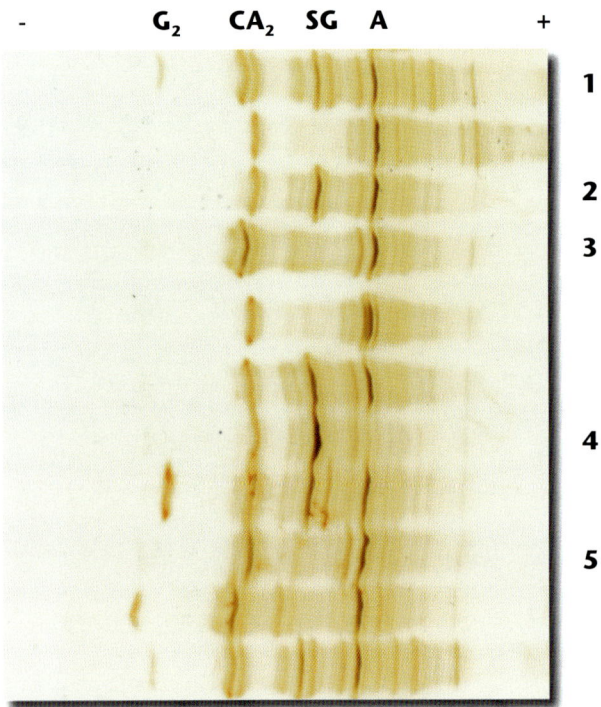

Figure 9.3
An example of Hb E trait by isoelectric focusing. 1-control, 2-Hb S trait, 3-Hb C trait, 4-Homozygous S, 5-Hb E trait.

Case 10

HISTORY
The patient is a 40-year-old Caucasian male who is asymptomatic. The physical examination is normal.

BLOOD COUNT DATA
RBC .... $6.0 \times 10^{12}/L$
Hb .... 15.0 g/dL
MCV .... 75.0 fL
WBC .... $6.3 \times 10^9/L$
Plt .... $250 \times 10^9/L$

PERIPHERAL BLOOD SMEAR
The peripheral blood smear is notable for microcytosis and mild hypochromia in the red blood cells with occasional target cells.

OTHER LABORATORY TESTS
The solubility test for sickling hemoglobin is negative.

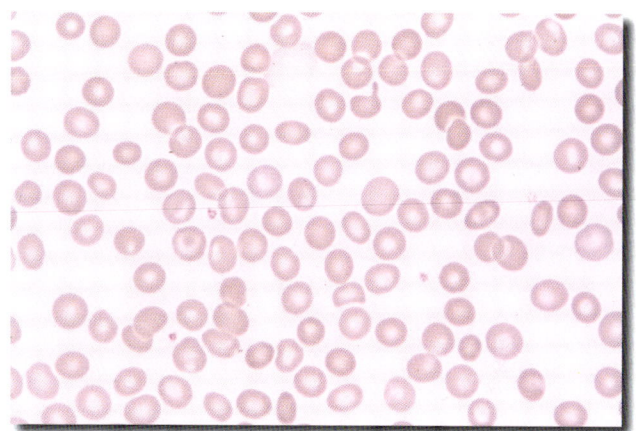

Alkaline Electrophoresis (pH 8.6)

Acid Electrophoresis (pH 6.2)

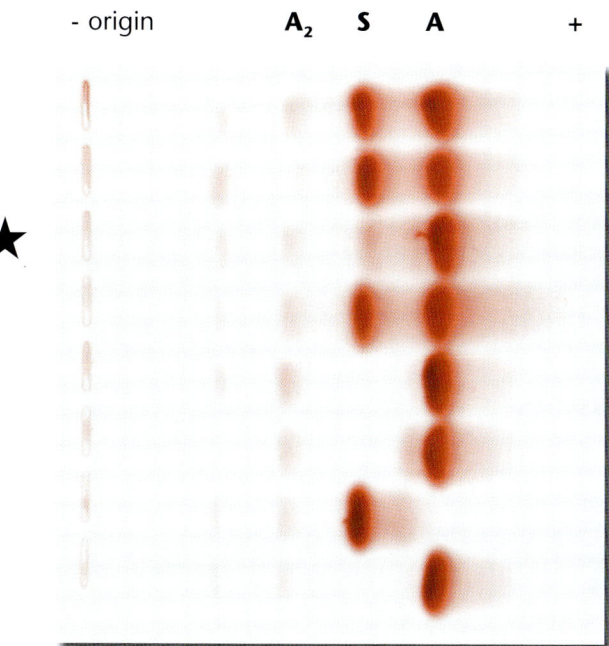
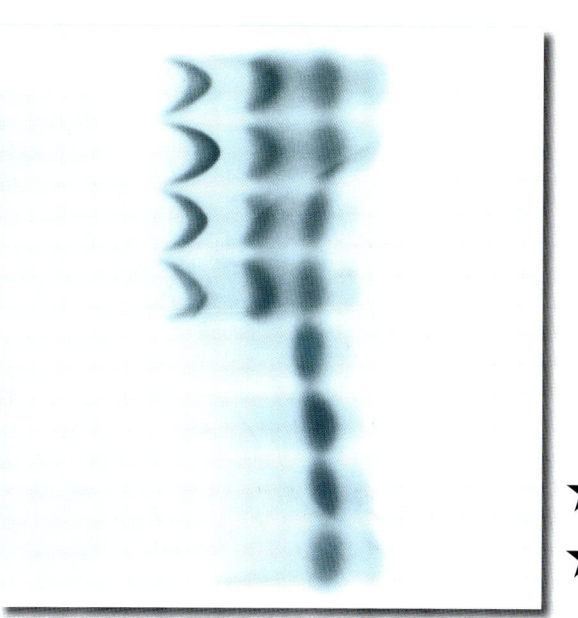

Case Studies 53

Case 10 Discussion

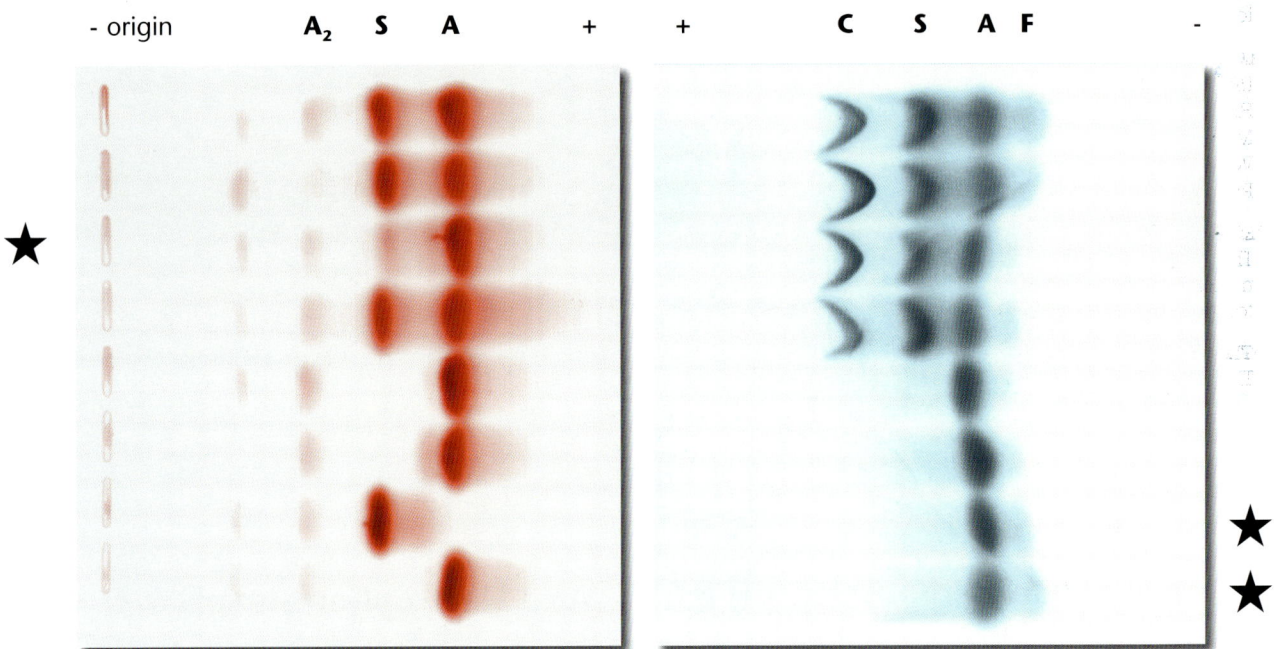

Interpretation
On alkaline electrophoresis, there is a band seen in the S position, which accounts for 10-15% of the total hemoglobin. The remainder is in the A position. On acid electrophoresis, there is only a band in the A position.

Diagnosis
Hb Lepore, probably Hb Lepore-Boston.

Performance
Hb Lepore has been used in the survey five times, with correct responses ranging from 59-77% with a gradual improvement in correct responses.

Discussion

Hb Lepore is a fusion hemoglobin that arose from a non-homologous meiotic crossover event between the β and δ genes. There are three different Hb Lepores described that differ in the precise fusion point of the β and δ genes. The most common of these is Hb Lepore-Boston [δ (1-87) β (115-146)] in which the hybrid globin chain is composed of the first 87 amino acids of delta chain and the last 32 amino acids of the beta chain. This variant has also been called Hb Lepore-Washington and Hb Lepore-Cyprus. The other two Lepores differ only in their breakpoints: Hb Lepore-Baltimore [δ (1-50) β (86-146)] and Hb Lepore-Hollandia [δ (1-22) β (50-146)]. The Hb Lepores are stable hemoglobins that are underproduced relative to normal β chains, and thus the Hb Lepore gene functions as a thalassemic allele. Hemoglobin Lepore-Boston is the only one found with any frequency. It is usually seen in people of Mediterranean descent, particularly in those of Greek, Italian, or Turkish ancestry. In southern Italy, Hb Lepore trait occurs once for every twenty-five cases of β-thalassemia minor. It is also found less frequently in those of northern European origin.

The presence of heterozygous Hb Lepore produces a state mimicking thalassemia minor due to the underproduction of Lepore δ/β hybrid (10-15% of normal). This includes microcytosis and increased target cells (Figure 10.1). There is some debate as to whether Hb Lepore trait can be associated with a mild anemia. Homozygous Hb Lepore produces a severe thalassemic disorder similar to β-thalassemia intermedia or major.

Hb Lepore represents 7-15% of total hemoglobin in the heterozygous state. It migrates in the S position on alkaline electrophoresis and in the A position on acid electrophoresis. Therefore, the differential diagnosis includes other variants with this pattern, the most common of which are Hb D and Hb G. The low proportion of the abnormal hemoglobin and the thalassemic peripheral blood picture allow a presumptive diagnosis of Hb Lepore. High performance liquid chromatography is very useful in the diagnosis of Hb Lepore, as it does not elute in the S window, but rather co-elutes with Hb A_2 (see Figure 10.2). Thus, a minor band in the Hb S position on alkaline electrophoresis with a negative sickle solubility test which co-elutes with Hb A_2 on HPLC is virtually diagnostic of Hb Lepore. An example of Hb Lepore trait on isoelectric focusing is shown in Figure 10.3.

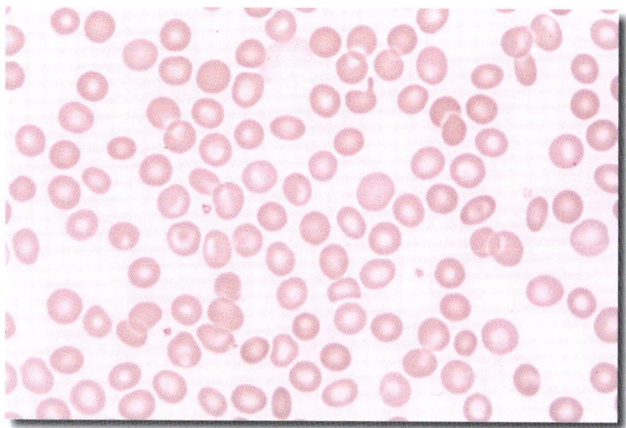

Figure 10.1 (Wright-Giemsa, 165x)
The peripheral blood smear from a patient with Hb Lepore trait. The findings are similar to those seen with β–thalassemia trait, including microcytosis and increased target cells.

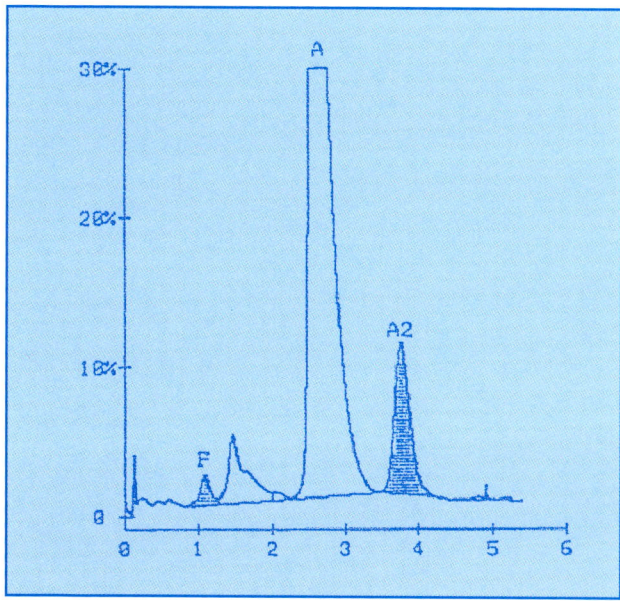

Figure 10.2
Results obtained by HPLC on a patient with Hb Lepore trait. (Originally included in survey set 1994 HG C [Specimen Hb 10].)

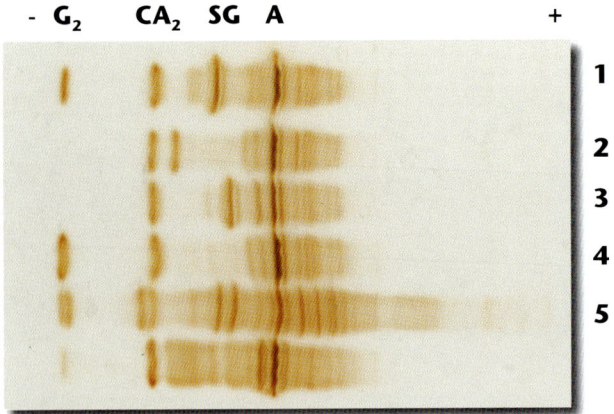

Figure 10.3
An example of Hb Lepore by isoelectric focusing (Lane 3). Hb Lepore migrates in the same position as Hb G-Philadelphia. 1-Hb Hasharon, 2-Hb A_2 Babinga, 4-Hb A_2', 5-control.

References

Baglioni C. The fusion of two peptide chains in hemoglobin Lepore and its interpretation as a genetic deletion. *Proc Natl Acad Sci USA.* 1962;48:1880-1886.

Bunn HF, Forget BG. *Hemoglobin: Molecular, Genetic and Clinical Aspects.* Philadelphia, PA: WB Saunders Co; 1986:297-298.

Duma H, Efremov G, Sadikario A, et al. Study of nine families with hemoglobin Lepore. *Br J Haematol.* 1968;15:161-172.

Fairbanks VF. *Hemoglobinopathies and Thalassemias.* New York, NY: Brian C. Decker; 1980:13,23.

Forget BG. Molecular mechanisms of beta-thalassemia. In: Steinberg MH, Forget BG, Higgs DR, Nagel RC, eds. *Disorders of Hemoglobin: Genetics, Pathophysiology and Clinical Management.* Cambridge, England: Cambridge University Press; 2001:264-265.

Weatherall DJ, Clegg JB. *The Thalassemia Syndromes.* Oxford, England: Blackwell Science, Ltd; 2001: 358-372.

Case 11

HISTORY
The patient is an asymptomatic 45-year-old man of English ancestry. No abnormalities were found on the physical examination.

BLOOD COUNT DATA
RBC .... 5.2×10^{12}/L
Hb .... 15.2 g/dL
MCV .... 87.0 fL
WBC .... 8.3×10^9/L
Plt .... 293×10^9/L

PERIPHERAL BLOOD SMEAR
No abnormalities.

OTHER LABORATORY TESTS
The solubility test for sickling hemoglobin is negative.

Alkaline Electrophoresis (pH 8.6)

- origin   A₂   S   A   +

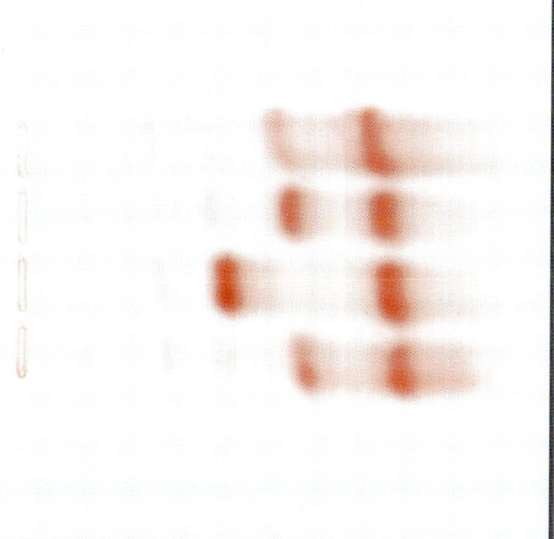

Acid Electrophoresis (pH 6.2)

+   C   S   A   F   -

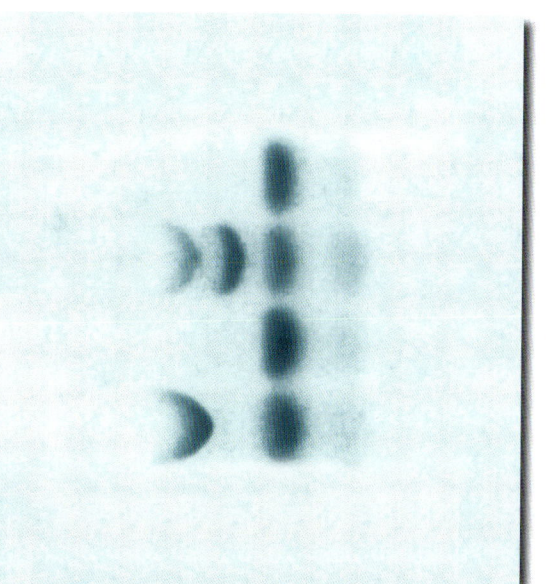

Case 11 Discussion

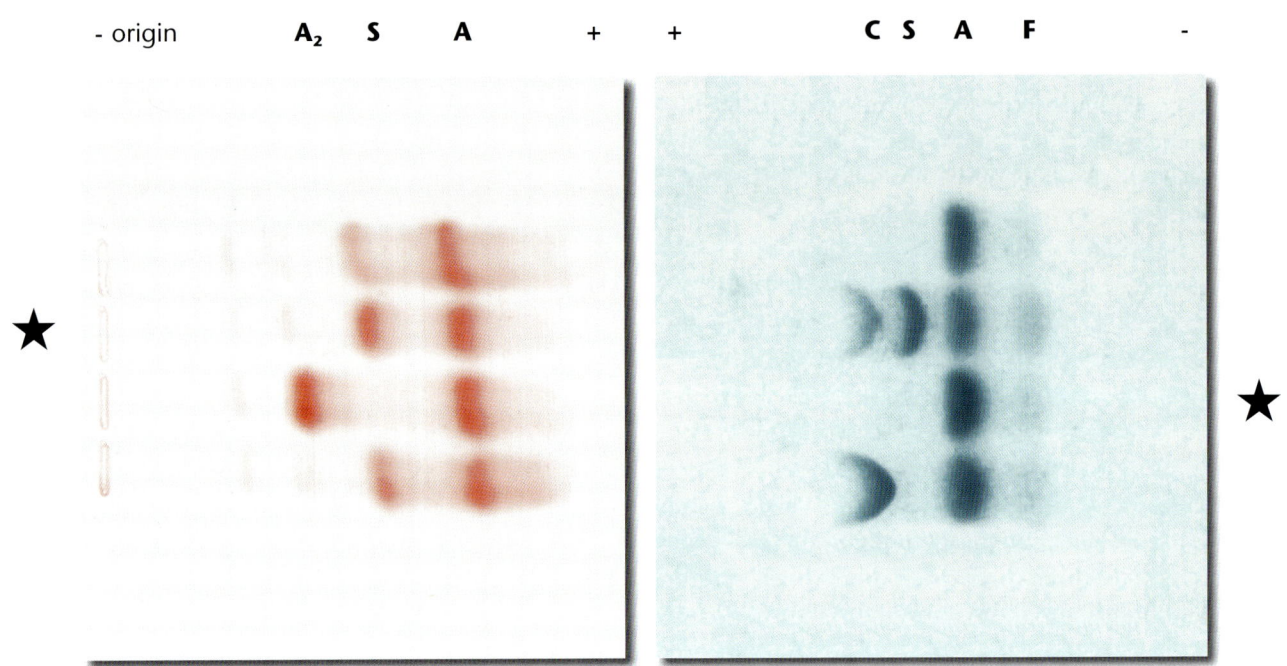

Interpretation

On alkaline electrophoresis, there are two bands present of roughly equal density: one in the A position and one in the S position. On acid electrophoresis, only a band in the A position is seen. Further testing, including isoelectric focusing, globin chain electrophoresis, and HPLC, identified the variant as Hb D-Los Angeles.

Diagnosis

Hb D-Los Angeles (D-Punjab).

Performance

Hb D-Los Angeles has been included in the survey nine times, with correct identifications ranging from 50.9–82%. However, in most cases, many laboratories were partially correct in answering Hb D or G β trait.

Discussion

Hb D-Los Angeles (D-Punjab) results from a substitution of glutamine for glutamic acid at the 121st position of the beta chain (β 121 Glu→Gln). This abnormal hemoglobin demonstrates no functional abnormalities. Worldwide, it is found in highest proportion in the Punjab region of India and Pakistan, where the prevalence of Hb D trait is 3%. In the United States, it is found in persons of North European ancestry, particularly English, where the prevalence is 1 in 10,000. It is also found in African Americans, with a prevalence of 1 in 30,000. Its presence in these two groups indicates some genetic heritage from India or Pakistan. In the English it is felt to be a result of the long British occupation of India.

Hb D-Los Angeles trait is a harmless condition. Patients homozygous for Hb D-Los Angeles have normal hemoglobin levels, normal RBC indices, and no evidence of hemolysis. This condition should be distinguished from Hb D in combination with $β^0$-thalassemia, in which patients have mild anemia and minimal hemolysis. Hb D-Los Angeles copolymerizes with Hb S to produce a severe sickling syndrome. This is felt to be due to enhancement of polymerization due to the Glu→Gln substitution at $β^{121}$, an important contact point for Hb S polymerization.

In the heterozygous state, Hb D-Los Angeles represents approximately 40% of total hemoglobin. Hb D-Los Angeles and Hb Korle-Bu [β 73 (Asp→Asn)] (see Case 20) have very similar electrophoretic mobilities. Therefore, it is often difficult, particularly in heterozygotes, to distinguish these two entities by the usual methods, such as alkaline electrophoresis, acid electrophoresis, globin chain electrophoresis, and isoelectric focusing (IEF). When either of these variants is present together with Hb S (i.e., no Hb A is present), this becomes easier on acid electrophoresis. Hb Korle-Bu migrates slightly anodic to Hb A (towards Hb S), whereas Hb D-Punjab migrates in the Hb A position. However, when Hb Korle-Bu is present together with Hb A, the two hemoglobins do not separate distinctly but rather form a somewhat broader band. High performance liquid chromatography (HPLC) can be very useful in distinguishing these two variants. As Figure 11.1 illustrates, Hb Korle-Bu elutes in the "A_2 window," whereas Hb D-Punjab has a longer retention time, eluting in "the D window." This distinction is of more than academic interest because, as mentioned, the combination of Hb S plus Hb D-Los Angeles causes a severe sickling disorder, whereas the combination of Hb S plus Hb Korle-Bu is equivalent to Hb S trait alone.

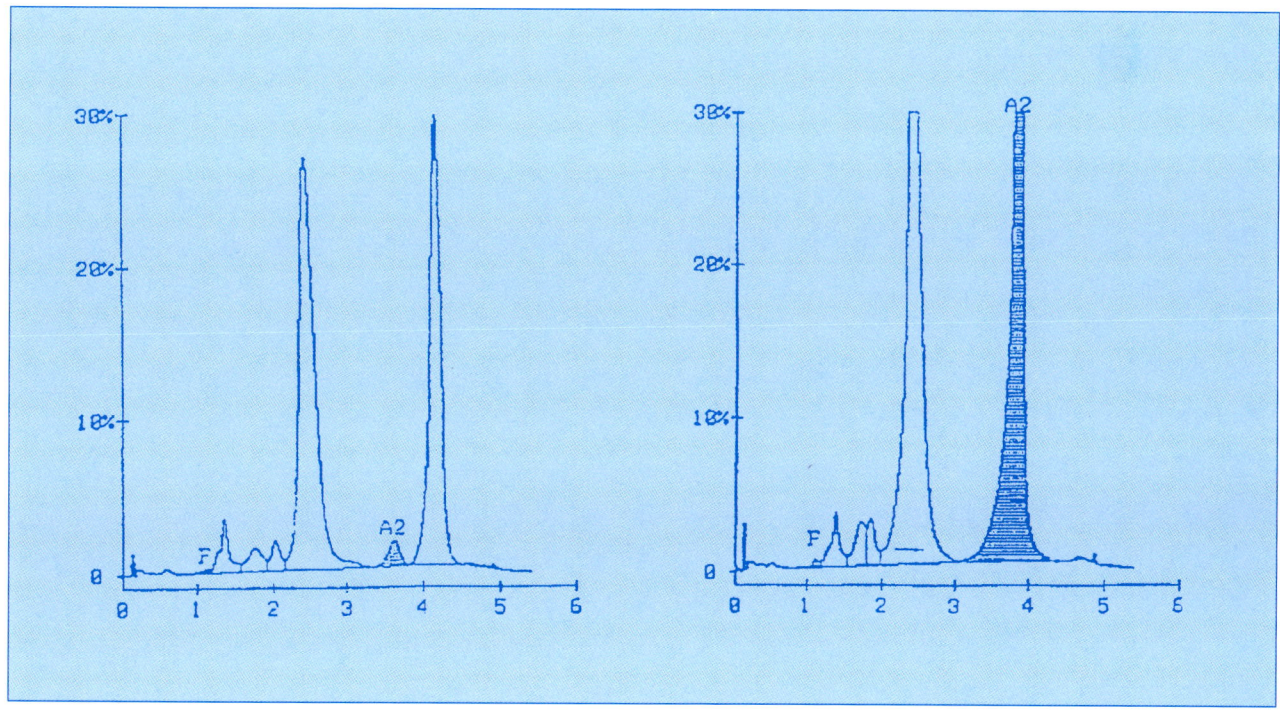

Figure 11.1
Retention times of Hb variants obtained by HPLC: (A) Hb D-Punjab and (B) Hb Korle-Bu. (Originally included in survey set 1996 HG C [Specimen Hb 10].)

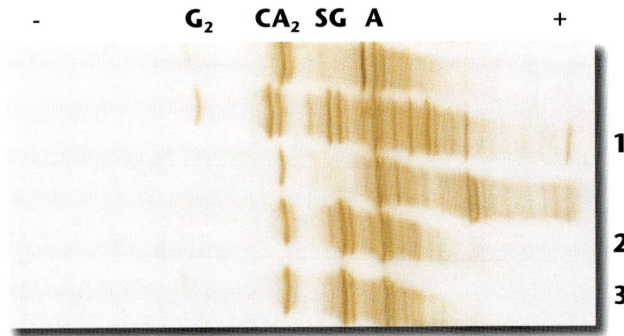

Figure 11.2
An example of Hb D-Los Angeles by isoelectric focusing. 1-control, 2-Hb D-Los Angeles, 3-Hb Korle Bu. As shown, Hb D-Los Angeles and Hb Korle Bu have virtually identical mobilities by isoelectric focusing. The smaller band seen in front of each major band in lanes 2 and 3 probably represents a small amount of glycosylated variant.

References

Babin DR, Jones RT, Schroeder WA. Hemoglobin D-Los Angeles: $\alpha_2^A\beta_2^{121\ GluNH}{}_2$. *Biochim Biophys Acta.* 1964;86:136:143.

Bird GWG, Lehman H. Haemoglobin D in India. *Br Med J.* 1956;1:514-515.

Bunn HF, Forget BG. *Hemoglobin: Molecular, Genetic and Clinical Aspects.* Philadelphia, PA: WB Saunders Co; 1986:425.

Chernoff AI. The hemoglobin D syndromes. *Blood.* 1958;13:116-127.

Itano HA. A third abnormal hemoglobin associated with hereditary hemolytic anemia. *Proc Nat Acad Sci USA.* 1951;7:775-784.

Tsistrakis GA, Scampardonis GJ, Clonizakis JP, et al. Hemoglobin D and D thalassemia: a family report, comprising 18 members. *Acta Haematol.* 1975;54:172-179.

Case 12

HISTORY
The patient is an asymptomatic 32-year-old African-American woman with a normal physical examination.

BLOOD COUNT DATA
RBC .... 4.9 x 10^{12}/L
Hb .... 14.1 g/dL
MCV .... 87.0 fL
WBC .... 3.9 x 10^9/L
Plt .... 272.0 x 10^9/L
Reticulocytes .... 50 x 10^9/L

PERIPHERAL BLOOD SMEAR
No abnormalities.

OTHER LABORATORY TESTS
A test for unstable hemoglobin was negative. A sickling test was negative.

Alkaline Electrophoresis (pH 8.6)

- origin   A₂   S   A   +

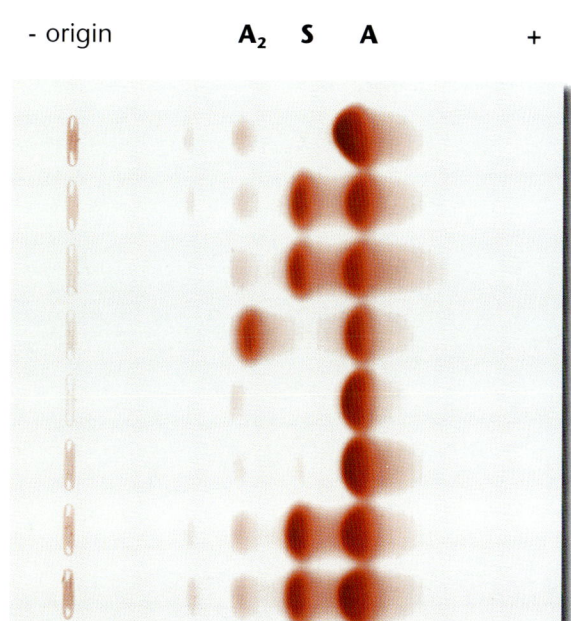

Acid Electrophoresis (pH 6.2)

+   C   S   A   F   -

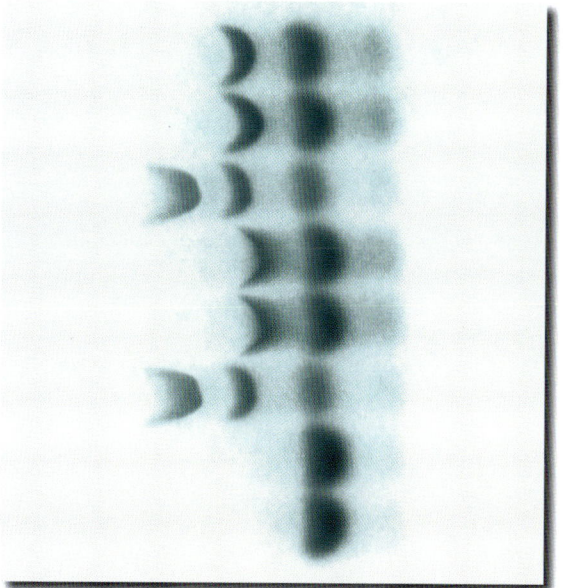

Case 12 Discussion

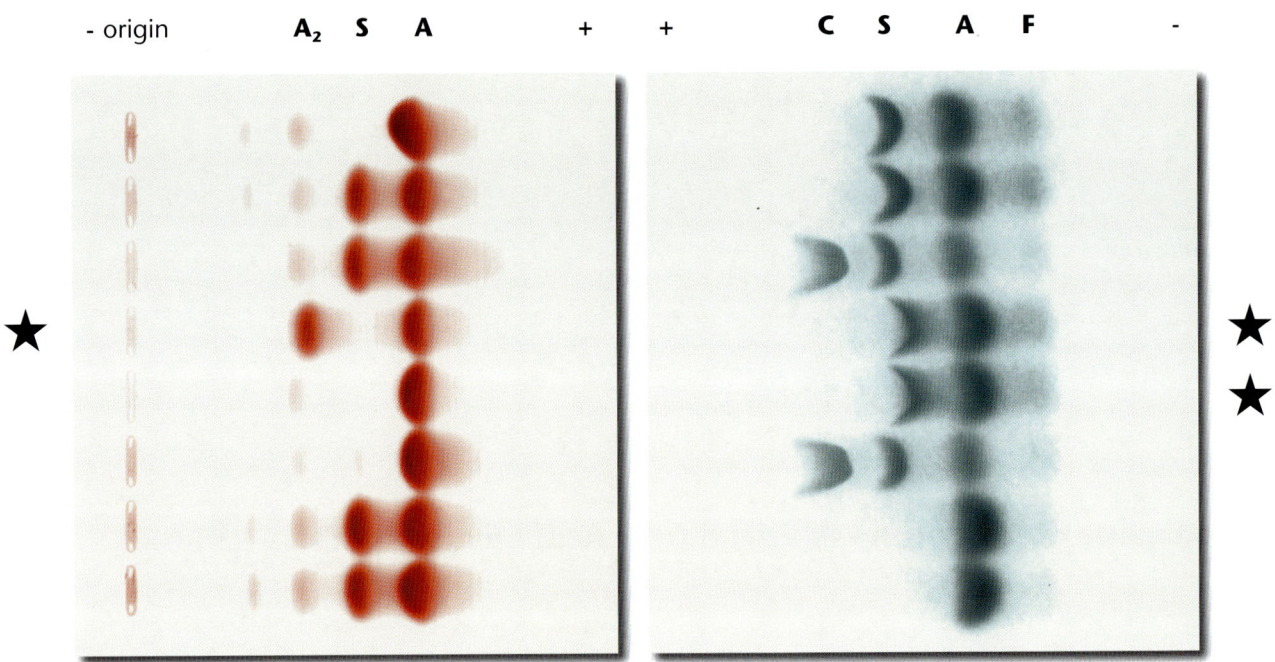

Interpretation

The alkaline electrophoresis gel demonstrates two distinct bands in the A and A₂/C positions, representing approximately 60% and 40% of the total hemoglobin, respectively. The acid electrophoresis demonstrates bands migrating in the A position and between A and S.

Diagnosis

Hb O-Arab trait.

Performance

Hb O-Arab trait has been used in the survey on three occasions. Among laboratories using alkaline and acid electrophoresis, isoelectric focusing, or HPLC, the diagnosis was made correctly by 67%, 69%, and 100% of participants. The most common misdiagnosis was Hb C-Georgetown (Harlem), which was submitted by 23%, 24%, and 0% of labs. Hemoglobin C trait was diagnosed by 5%, 7%, and 0% of labs.

Discussion

Hemoglobin O-Arab results from a glutamic acid to lysine substitution at the 121st amino position of the β globin chain (β121 Glu→Lys). This substitution results in migration to the A_2/C position on alkaline electrophoresis. Hemoglobin O-Arab has a wide geographic distribution but occurs most commonly in the African-American population, with a prevalence of approximately 1 in 30,000. Interestingly, it is most commonly found in Bulgaria, but it is actually rare in Arabs.

Hemoglobin O-Arab causes no hematologic abnormalities in heterozygotes and a mild anemia in homozygotes. It is clinically significant only when seen in the double heterozygous state with hemoglobin S. Despite the fact that it is not in itself a sickling hemoglobin (in that it lacks the $β^{6Val}$ substitution), it co-polymerizes with hemoglobin S and produces a disorder similar to SS disease, with prominent vasoocclusive phenomena and moderately severe anemia, although the hemolysis tends to be slightly less severe than in SS disease. This property appears to derive from the presence of an amino acid substitution at β121, an important intermolecular contact site; this feature is also shared by hemoglobin D-Los Angeles (Punjab).

Hemoglobin O-Arab is easily distinguished from Hb A_2 because it represents greater than 10% of the total hemoglobin (which A_2 virtually never does). After identification of an abnormal hemoglobin migrating in the A_2/C position on alkaline electrophoresis, additional studies are needed to further characterize this and differentiate it from other hemoglobins migrating in the C position of alkaline gels, most notably Hb C, Hb E, and Hb C-Harlem. On acid gels, Hb O-Arab migrates between hemoglobins S and A, in contrast to Hb C-Harlem, which migrates with Hb S, and Hb E, which migrates with Hb A. Because Hb O-Arab can migrate very close to Hb S on acid gels, additional information may be needed to firmly differentiate it from Hb C-Harlem. In this case, the negative sickling test rules out Hb C-Harlem. Note that hemoglobins O-Arab, E, and C-Harlem show identical migration patterns on isoelectric focusing. An example of Hb O-Arab trait on HPLC and IEF are shown in figures 12.1 and 12.2.

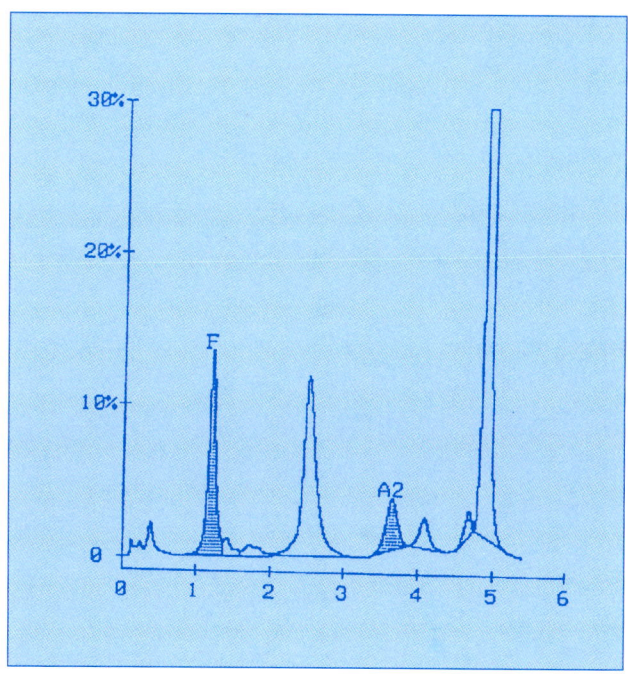

Figure 12.1
An example of Hb O-Arab trait by HPLC. There is a prominent peak present with a retention time that is between the S window and C window. This peak elutes slightly less than five minutes. The increased amount of Hb F is due to this patient's young age.

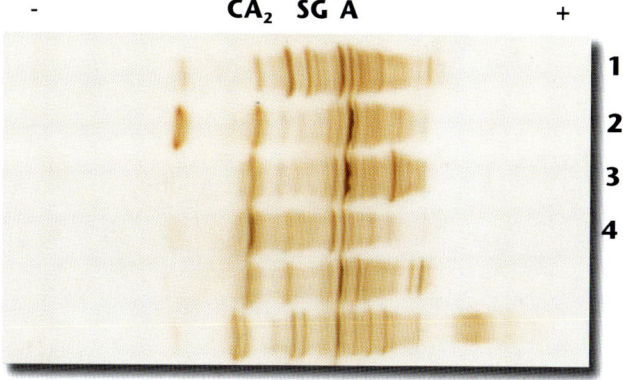

Figure 12.2
An example of Hb O-Arab trait by isoelectric focusing. Hb O-Arab migrates in the A_2 position and is shown in lane 4. Other hemoglobins included on this gel include: 1-Hb Stanleyville, 2-Hb A_2', 3-Hb I trait.

References

Baglioni C, Lehmann H. Chemical heterogeneity of hemoglobin O. *Nature.* 1962:196:229.

Ibrahim SA, Mustafa D, Mohamed AO, Mohen MB. Homozygous hemoglobin O disease and conjugated hyperbilirubinemia in a Sudanese family. *Br J Med.* 1992;304:27.

Milner PF, Miller C, Grey R, et al. Hemoglobin O Arab in four negro families and its interaction with hemoglobin S and hemoglobin C. *N Engl J Med.* 1970;283:1417.

Ramot B, Fisher S, Remez D, et al. Hemoglobin O in an Arab family: sickle cell hemoglobin O trait. *Br Med J.* 1960;2:1262.

Zimmerman SA, O'Branski EE, Rosse WF, Ware RE. Hemoglobin S/O(Arab): thirteen new cases and review of the literature. *Am J Hematol.* 1999;60:279-284.

Case 13

HISTORY
The patient is an 18-year-old African-American male who was evaluated for mild microcytosis. The physical examination is unremarkable.

BLOOD COUNT DATA
RBC................................6.3 x 10^{12}/L
Hb..................................14.2 g/dL
MCV...............................68.0 fL
WBC...............................5.8 x 10^9/L
Plt...................................319 x 10^9/L

PERIPHERAL BLOOD SMEAR
The red blood cells show mild hypochromia and microcytosis with occasional target cells and cells with basophilic stippling.

OTHER LABORATORY TESTS
Serum ferritin 272 µg/L.
Test for unstable hemoglobin was negative.
The solubility test for sickling hemoglobin was negative.

Alkaline Electrophoresis (pH 8.6)

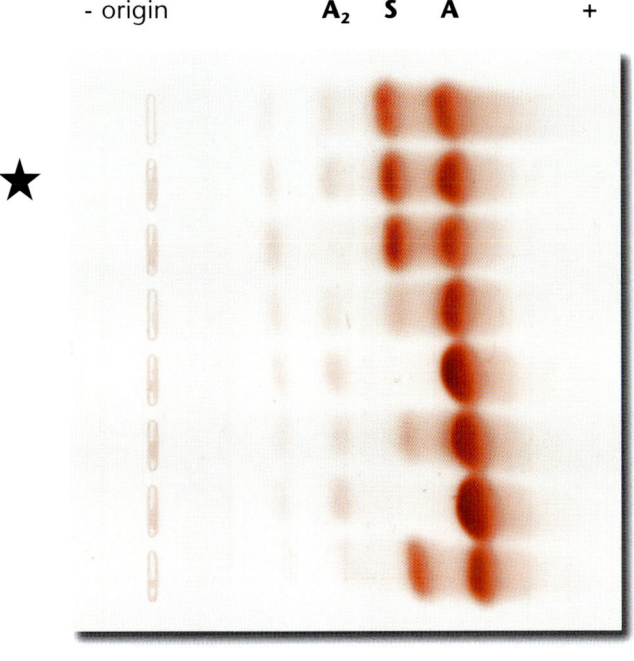

Acid Electrophoresis (pH 6.2)

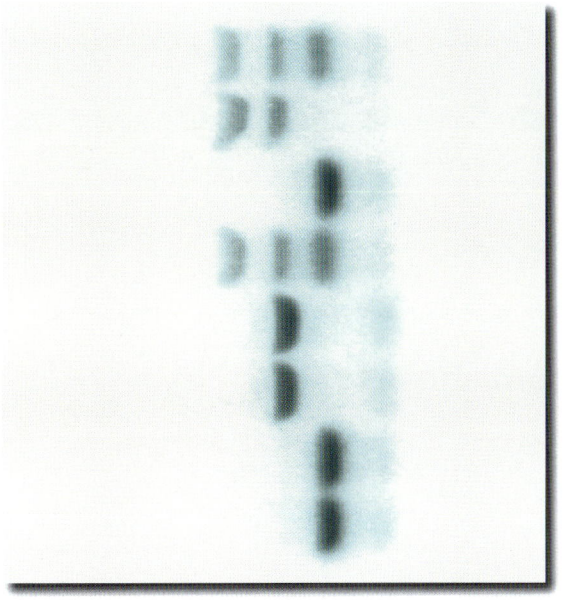

Case 13 Discussion

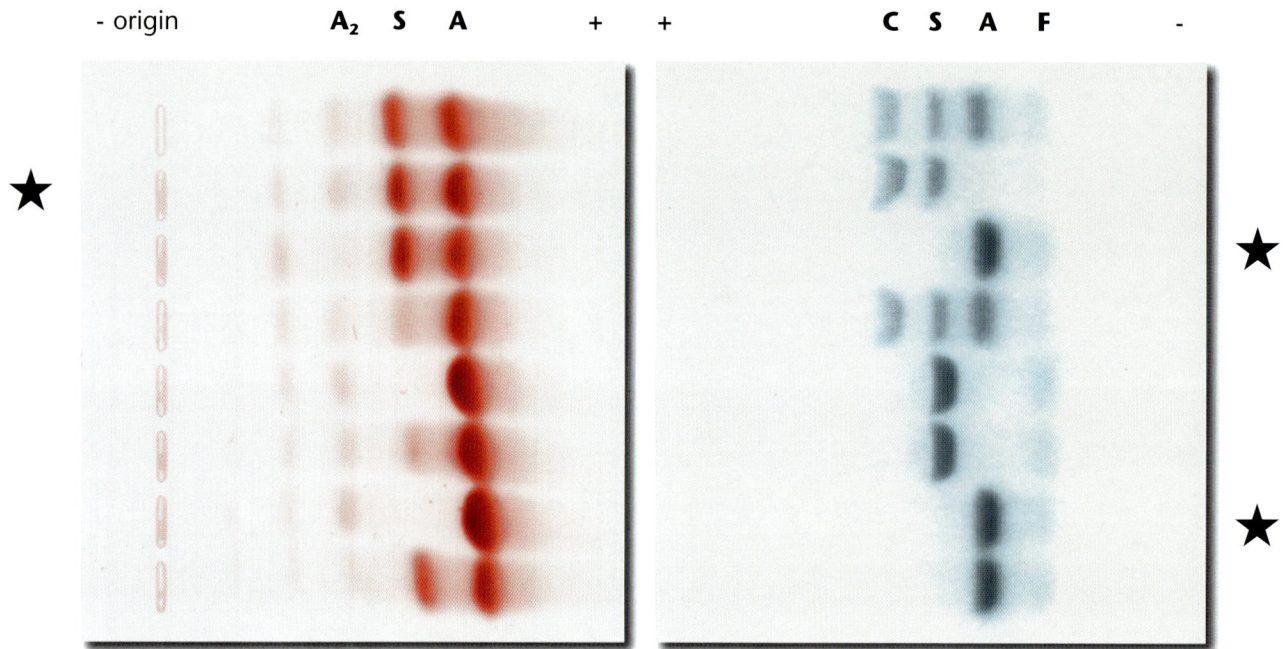

Interpretation

On alkaline electrophoresis, there are two major bands seen; one in the A position, and one in the S position, which accounts for 45% of the total hemoglobin. On acid electrophoresis, there is only a band in the A position. Other techniques, such as isoelectric focusing, globin chain electrophoresis, and HPLC, identify the variant as Hb G-Philadelphia.

Diagnosis

Hb G-Philadelphia, with homozygous α-thalassemia-2.

Performance

Hb G-Philadelphia has been included in the survey twice; the correct identification of Gα trait was given by 53.9% and 60.2% of laboratories.

Discussion

Hb G-Philadelphia results from an asparagine to lysine substitution at the 68th position of the α globin chain (α 68 Asn→Lys). It is the commonest α variant seen in the US, and it is found primarily in African Americans, with a prevalence of 1 in 5000. It has also been reported in Italians and rarely in Chinese. Hb G-Philadelphia has no clinical or hematological effects. Because it is found primarily in African Americans, it can be seen in combination with β globin chain variants such as Hb S and Hb C. This combination of an α and β chain variant can give a bewildering array of bands (see Case 19, page 93).

Hb G-Philadelphia needs to be differentiated from other variants that migrate in the S position, particularly β chain variants. A helpful feature is the presence of Hb G_2, which results from the G-Philadelphia α chains in combination with normal δ chains. On alkaline electrophoresis, Hb G_2 is seen near the carbonic anhydrase position. However, it is often difficult to visualize. It is much more easily seen on isoelectric focusing (Figure 13.2) and is also seen on HPLC (Figure 13.1).

When seen in African Americans, Hb G-Philadelphia is usually associated with the 3.7 Kb α-thalassemia-2 deleteion (-$α^G$) (see *A Closer Look At...Alpha-Thalassemia*, page 18). Because there are only three functional alpha globin genes present, Hb G-Philadelphia accounts for approximately 30% of total hemoglobin. α-thalassemia-2 trait is very common in African Americans (found in approximately 1/3 of individuals); when an α-thalassemia deletion is present on both chromosome 16's, there are only two functioning α-globin genes (-$α^G$/-α) and so Hb G-Philadelphia accounts for 35-40% of the total hemoglobin, as is seen in this case. When Hb G-Philadelphia is seen in Italians, it is not associated with α-thalassemia-2 trait.

A summary of the different combinations is given below.
1. No α gene deleted, Hb G trait; 20-25% Hb G; no hematologic effect.
2. One α gene deleted (α-thalassemia-2 trait), Hb G-trait; 25-35% Hb G; usually no hematologic effect.
3. Two α genes deleted (homozygous α-thalassemia-2), Hb G-trait; 35-45% Hb G; microcytosis.
4. Two α genes deleted (homozygous α-thalassemia-2), Homozygous Hb G; 95% Hb G; microcytosis.

Table 13.1 is a summary of other hemoglobin variants associated with α-thalassemia.

Table 13.1 α Chain Variants Associated with Deletional Forms of α–Thalassemia

Hb Variant	Substitution	Deletion	Ethnic Group
Hb Evanston	$α^{14}$Trp→Arg	-$α^{3.7}$	African
Hb Hasharon	$α^{47}$Asp→His	-$α^{3.7}$ and αα	Mediterranean, Ashkenazic Jews
Hb G-Philadelphia	$α^{68}$Asn→Lys	-$α^{3.7}$ and αα	African, Mediterranean, Melanesian
Hb Q-Thailand	$α^{74}$Asp→His	-$α^{4.2}$	Southeast Asian
Hb Duan	$α^{75}$Asp→Ala	-$α^{4.2}$	Chinese
Hb Nigeria	$α^{81}$Ser→Lys	Not determined	African
Hb J-Capetown	$α^{92}$Arg→Gln	-$α^{3.7}$	South African
Hb J-Tongariki	$α^{115}$Ala→Asp	-$α^{3.7}$	Melanesian

Modified from Higgs DR, et al. A review of the molecular genetics of the human alpha-globin gene cluster. Blood. 1989;73(5):1091.

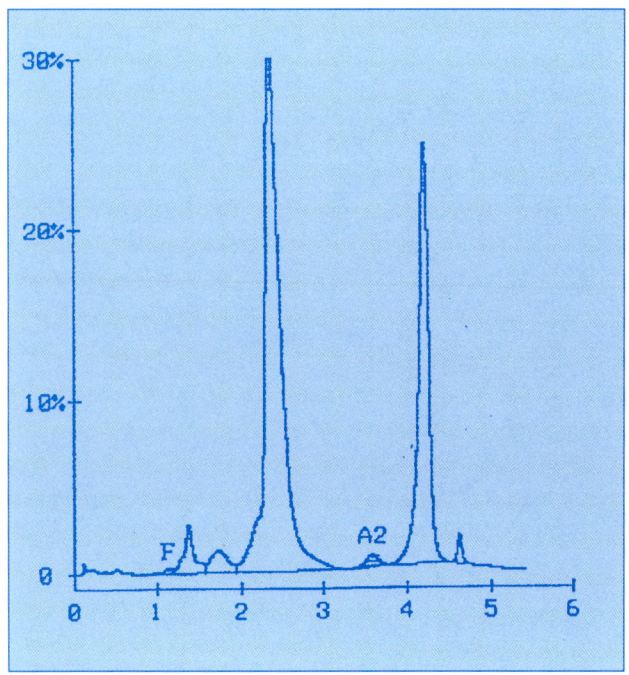

Figure 13.1
An example of Hb G-Philadelphia trait by HPLC. There is a prominent peak seen accounting for approximately 30% of the hemoglobin, which elutes in the D window (3.9-4.2 minutes). The G_2 variant is seen as a small peak at 4.6-4.7 minutes.

Figure 13.2
An example of Hb G-Philadelphia trait by isoelectric focusing (lane 1). In addition to the Hb G-Philadelphia band, there is a band cathodal to Hb A_2 which represents the G_2 variant ($\alpha^G_2\delta_2$). Lane 2-control specimen consisting of a mixture of Hb C, Hb S, Hb G-Philadelphia, Hb J, and Hb I.

References

Baine BM, Rucknagel DL, Dublin DA Jr, Adams JG III. Trimodality in the proportion of hemoglobin G-Philadelphia in heterozygotes: evidence of heterogeneity in the number of human alpha chain locations. *Proc Natl Acad Sci.* 1976;73:3633-3636.

Blackwell RQ, Wang CL, Liu CS, Shih TB. Haemoglobin G-Philadelphia alpha 68, (alpha E17) asn→lys, in a Chinese subject in Taiwan. *Vox Sang.* 1973;25: 184-186.

Milner PF, Huisman TH. Studies of the proportion and synthesis of haemoglobin G-Philadelphia in red cells of heterozygotes, a homozygote, and a heterozygote for both haemoglobin G and alpha thalassemia. *Br J Haematol.* 1976;34:207-220.

Reider RF, Woodbury DH, Rucknagel DL. The interaction of α-thalassemia and hemoglobin G-Philadelphia. *Br J Haematol.* 1976;32:159-165.

Sciarratta GV, Sansone G, Ivaldi G. Alternate organization of α G-Philadelphia globin genes among US Black and Italian Caucasian heterozygotes. *Hemoglobin.* 1984;8:537-547.

Case 14

HISTORY
The patient is a 38-year-old male of Southeast Asian origin who is asymptomatic. The physical examination shows no abnormalities.

BLOOD COUNT DATA
RBC.................................6.5×10^{12}/L
Hb...................................13.6 g/dL
MCV................................65.0 fL
WBC................................8.9×10^9/L
Plt....................................234×10^9/L

PERIPHERAL BLOOD SMEAR
Moderate hypochromia and microcytosis; increased numbers of target cells. No polychromasia.

OTHER LABORATORY TESTS
Reticulocytes: 1.2% (absolute= 78×10^9/L)
Test for unstable Hb (isopropanol test) was positive.

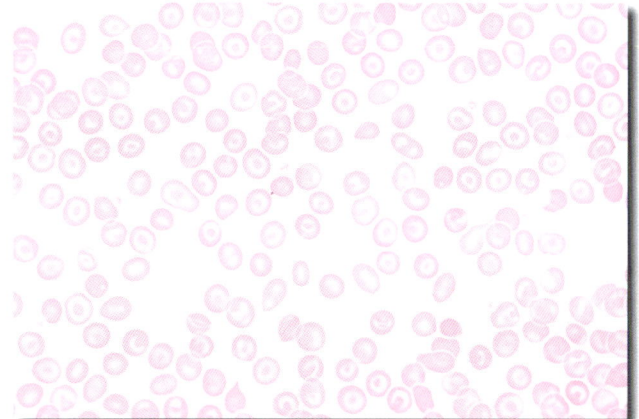

Alkaline Electrophoresis (pH 8.6)

- origin   A₂   S   A   J   +

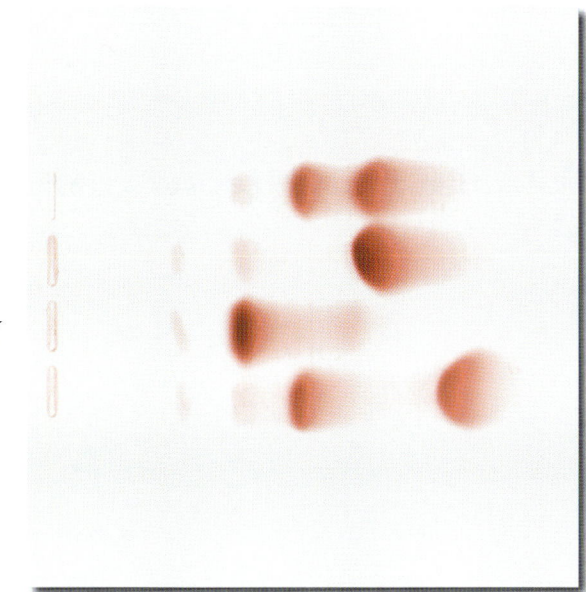

Acid Electrophoresis (pH 6.2)

+   C   S   A   F   -

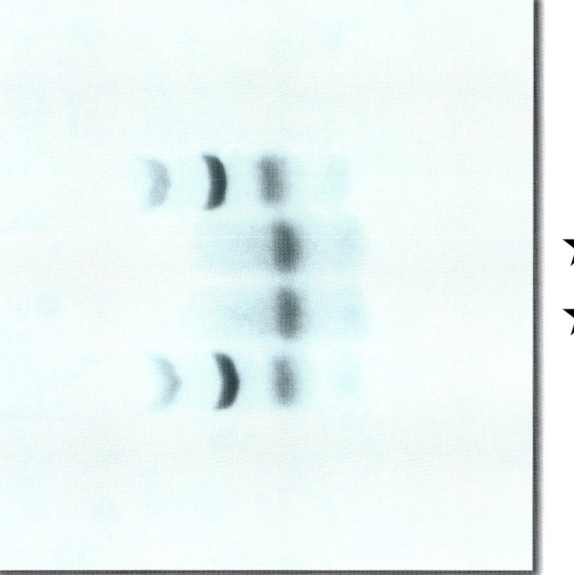

Case Studies

Case 14 Discussion

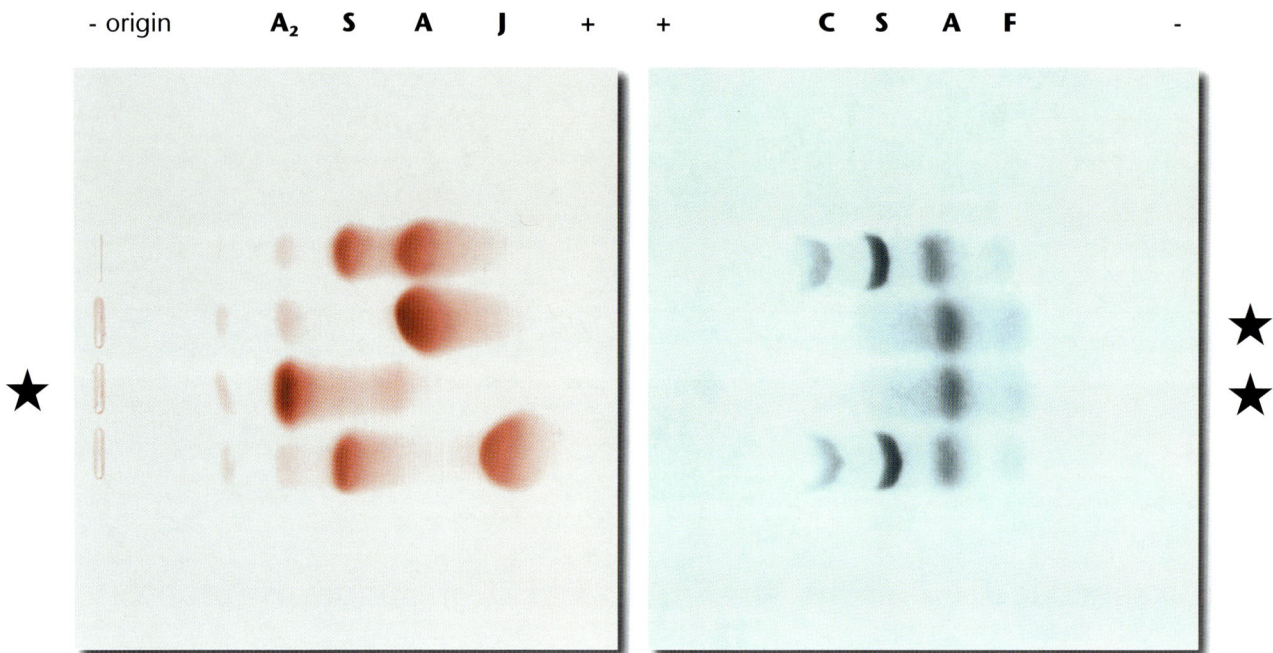

Interpretation

On alkaline electrophoresis, there is no Hb A present. There is a major band seen in the Hb A_2 (CEO) position. On acid electrophoresis, this band is in the A position. Both alkaline and acid electrophoresis show a small amount of Hb F.

Diagnosis

Homozygous Hb E.

Performance

Homozygous Hb E has been included twice in the survey, with correct identifications of 80% and 88%.

Discussion

Homozygous Hb E results from inheritance of two Hb E alleles (see Case 9). All published cases of homozygous Hb E (with the exception of one consanguineous pair in Italy) are Southeast Asians. This disorder has an estimated 4% frequency among Khmer (Cambodians) and a much higher frequency (25%) in certain tribal groups in northeastern India.

Homozygous hemoglobin E is a clinically insignificant disorder characterized mainly by microcytosis (average MCV of 67 fL); there is no associated hemolysis. As in this case, males generally do not have anemia. Women with homozygous Hb E may have mild anemia, but the hemoglobin concentration is generally above 11 g/dL. The peripheral blood smear shows abundant target cells with little anisopoikilocytosis (Figure 14.1). Intra-erythrocyte inclusions are not present.

Homozygous hemoglobin E may be confused hematologically with iron deficiency and β-thalassemia trait (which it closely resembles). The electrophoretic findings easily discriminate homozygous Hb E from both of these disorders. On an electrophoretic basis, the primary differential diagnoses are homozygous Hb C and Hb E/β-thalassemia. The migration with Hb A on acid electrophoresis rules out Hb C. In Hb E/β-thalassemia, there is a moderate to severe anemia, as well as icterus and splenomegaly. Furthermore, on electrophoresis, Hb E ranges from 40-70% of total hemoglobin, and Hb F represents 30-60%. In contrast, in homozygous Hb E disease, Hb F is usually normal and should not exceed 5% of total hemoglobin in adults; Hb E will comprise 95-97% of total hemoglobin. An example of homozygous Hb E on HPLC is shown in Figure 14.2.

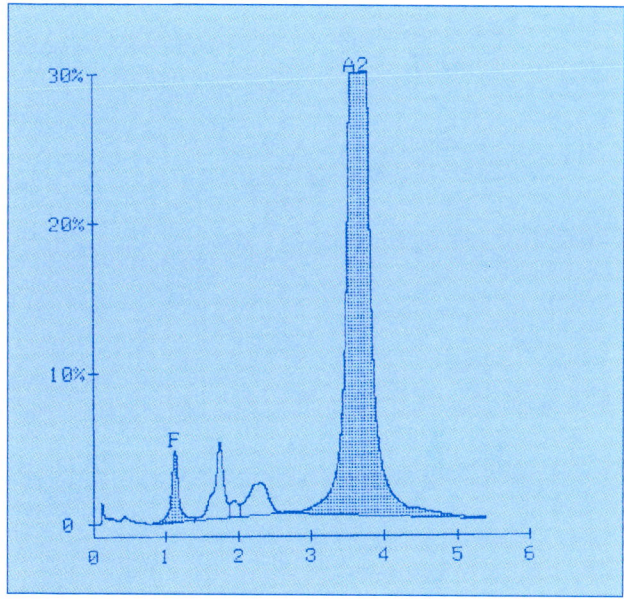

Figure 14.2
An example of Homozygous Hb E by HPLC. There is a very prominent peak in the A_2 window, which accounts for virtually all of the total hemoglobin. There is a small amount of Hb F present as well. The small peak seen at just after 2 minutes does not represent Hb A, as no Hb A was seen by alkaline electrophoresis or isoelectric focusing.

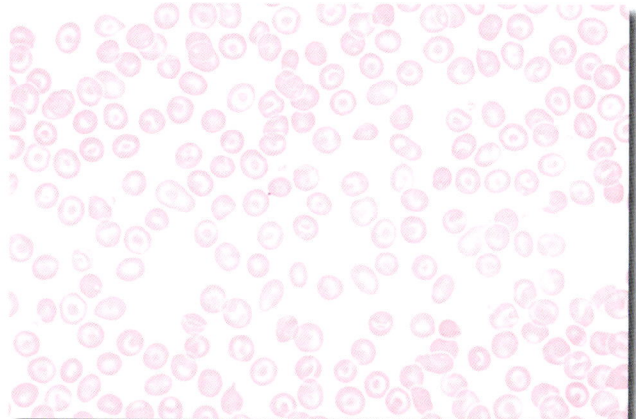
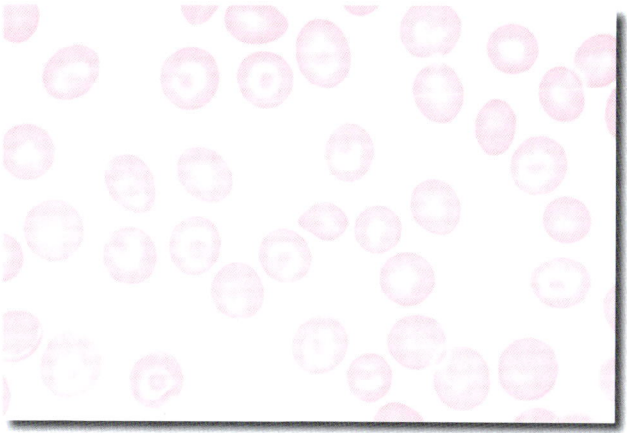

Figure 14.1 (Wright-Giemsa, 160x and 400x)
Low- and high-power views of the peripheral blood smear in a patient with homozygous Hb E. The red blood cells are more microcytic than seen in Hb E trait, and more target cells are present. Anisocytosis is slight.

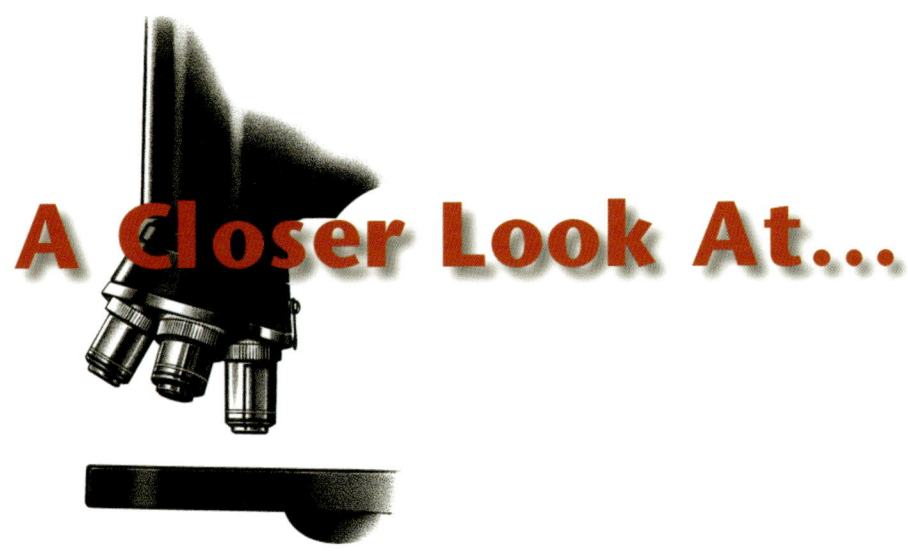

Hb E-Associated Disorders

In addition to Hb E, several other disorders of hemoglobin are prevalent in the Southeast Asian population. Therefore, Hb E may be encountered in conjunction with another abnormality. A description of the various Hb E-associated disorders is provided below. Figure 14.3 summarizes the electrophoretic patterns of these disorders.

1. Hb E trait. A harmless condition characterized by mild microcytosis and often by erythrocytosis. No icterus, no splenomegaly, no anemia. MCV about 75 fL (adult). Electrophoresis: Hb E 30-35%, Hb A 65-70%, Hb F <2%.
2. Homozygous Hb E. A harmless condition characterized only by mild microcytosis and erythrocytosis. No icterus, no splenomegaly, no anemia (hemoglobin concentration >11 g/dL in females, >14 g/dL in males). MCV about 67 fL (adults). Electrophoresis: Hb E about 99%, the rest Hb F.
3. Hb E trait/α-thalassemia. (See Case 34, page 155.) This combination results in microcytosis, but usually no other adverse effects (no anemia, no splenomegaly, no icterus). Serum ferritin assay is required to differentiate this condition from Hb E trait/iron deficiency. Electrophoresis (1 α gene deletion): Hb E 25-30%; remainder Hb A; Hb F normal. Electrophoresis (2 α gene deletion): Hb E 20-25%; remainder Hb A; Hb F normal. Since Hb E and Hb A_2 co-migrate in all electrophoresis media and co-elute from chromatography columns, a common laboratory error is to ascribe the electrophoresis findings to β-thalassemia trait. However, in the latter, Hb A_2 is always <10%.
4. Hb E trait/Hb H disease. In this disorder, Hb E trait is inherited in conjunction with a three locus α gene deletion. This is a moderately severe thalassemic disorder with features identical to Hb H disease. However, electrophoresis does not reveal Hb H. Instead, Hb E represents about 10-15% of hemoglobin; most of the remainder is Hb A. This paradox is due to reduced total synthesis of β globin chains. As a result, not enough surplus β chains are present to form β tetramers (Hb H). Instead, Hb Bart's is present. (Thus, this condition has also been called "Hb A + E + Bart's Disease.")
5. Homozygous Hb E/Hb H disease. This disorder has the same features as Hb H disease. However, electrophoresis reveals mostly Hb E (about 95%) and a small proportion of Hb F. It is believed that in this condition, the β^E tetramers co-migrate with Hb E in all electrophoresis media.
6. Hb E trait/α-thalassemia/Hb Constant Spring. Features are the same as 4 and 5 above, except for faint additional hemoglobin bands (as many as five) between the positions of Hb E and the site of application. These additional faint bands represent Hb Constant Spring.
7. Hb E trait/iron deficiency. A benign condition characterized by microcytosis, often erythrocytosis, and anemia. The anemia is due to iron deficiency and thus may be minimal to severe. There is no icterus and no splenomegaly. Electrophoresis shows the same pattern as Hb E trait/α-thalassemia. The combination should be suspected in an anemic patient with a "Hb

A_2'' concentration of 10-20%. The diagnosis is confirmed by a serum ferritin assay. Following treatment, repeat electrophoresis will show Hb E representing 30-35% of total (unless the patient also has Hb E trait/α-thalassemia).

8. **Hb E/β⁰-thalassemia.** This is a serious thalassemic disorder due to compound heterozygosity for both Hb E trait and β-thalassemia trait. Characteristics are severe anemia, icterus, marked splenomegaly, and microcytosis. Affected children suffer all the problems of β-thalassemia major. Most require frequent transfusions and should also receive iron chelation therapy. This is the most common severe thalassemia of Southeast Asians. Neurologic manifestations are often reported that are due to brain or spinal cord compression by extramedullary hematopoietic tumors, which may cause paraplegia. The tumors respond to radiotherapy. Electrophoresis: Hb E is 40-90% of total; the rest is Hb F. (Note: Because these patients usually require transfusion, Hb A may be present from donor blood). It should be pointed out that it is not necessary to document elevated Hb A_2 levels to establish a diagnosis of Hb E/β⁰-thalassemia. The diagnosis is easily established on the basis of a Hb E concentration >40% with the remainder representing Hb F (usually 30-60%) and an absence of Hb A.

9. **Hb E/β⁰-thalassemia, post-splenectomy.** Same condition as 11 above, but often confusing in laboratories. Splenectomy is a common treatment in Hb E/β⁰-thalassemia and is reputed to be beneficial for those with severe anemia. The post-splenectomy blood picture is characterized by marked normoblastemia and a positive solubility test for sickling hemoglobin. The latter is due to the large number of normoblast nuclei causing strong persistent turbidity. Pulmonary artery occlusion is a common complication in splenectomized patients with Hb E/β⁰-thalassemia. Prophylactic therapy with daily doses of aspirin or dipyridamole is indicated for all patients with this disorder who have been splenectomized.

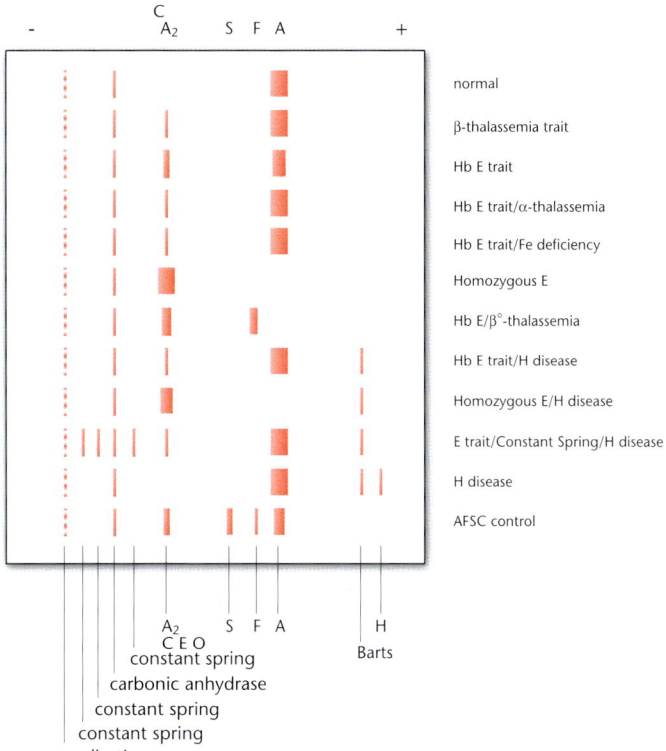

Figure 14.3
Hemoglobin E-related disorders: characteristic electrophoretic patterns (cellulose acetate, pH 8.6).

References

Anderson HM, Ranney HM. Southeast Asian immigrants: the new thalassemias in Americans. *Semin Hematol.* 1990;27:239-246.

Fairbanks VF, Gilchrist GS, Brimhall B, et al. Hemoglobin E trait reexamined: a cause of microcytosis and erythrocytosis. *Blood.* 1979;53:109-115.

Fairbanks VF, Oliveros R, Brandabur JH, et al. Homozygous hemoglobin E mimics β-thalassemia minor without anemia or hemolysis: hematologic, functional, and biosynthetic studies of first North American cases. *Am J Hematol.* 1980;8:109-121.

Fucharoen S. Hemoglobin E disorders. In: Steinberg MH, Forget BG, Higgs DR, Nagel RL, eds. *Disorders of Hemoglobin: Genetics, Pathophysiology and Clinical Management.* Cambridge, England: Cambridge University Press; 2001:1139-1154.

Monzon CM, Fairbanks VF, Burgert EO Jr, et al. Hematologic genetic disorders among Southeast Asian refugees. *Am J Hematol.* 1985;19:27-36.

Sandhaus LM, Smith CM Jr, Peterson L. Hemoglobin E disorders in a Minnesota Southeast Asian immigrant population: morphology, indices, electrophoretic patterns, and clinical manifestations. *Minn Med.* 1983;66:163-166.

Wasi P. Hemoglobinopathies including thalassemias, part 1: tropical Asia. *Clin Haematol.* 1981;10:707-729.

Case 15

HISTORY
The patient is a 56-year-old African-American female who is asymptomatic. The physical examination is notable for mild splenomegaly.

BLOOD COUNT DATA
RBC .... 5.38 x10^{12}/L
Hgb .... 13.3 g/dL
MCV .... 74.9 fL
WBC .... 6.7 x 10^9/L
Plt .... 198 x 10^9/L

PERIPHERAL BLOOD SMEAR
The peripheral blood smear shows polychromasia, target cells, and spherocytes.

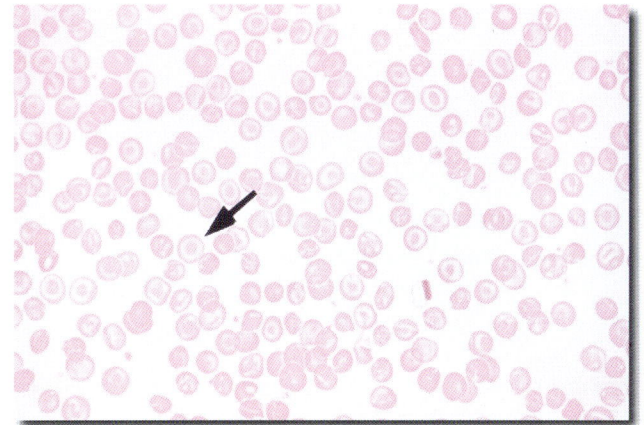

Alkaline Electrophoresis (pH 8.6)

- origin   A$_2$ S   A   +

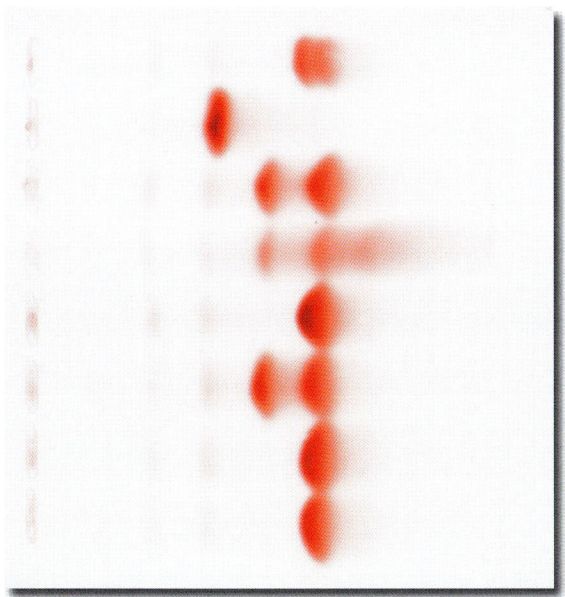

Acid Electrophoresis (pH 6.2)

+   C   S   A   F   -

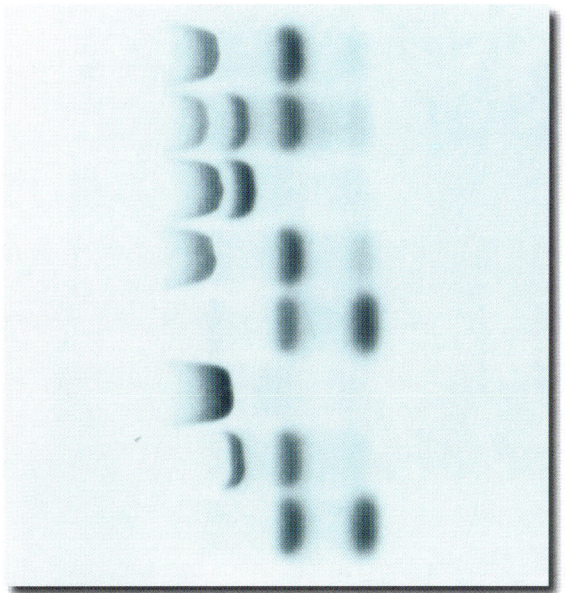

Case 15 Discussion

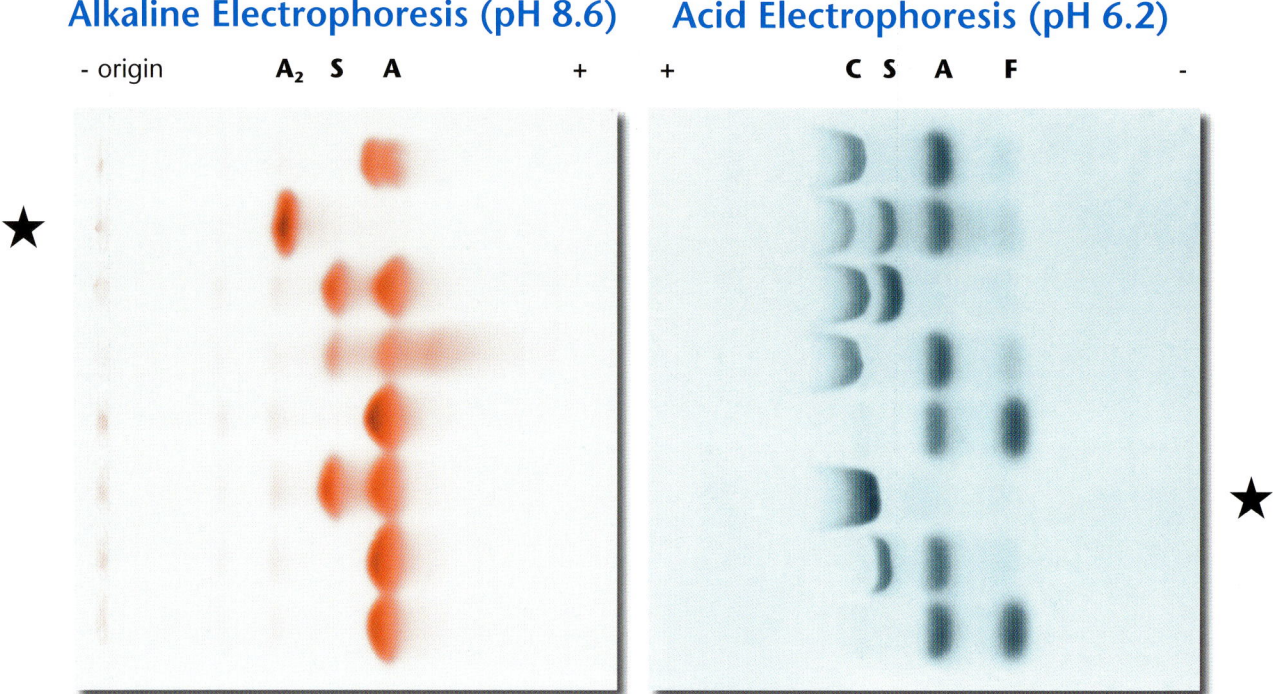

Interpretation

On alkaline electrophoresis, there is no Hb A band, only a major band in the A_2 position. Acid electrophoresis shows a major band in the C position. There is no Hb A present.

Diagnosis

Homozygous Hb C.

Performance

Homozygous Hb C has appeared in the survey once, with 97.4% of participants giving a correct identification.

Discussion

Hb C results from an amino acid substitution of lysine for glutamic acid at the sixth position of the β chain (β 6 Glu→ Lys). Heterozygous Hb C (Hb C trait) is a clinically benign disorder and has been presented in Case 8. The epidemiology of Hb C has also been discussed in that case. Although homozygous Hb C does not produce a serious clinical disorder like that of homozygous Hb S, Hb C is less soluble than Hb A and crystallizes within the red cell. In contrast to Hb S, in which hemoglobin polymerizes when the red cells become deoxygenated, Hb C crystals are formed in the oxygenated state. It is not clear whether the intraerythrocytic crystals contribute significantly to the hemolysis in this disorder. It is felt by some authors that cellular dehydration due to increased potassium efflux is the major determinant of hemolysis. Red cell life span in homozygous Hb C disease is decreased to 30-35 days. Hb C interacts with Hb S to produce a sickling disorder (see Case 17, page 85).

Patients who are homozygous for Hb C generally have a mild to moderate hemolytic anemia with a mild microcytosis (MCV approximately 70-72 fL). However, as demonstrated in this patient, the hemolysis is usually well compensated, and anemia may not be present. There is generally some splenomegaly present, but apart from this, the patients are largely asymptomatic. The peripheral blood shows characteristic findings, with numerous small target cells and microspherocytes. Hb C crystals may be identified. These are dense polyhedral crystals that can be seen either intra- or extra-cellularly (Figure 15.1).

Homozygous Hb C appears identical to homozygous Hb E on alkaline electrophoresis but can be easily differentiated by acid electrophoresis (Hb E migrates in the A position in this medium). Homozygous Hb C should be differentiated from Hb C/β⁰-thalassemia (see Case 30). In Hb C/β⁰-thalassemia, the cells are more microcytic (MCV 55-70 fL), and the anemia and splenomegaly are often more severe. The Hb F level commonly exceeds 5%, whereas in homozygous Hb C, the Hb F seldom exceeds 3%. Family studies will also help to distinguish between these two conditions. Examples of homozygous Hb C on HPLC and isoelectric focusing are shown in Figures 15.2 and 15.3.

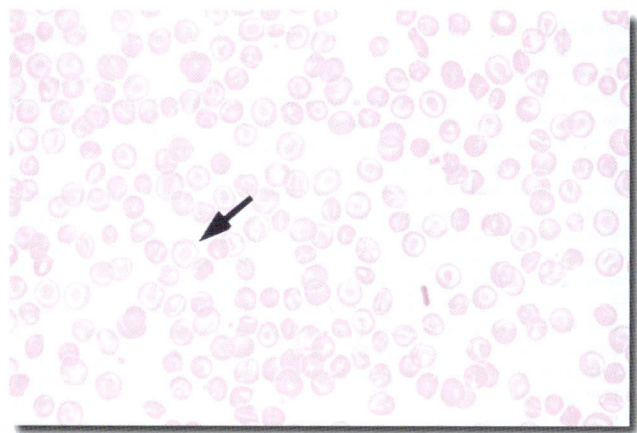
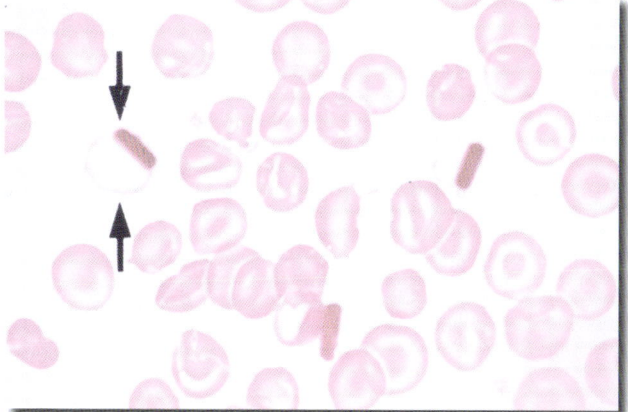

Figure 15.1 (Wright-Giemsa, 160x and 400x)
Low- and high-power views of the peripheral blood smear of a patient with homozygous Hb C. Abundant target cells are seen; the red blood cells show only slight anisocytosis. Several Hb C crystals are present.

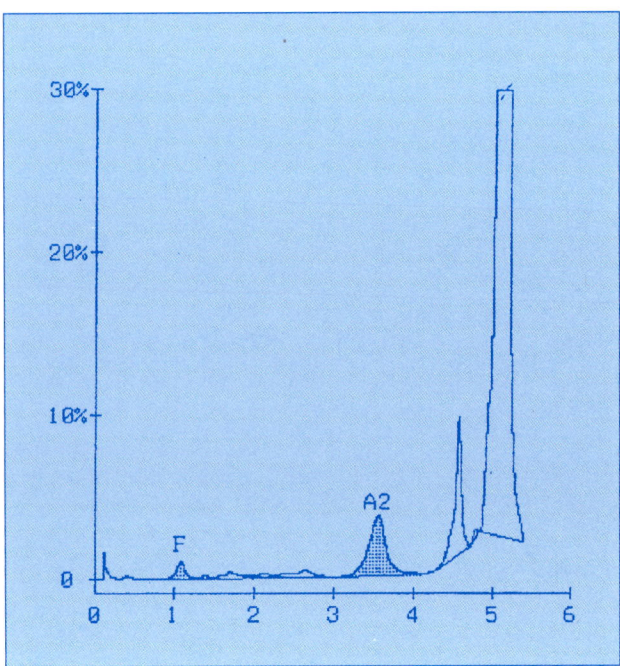

Figure 15.2
An example of Homozygous Hb C by HPLC. There is a prominent peak migrating in the C window (4.85-5.15 minutes) which accounts for almost all of the total hemoglobin.

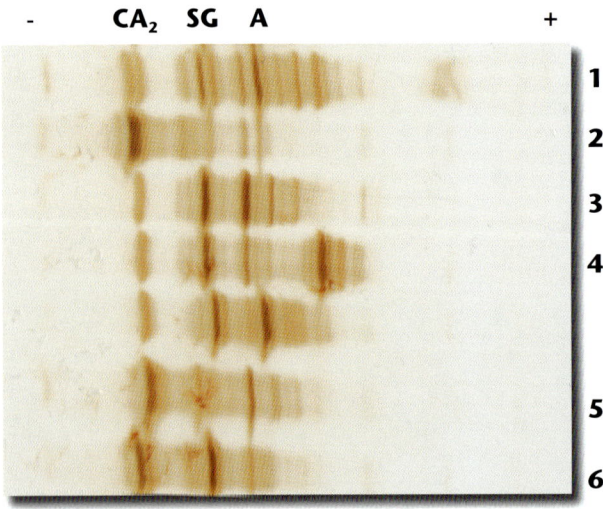

Figure 15.3
An example of homozygous Hb C by isoelectric focusing (lane 2). 1-control, 3-Hb S/HPFH, 4-Hb S/Hb N-Baltimore, 5-Hb E/β^0-thalassemia, 6-Hb S/C.

References

Brugnara C, Kopin AS, Bunn HF, Tosteson DC. Regulation of cation content and cell volume in hemoglobin erythrocytes from patients with homozygous hemoglobin C disease. *J Clin Invest.* 1985;75:1608-1617.

Bunn HT, Forget BG. *Hemoglobin: Molecular, Genetic and Clinical Aspects.* 1st ed. Philadelphia, PA: WB Saunders Co; 1986:421-425.

Dover GJ, Platt OS. Sickle cell disease. In: Nathan DG, Orkin SH, eds. *Hematology of Infancy and Childhood.* 5th ed. Philadelphia, PA: WB Saunders Co; 1998:762-809.

Fairbanks VF. *Hemoglobinopathies and Thalassemias.* New York, NY: Brian C. Decker; 1980:153-156.

Lukens JN. The abnormal hemoglobins: general principles. In: Lee GR, Foerster J, Lukens J, et al, eds. *Wintrobe's Clinical Hematology.* 10th ed. Baltimore, MD: Williams and Wilkins; 1999:1329-1345.

Nagel RL, Steinberg MH. Hb S/C disease and Hb C disorders. In: Steinberg MH, Forget BJ, Higgs DR, Nagle RL, eds. *Disorders of Hemoglobin: Genetics, Pathophysiology and Clinical Management.* Cambridge, England: Cambridge University Press; 2001:756-785.

Smith TW, Krevans JR. Clinical manifestations of hemoglobin C disorders. *Bull Johns Hopkins Hosp.* 1959;104:17.

Terry DW, Motulsky AG, Rath CE. Homozygous hemoglobin C: a new hereditary hemolytic disease. *N Engl J Med.* 1954;251:365.

Case 16

HISTORY
The patient is a 16-year-old African-American male who had a long history of recurrent abdominal and joint pain, often requiring narcotics for relief. The physical examination revealed a slender, black male in acute distress from abdominal pain. There was moderate scleral icterus and pale conjunctivae and mucous membranes. The spleen was not palpable.

BLOOD COUNT DATA
RBC.................................1.6×10^{12}/L
Hb...................................5.4 g/dL
MCV................................85.0 fL
WBC................................12.9×10^9/L
Plt....................................253×10^9/L

PERIPHERAL BLOOD SMEAR
Crescentic shaped RBCs, target cells, and Howell-Jolly bodies.

OTHER BLOOD COUNT DATA
The solubility test for sickling hemoglobin is positive.

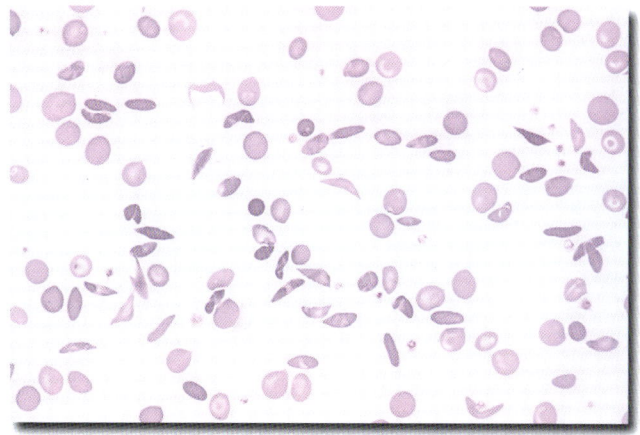

Alkaline Electrophoresis (pH 8.6)

- origin   A₂   S   A   +

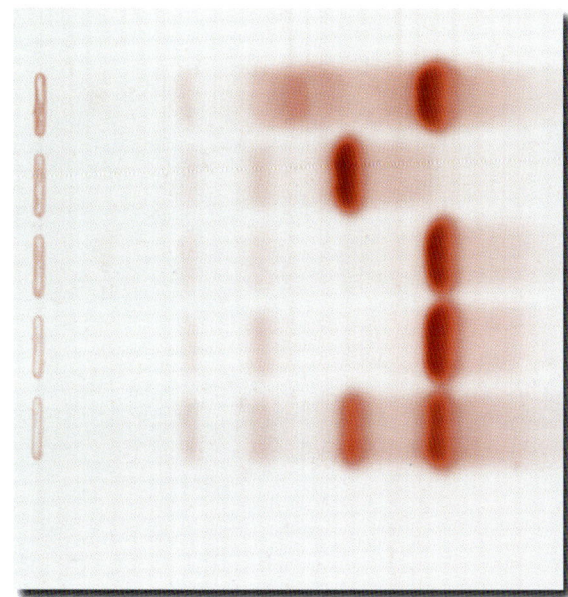

Acid Electrophoresis (pH 6.2)

+   C   S   A   F   -

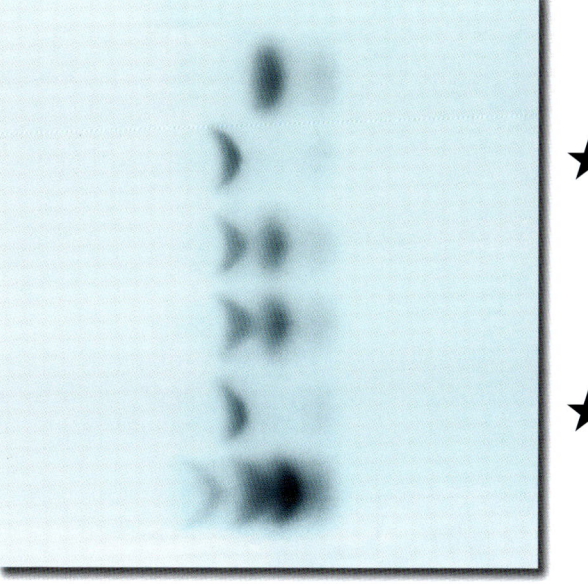

Case Studies

Case 16 Discussion

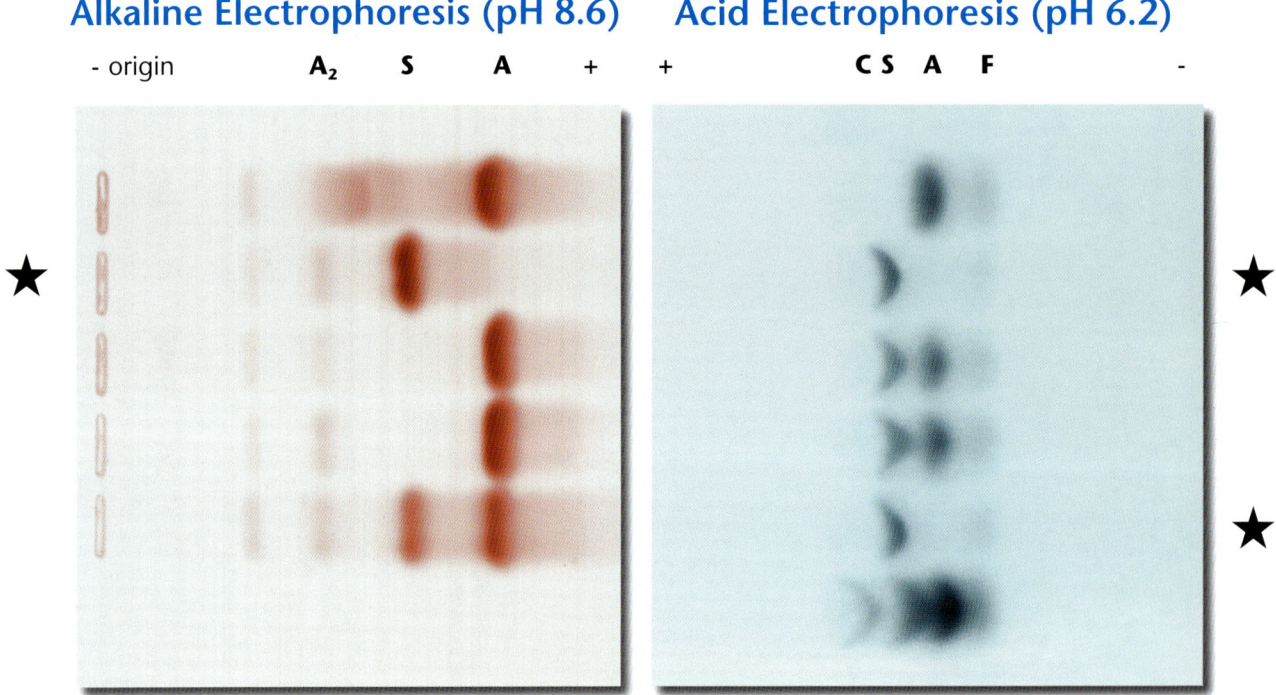

Interpretation

Both the alkaline and acid electrophoretic gels demonstrate a single dominant band at the S position. There is no Hb A present.

Diagnosis

Homozygous hemoglobin S.

Performance

Homozygous hemoglobin S (SS disease) has been used in the survey on only one occasion. Of laboratories using both alkaline and acid electrophoresis, isoelectric focusing, or HPLC, 99% correctly reported the presence of hemoglobin S, and 95.3% correctly interpreted this as homozygous hemoglobin S.

Discussion

Hemoglobin S results from a glutamic acid to valine substitution at the sixth amino acid position of the β globin chain (β6 Glu→Val). The $β^{6Val}$ amino acid substitution results in decreased solubility of de-oxygenated hemoglobin. De-oxygenated hemoglobin S forms rigid polymers that distort red cells into the characteristic sickled shape. While this is an initially reversible phenomenon, repeated bouts of sickling and unsickling result in permanent membrane damage and irreversible sickling. These irreversibly sickled cells are less deformable than normal RBCs and are removed from circulation by the mononuclear phagocyte system in various organs. The tendency of a cell to sickle is in large part determined by the concentration of hemoglobin S. Thus, homozygous SS cells begin to sickle at oxygen tensions encountered in the normal physiologic state (approximately 40 mm of Hg), whereas S-trait cells only sickle at much lower partial pressures of oxygen, which are not normally encountered in the vascular system. The sickling process is time dependent, so prolonged exposure of blood to low oxygen areas (e.g., vascular stasis) will also produce increased sickling. In addition, factors which enhance oxygen unloading (i.e., shift of the oxygen dissociation curve to the right), such as decreased pH, will also increase the sickling process. The myriad clinical manifestations of sickle cell disease result from the two major consequences of the sickling process: chronic hemolysis and microvascular occlusion. The degree of hemolysis is directly related to the number of irreversibly sickled cells in the blood. Vaso-occlusive phenomena, however, are not directly related to the presence of irreversibly sickled cells but instead appear to be due to increased red cell adhesion to endothelium because of membrane damage. The property of sickling is absolutely dependent on the presence of the $β^{6Val}$ mutation; thus the rare C Harlem ($β^{6Val,73Asn}$) and S Antilles ($β^{6Val,23\,Ile}$) are also sickling hemoglobins.

In the United States, the $β^S$ gene has an allelic frequency of about 4% in the African-American population but is rare in other ethnic groups (see Case 7). It may be inherited in heterozygous fashion (S-trait), in a double heterozygous state with another abnormal hemoglobin or thalassemia gene (e.g., SC disease, S/β-thalassemia), or in the homozygous state. The high frequency of this gene in individuals of African descent is attributed to a protective effect against malaria in the heterozygous state.

SS disease is a severe, debilitating illness. The hemolytic component of the disease is only partially compensated, with steady-state hemoglobin levels of 6-10 g/dL (average 8 g/dL). Typical peripheral blood findings include sickled cells, target cells, polychromasia, circulating normoblasts, and signs of hyposplenism such as Howell-Jolly bodies and Pappenheimer bodies in adult patients (Figure 16.1). As with other chronic hemolytic processes, patients with SS disease are prone to the development of pigment gallstones. Common clinical manifestations related to microvascular occlusion include incapacitating pain crises, cerebrovascular accidents, skin ulcers, and aseptic hip necrosis. Autosplenectomy from repeated episodes of splenic infarction is a nearly constant feature in adult patients with SS disease. This complication is largely responsible for the increased susceptibility to bacterial infection seen in these patients; infection is the most common cause of death in children with SS disease. Factors known to precipitate vaso-occlusive phenomena include acidosis, infection, hypoxia, and cold exposure. The overall life expec-

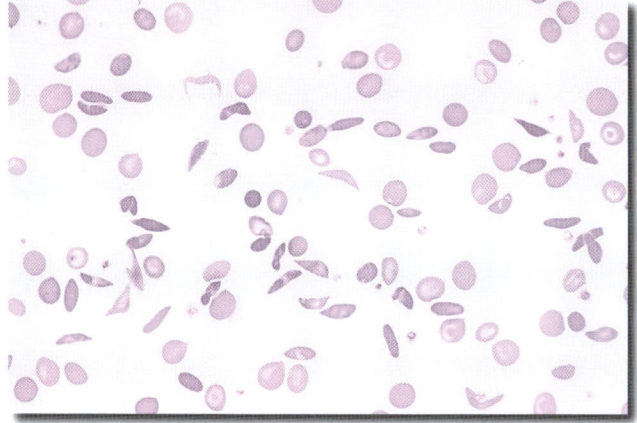 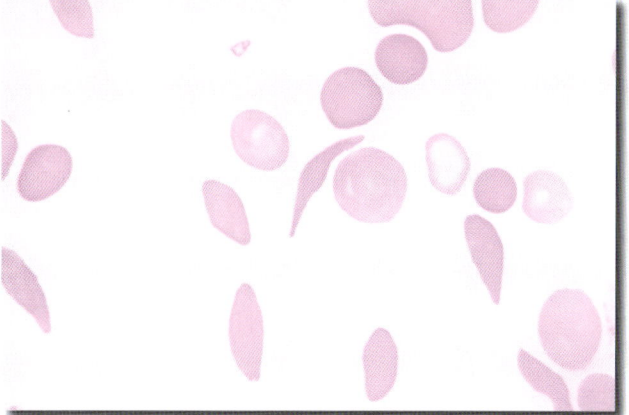

Figure 16.1 (Wright-Giemsa, 160x and 400x)
Low- and high-power views of the peripheral blood smear from a patient with homozygous Hb S. There are abundant sickle cells (drepanocytes) present. The presence of target cells and Howell-Jolly bodies indicates autosplenectomy.

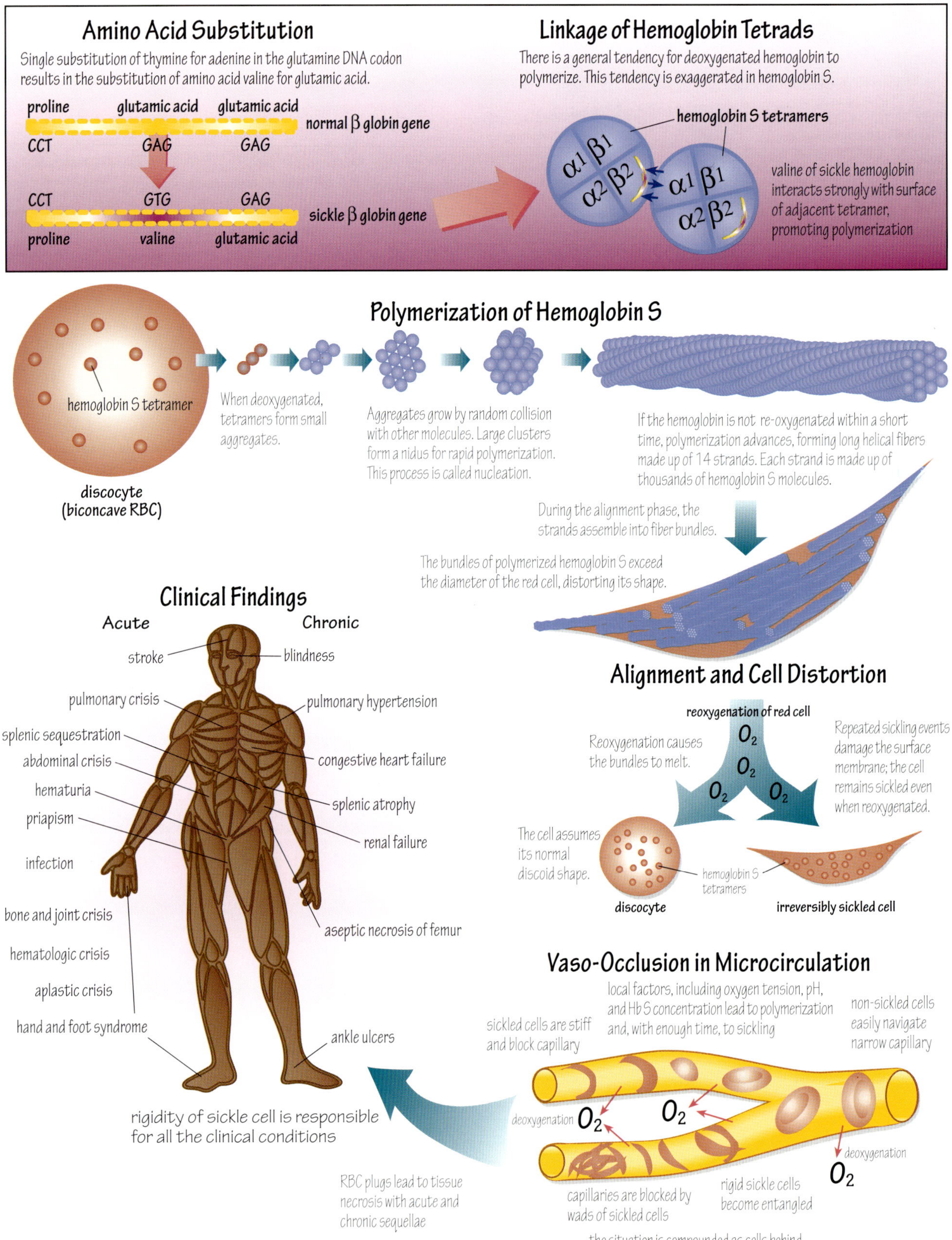

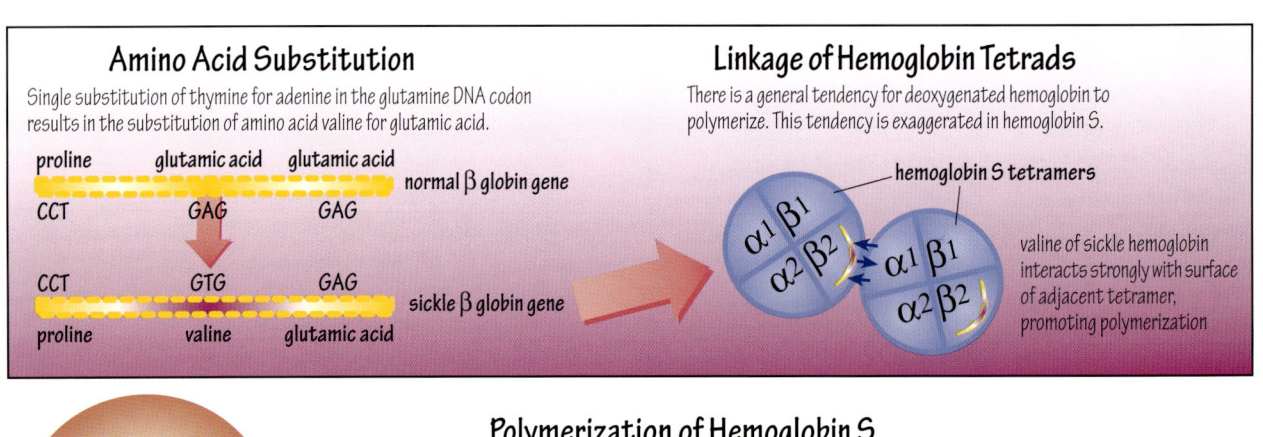

Figure 16.2
Sickle Cell Anemia Summary
Adapted from Glassy EF, ed. Color Atlas of Hematology. *Northfield, IL: College of American Pathologists; 1998:99.*

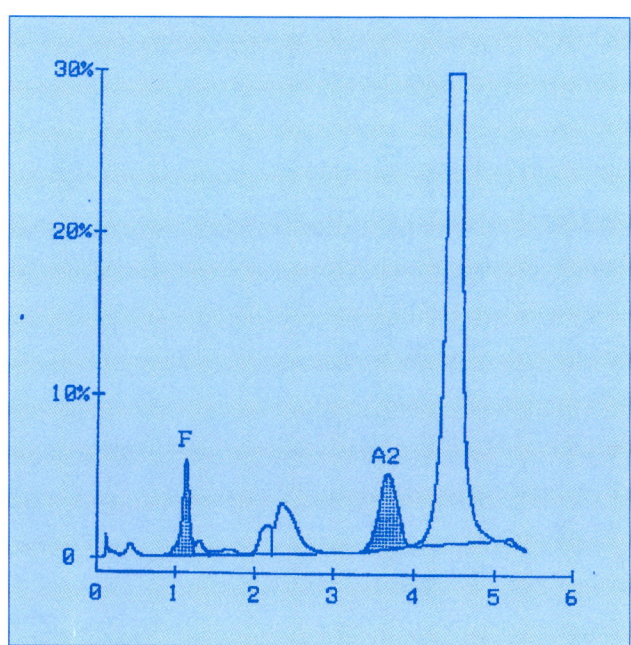

Figure 16.3
An example of homozygous Hb S by HPLC. There is a major peak eluting in the S window, which comprises the majority of the hemoglobin present. There is a slight increase in Hb F. Similar to Hb S trait, the Hb A_2 peak appears slightly elevated.

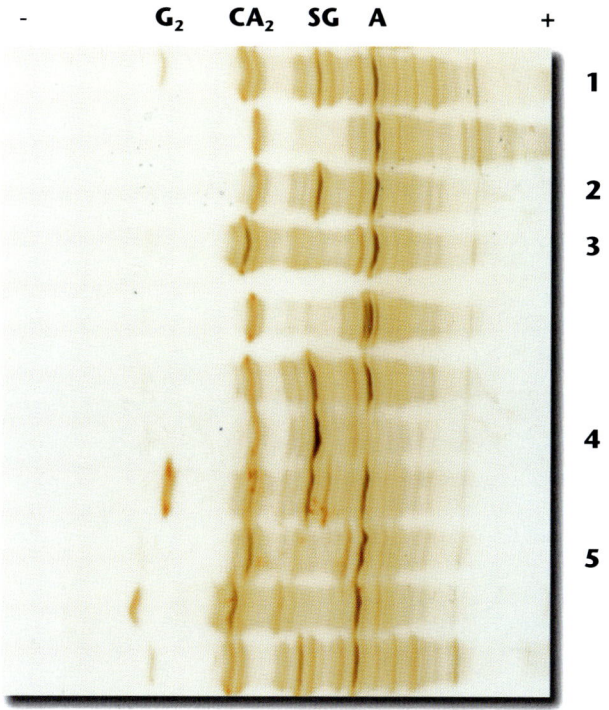

Figure 16.4
An example of homozygous S by isoelectric focusing. 1-control, 2-Hb S trait, 3-Hb C trait, 4-Homozygous S, 5-Hb E trait.

tancy of patients with SS disease is decreased, with a median age of death of 42 years for males, and 48 years for females. Figure 16.2 summarizes the clinical and pathophysiologic processes in sickle cell anemia.

The diagnosis of hemoglobin S is straightforward when both alkaline and acid electrophoresis are employed, as it migrates to characteristic positions distinct from hemoglobin A at both pH levels. On alkaline electrophoresis, hemoglobins D, G, and Lepore migrate with S, so this study alone is insufficient to identify the presence of hemoglobin S. A rapid test for sickling hemoglobins (such as the sickle solubility test or the sodium metabisulfite test) may be used to confirm the presence of hemoglobin S but will not distinguish SS disease from S/D, S/G, or S/Lepore. Therefore, acid electrophoresis or techniques such as isoelectric focusing or HPLC are necessary to confirm the homozygous state. (See Figures 16.3 and 16.4) On acid electrophoresis, D, G, and Lepore all migrate with hemoglobin A. Note that HbS may give a false-positive result on the isopropanol stability test for unstable hemoglobins, as in the current case.

References

Beutler E. The sickle cell diseases and related disorders. In: Beutler E, Lichtman MA, Coller BS, Kipps TJ, Seligsohn U, eds. *Williams Hematology.* 6th ed. New York, NY: McGraw-Hill; 2000:581-606.

Dover GJ, Platt OS. Sickle cell disease. In: Nathan DG, Orkin SH, eds. *Hematology of Infancy and Childhood.* 5th ed. Philadelphia, PA: WB Saunders; 1998:762-809.

Nagel RC, Platt VS. General pathophysiology of sickle cell anemia. In: Steinberg MH, Forget BJ, Higgs DR, Nagle RL, eds. *Disorders of Hemoglobin: Genetics, Pathophysiology and Clinical Management.* Cambridge, England: Cambridge University Press; 2001:494-526.

Wang WC, Lukens JN. Sickle cell anemia and other sickling syndromes. In: Lee GR, Foerster J, Lukens J, et al, eds. *Wintrobe's Clinical Hematology.* 10th ed. Baltimore, MD: Williams and Wilkins; 1999: 1346-1397.

Case 17

HISTORY
The patient is a 21-year-old African-American woman with recurrent episodes of joint pain.

BLOOD COUNT DATA
RBC .... 4.06×10^{12}/L
Hb .... 11.6 g/dL
MCV .... 87.0 fL
WBC .... 9.2×10^9/L
Plt .... 198×10^9/L

PERIPHERAL BLOOD SMEAR
There are many target cells and a few "boat-shaped" cells.

OTHER LABORATORY TESTS
The solubility test for sickling hemoglobin is positive.

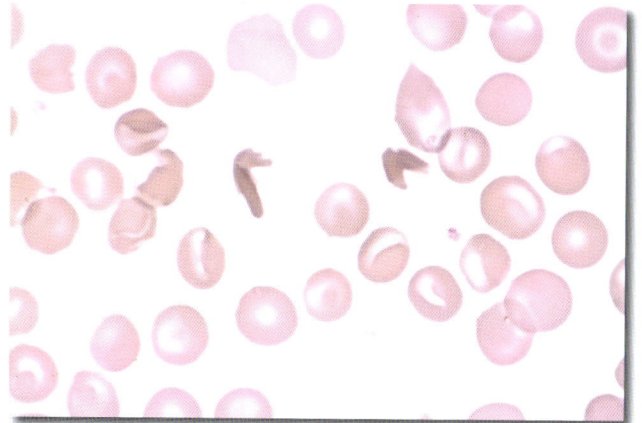

Alkaline Electrophoresis (pH 8.6)

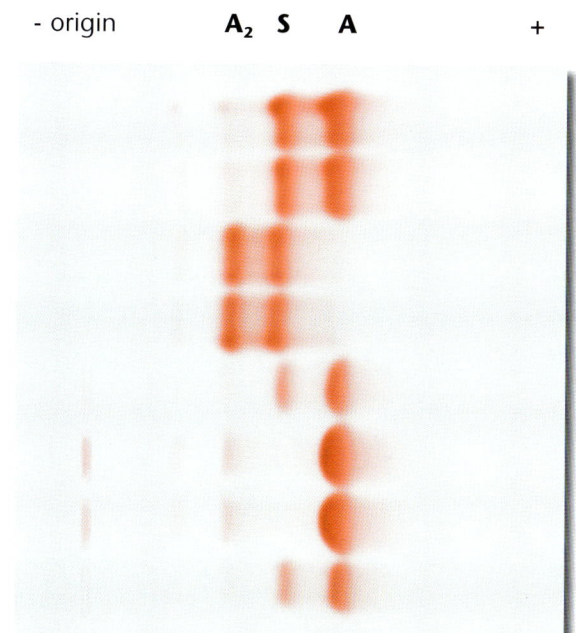

Acid Electrophoresis (pH 6.2)

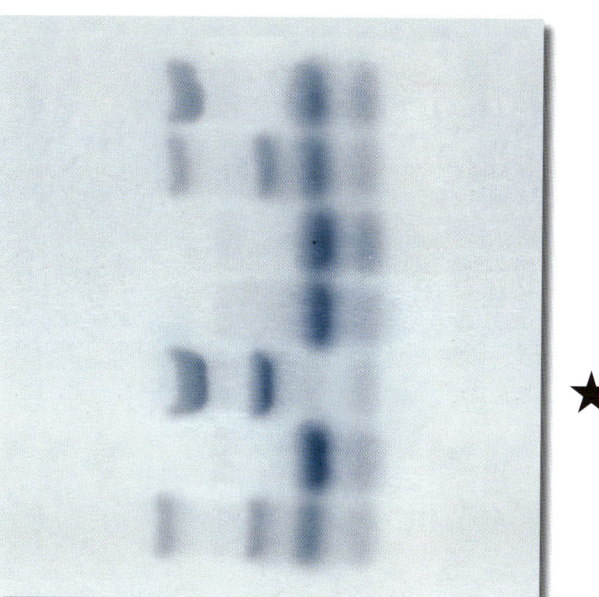

Case Studies

Case 17 Discussion

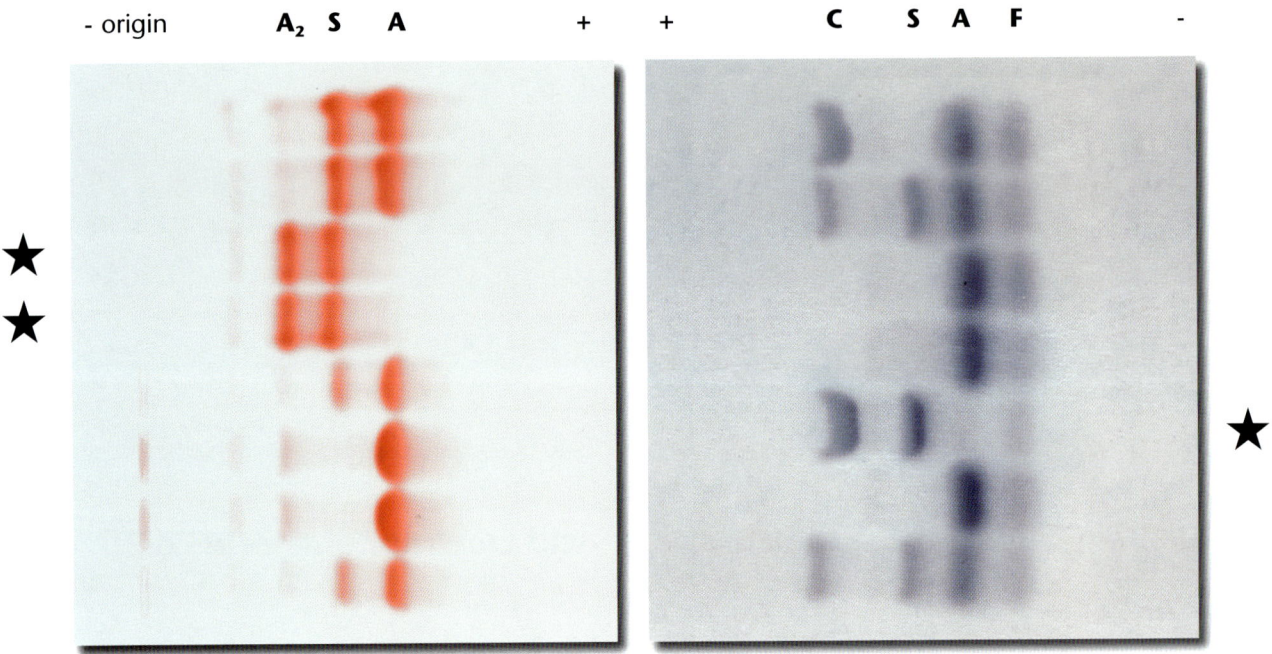

Interpretation

On alkaline electrophoresis, no Hb A is observed. There are two major bands present, one in the S position and one in the A$_2$ (CEO) position. Likewise, on acid electrophoresis, there are bands in the S and C positions.

Diagnosis

Hb S/C disease.

Performance

Hb S/C disease has been included in the survey twice, with correct identification by 97.2% and 90% of participants.

Discussion

The amino acid substitutions and geographic distribution of Hb S and Hb C have been discussed in Cases 7 and 8. The prevalence of Hb S/C disease in African Americans is 0.13%.

The pathogenesis of sickling manifestations in S/C disease is controversial. While it is commonly stated that hemoglobins S and C co-polymerize, it is felt by some experts that this is not the case. Bunn et al demonstrated that the characteristics of mixtures of Hb S and Hb C are identical to mixtures of Hb S and Hb A. Thus, the fact that sickling occurs in S/C disease but not S trait requires explanation. Sickling phenomena in S/C disease have been attributed to two factors. First is the increased percentage of Hb S in S/C disease compared to S trait (approximately 50% vs. 40%). The second is the cellular dehydration that occurs as a consequence of the presence of Hb C, thus increasing the intracellular concentration of Hb S.

Hb S/C produces a sickling syndrome with clinical manifestations that are milder than those of SS disease. The hemolytic anemia is mild to moderate (the hemoglobin levels are usually above 10), and complications from the hemolytic anemia (cholelithiasis, leg ulcers, hepatomegaly, and cardiomegaly) are less frequent. Growth development, sexual maturation, and body habitus are usually normal; life expectancy is usually only slightly shortened. Painful vaso-occlusive crises (abdominal, musculoskeletal, neurologic) are less frequent, and infarctive damage (e.g., bone, lung) is usually less disabling. Approximately half of patients have splenomegaly. Although asplenia occurs in only 25% of patients, painful splenic infarcts are common, and acute splenic sequestration crisis may also occur. Because the function of the spleen is usually intact, the frequency of pneumococcal infections (meningitis, sepsis) is not increased. The frequency of cerebrovascular accidents is about equal to that of sickle cell anemia patients. Interestingly, thromboembolic complications, renal papillary necrosis, and proliferative retinopathy are more frequent in S/C disease than in sickle cell anemia. Aseptic necrosis of the femoral head is about half as frequent as in sickle cell anemia; however, aseptic necrosis of the humoral head is more common. Although there are fewer complications at the time of delivery, pregnant women with S/C disease have a high rate of spontaneous early abortions.

The peripheral blood findings in Hb S/C disease are characteristic. True sickle cells are rare; there are usually irregularly shaped cells, which appear to contain misshapen crystals, which have been called "S/C poikilocytes." Other cells have a "clam" or "boat-shaped" appearance. Although S/C poikilocytes appear to contain crystals, classic polyhedral Hb C crystals are unusual. Target cells are usually increased (Figure 17.1).

Although Hb S/C disease in general follows a milder course than sickle cell anemia, there is a wide spectrum of severity. Some individuals may be almost completely asymptomatic, while others have a more complicated course with frequent crises and severe sequelae. The reason for this variability is not known. One possible modifier may be the co-inheritance of α-thalassemia, which is also common in blacks. It is well known that coexistent α-thalassemia has a moderating effect on the severity of the hemolytic anemia in sickle cell anemia, and the same may be true for S/C disease.

Hb S/C demonstrates a 1:1 ratio of Hb S to Hb C bands on alkaline electrophoresis. However, since Hb A_2 migrates with Hb C, there is actually slightly more Hb S present. The combination of Hb S and Hb C will look identical to Hb S/Hb E and Hb S/Hb O-Arab on alkaline electrophoresis. Other methods such as acid electrophoresis, HPLC, globin chain electrophoresis, or isoelectric focusing will easily differentiate these combinations. (See Figures 17.2 and 17.3.)

Figure 17.1 (Wright-Giemsa, 400x)
The peripheral blood smear from a patient with Hb S/C disease. In addition to increased target cells, there are irregularly shaped cells (SC poikilocytes). These contain misshapen crystals. However, polyhedral Hb C crystals are not seen. True sickle cells are not present.

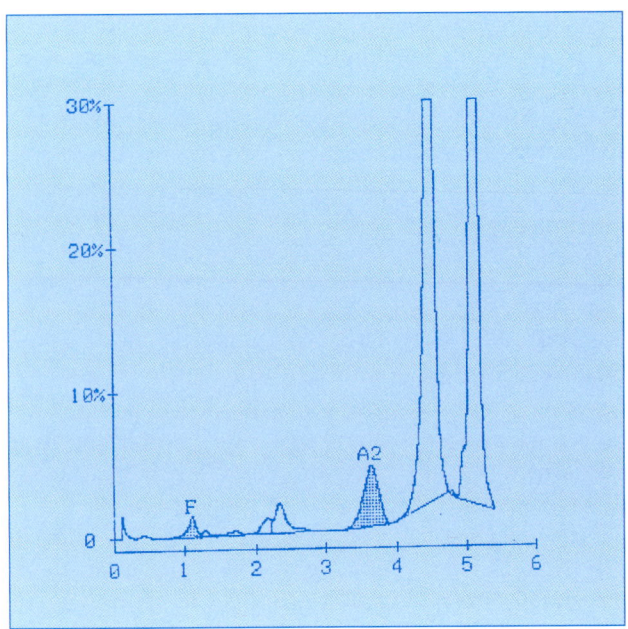

Figure 17.2
An example of Hb SC disease by HPLC. There are two major peaks seen in the S window and C window respectively.

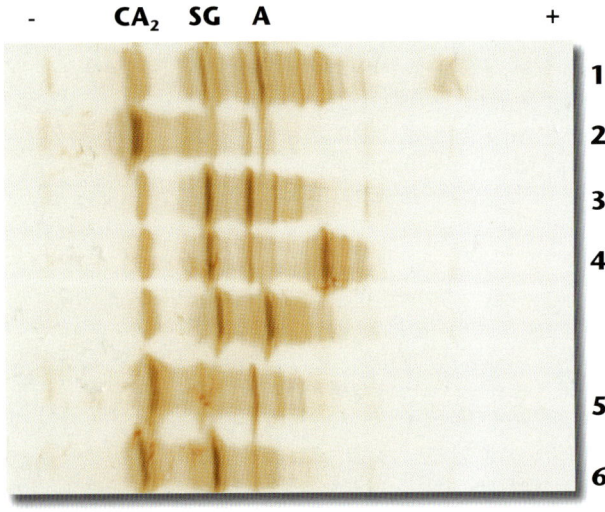

Figure 17.3
An example of Hb S/C disease by isoelectric focusing (lane 6). 1-control, 2-homozygous C, 3-Hb S/HPFH, 4-Hb S/Hb N-Baltimore, 5-Hb E/β^0 thalassemia.

References

Bain BA. Blood film features of sickle cell-haemoglobin C disease. *Br J Haematol.* 1983:53:516-518.

Ballas SK, et al. Clinical, hematological, and biological features of Hb S/C disease. *Am J Hematol.* 1982;13: 37-51.

Bunn HF, Forget BG. *Hemoglobin: Molecular, Genetic and Clinical Aspects.* 1st ed. Philadelphia, PA: WB Saunders Co; 1986:533-536.

Bunn HF, Noguchi CT, Hofrichter J, Schechter GP, Schechter AN, Eaton WA. Molecular and cellular pathogenesis of hemoglobin S/C disease. *Proc Natl Acad Sci USA.* 1982;79:7527-7531.

Dover GJ, Platt OS. Sickle cell disease. In: Nathan DG, Orkin SH, eds. *Hematology of Infancy and Childhood.* 5th ed. Philadelphia, PA: WB Saunders Co; 1998:762-809.

Jandl JF. *Blood: A Textbook of Hematology.* 1st ed. Boston, MA: Little, Brown, and Co; 1987:385-386.

Lawrence C, Fabry ME, Nagel RL. The unique red cell heterogeneity of S/C disease: crystal formation, dense reticulocytes, and unusual morphology. *Blood.* 1991;78:2104-2112.

Nagel RL, Steinberg MH. Hb S/C disease and Hb C disorders. In: Steinberg MH, Forget BJ, Higgs DR, Nagle RL. *Disorders of Hemoglobin: Genetics, Pathophysiology and Clinical Management.* Cambridge, England: Cambridge University Press; 2001:756-785.

River GL, Robbins AB, Schwartz SO. S/C hemoglobin: a clinical study. *Blood.* 1961;18:385-416.

Case 18

HISTORY
A 25-year-old woman was incidentally discovered to have microcytosis and erythrocytosis. She was asymptomatic with a normal physical examination. There was no history of anemia.

BLOOD COUNT DATA
RBC .... 6.9 x 10^{12}/L
Hb .... 14.2 g/dL
MCV .... 66.2 fL
WBC .... 7.3 x 10^9/L
Plt .... 223 x 10^9/L

PERIPHERAL BLOOD SMEAR
Moderate poikilocytosis, microcytosis, and occasional target cells.

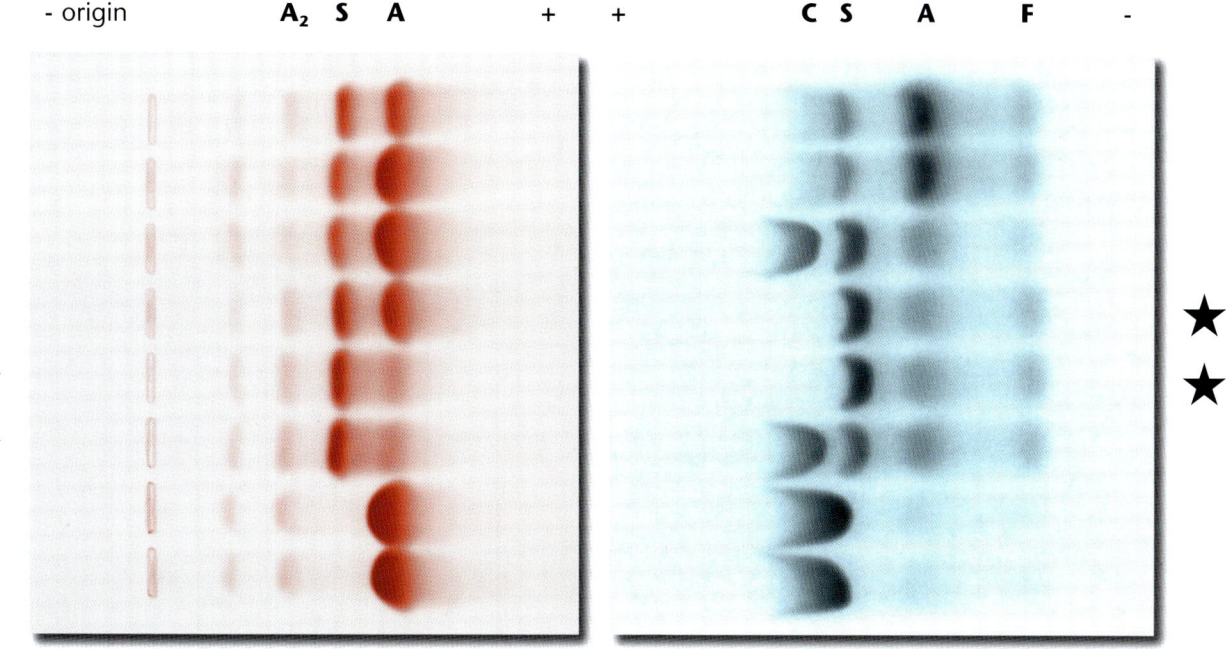

Alkaline Electrophoresis (pH 8.6)   Acid Electrophoresis (pH 6.2)

Case 18 Discussion

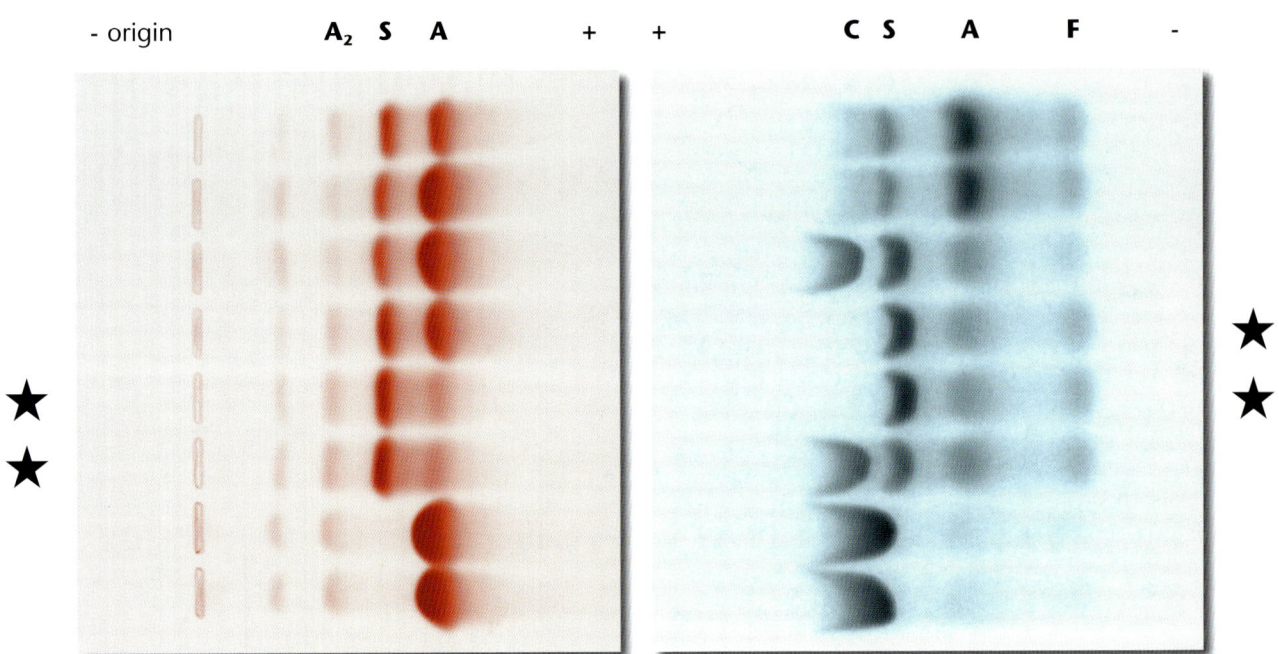

Interpretation

The alkaline electrophoresis gel demonstrates two major bands at the A and S positions, comprising 27% and 63% of the total hemoglobin, respectively. These were accompanied by a minor band between the A and S positions, likely corresponding to increased hemoglobin F, and a slightly more intense band at the A_2 position than in the other lanes. The acid electrophoresis demonstrates bands migrating in the F, A, and S positions.

Additional tests for quantification of Hb F and Hb A_2 yielded results of 4.6% and 5.4%.

Diagnosis

Hb S/β+-thalassemia.

Performance

Hb S/β+-thalassemia has been used only once in the survey. 98% of participants correctly identified the presence of Hb S A, S, and F. 92% correctly diagnosed the case as Hb S/β+-thalassemia.

Discussion

Given that β-thalassemia minor occurs in approximately 1% of African Americans, the combination of Hb S and β-thalassemia is encountered relatively frequently (approximately 1 in 625 black individuals). In contrast to the $β^0$-thalassemia (no output from affected β gene) that is common in Mediterranean and Asian peoples, the β-thalassemia in those of African heritage is most commonly a mild $β^+$-thalassemia in which β chain output from the affected allele is only modestly decreased. Molecular studies have shown that these mild forms of β-thalassemia that are typically encountered in black Americans are due to mutations in the promoter region 5' to (upstream from) the first exon of the β globin gene (see *A Closer Look At...Beta-Thalassemia*, page 24). The combination of a $β^+$ mutation *trans* to a $β^S$ mutation results in decreased normal β chains compared to $β^S$ chains, and thus less Hb A than Hb S. A hallmark of β-thalassemia is increased production of Hb A_2; this also occurs in Hb S/$β^+$-thalassemia. Two rather mild forms of Hb S/$β^+$-thalassemia occur in individuals of African descent: Hb S/$β^+$-thalassemia type 1, in which Hb A represents 5-15% of total hemoglobin; and S/$β^+$-thalassemia type 2, in which Hb A represents 20-30% of total. (The latter has also been called Hb S/$β^{++}$-thalassemia, but this notation is now rarely used.) The current case is an example of Hb S/$β^+$-thalassemia type 2.

The clinical consequences of S/β-thalassemia depend largely on the relative proportions of Hb A and Hb S. Patients with S/$β^0$-thalassemia will have a similar clinical course to patients with SS, although they have less hemolysis and a slightly higher hemoglobin level. This mild ameliorative effect may be based on a relatively decreased concentration of Hb S per cell because of the hypochromia resulting from the deficient β chain production. However, these patients may suffer from most of the other disease-related complications seen in SS disease. An exception to this is that S/$β^0$-thalassemia patients commonly have splenomegaly beyond childhood, in contrast to the early autosplenectomy seen in SS disease. Because of this, they may experience splenic sequestration crisis in adult life, in contrast to patients with SS disease. Patients with S/$β^+$-thalassemia will generally have a milder clinical course than those with S/$β^0$-thalassemia because of the beneficial effects of Hb A in the prevention of sickling. They may in fact be asymptomatic, as in the current case. However, splenomegaly is common in these patients as well.

As the performance data for this case indicated, the definitive identification of the presence of Hb S and Hb A are straightforward based on the relative mobilities on the alkaline and acid gels. The key to making the correct diagnosis in this case is the recognition that Hb S is present in larger amounts than Hb A. In uncomplicated S-trait, Hb A is *always* greater than Hb S. Essentially the only situations in which the S band is larger than the A band on routine alkaline electrophoresis are Hb S/$β^+$-thalassemia, transfused SS disease and, rarely, Hb S/G-Philadelphia (see Case 19, page 93). The microcytosis and mild elevation of Hb F are also characteristic of this disorder.

References

Pearson HA. Hemoglobin S-thalassemia syndrome in Negro children. *Ann N Y Acad Sci.* 1969;165:83-92.

Serjeant GR, Ashcroft MT, Serjeant BE. The clinical features of haemoglobin SC disease in Jamaica. *Br J Haematol.* 1973;24:491-501.

Stevens MC, Maude GH, Beckford M, et al. Haematological change in sickle cell-haemoglobin C disease and in sickle cell-beta thalassaemia: a cohort study from birth. *Br J Haematol.* 1985;60:279-292.

Steinberg, MH. Compound heterozygous and other sickle hemoglobinopathies. In: Steinberg MH, Forget BJ, Higgs DR, Nagle RL. *Disorders of Hemoglobin: Genetics, Pathophysiology and Clinical Management.* Cambridge, England: Cambridge University Press; 2001:786-792.

Weatherall DJ. Biochemical phenotypes of thalassemia in the American negro population. *Ann N Y Acad Sci.* 1964;119:450-462.

Weatherall DJ, Clegg JB. *The Thalassemia Syndromes.* 4th ed. Oxford, England: Blackwell Science, Ltd; 2001:393-411.

Case 19

HISTORY
The patient is a 39-year-old black woman who is asymptomatic.

BLOOD COUNT DATA
RBC.....................4.0 x 10^{12}/L
Hb........................14.2 g/dL
MCV......................97.5 fL
WBC.....................3.9 x 10^9/L
Plt.........................197 x 10^9/L
Reticulocytes.........1.4%

PERIPHERAL BLOOD SMEAR
No abnormalities

OTHER LABORATORY TESTS
A test for unstable hemoglobin was negative.

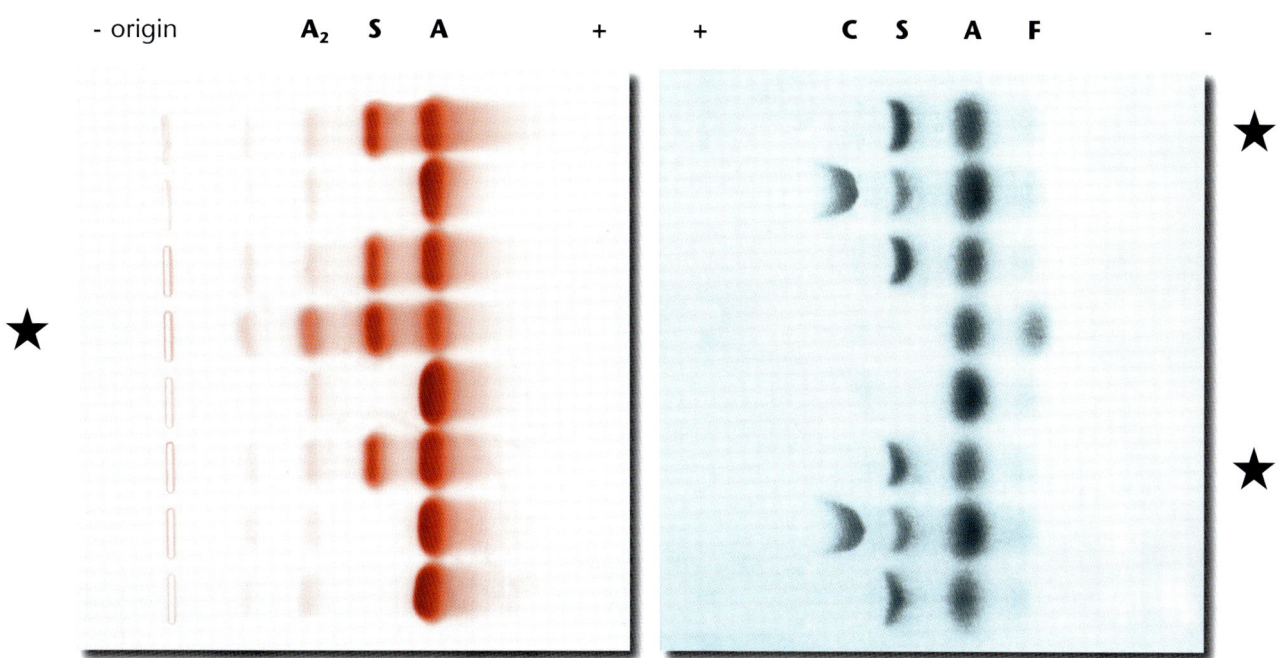

Alkaline Electrophoresis (pH 8.6)

Acid Electrophoresis (pH 6.2)

Case 19 Discussion

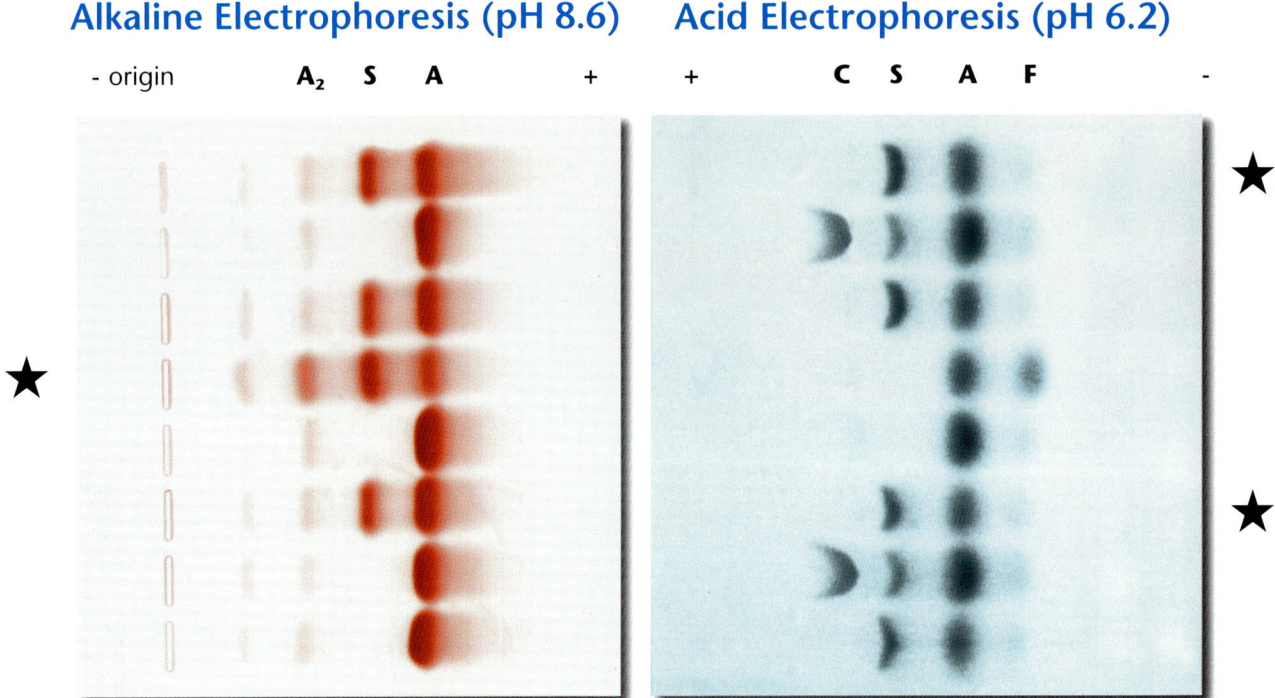

Interpretation

The alkaline electrophoresis gel demonstrates three distinct bands in the A, S, and A$_2$ positions, representing approximately 37%, 47%, and 15% of the total hemoglobin, respectively. In addition, a very faint band may be appreciated cathodal to the hemoglobin A$_2$ position, near carbonic anhydrase. The acid electrophoresis demonstrates bands migrating in the A and S positions.

Diagnosis

Hb S trait with Hb G-Philadelphia trait.

Performance

The double heterozygous state for hemoglobin S and hemoglobin G-Philadelphia has been used in the survey three times. On the occasion of the first challenge, S/G-Philadelphia was correctly identified by only 34% of laboratories using alkaline and acid electrophoresis or isoelectric focusing. On subsequent challenges, this rose to 62.4% and 64.5%.

Discussion

Hemoglobin G-Philadelphia results from the substitution of lysine for asparagine at the 68th amino acid position of the α globin chain (α68 Asn→Lys) (see Case 13). It is the most frequently encountered α variant, and is seen most commonly in African Americans (1 in 5000 frequency). Double heterozygosity for Hb S and Hb G-Philadelphia is seen in approximately 1 in 125,000 blacks. Hb G-Philadelphia is stable and functionally normal, so it does not produce any hematologic abnormalities. Thus, S/G-Philadelphia is equivalent to S trait and is accompanied by virtually no hematologic or clinical manifestations. As detailed in Case 13, in the black population the Hb G-Philadelphia mutation is accompanied by an α gene deletion in *cis* to the mutated allele (-$α^G$/ αα). Therefore, approximately 1/3 of the α chain output will consist of $α^G$, (instead of 1/4). Therefore, in the present case, one would expect Hb G and Hb S/G to total 25-35%.

This example of the double heterozygous state for hemoglobins S and G-Philadelphia demonstrates the potentially confusing consequences of the simultaneous presence of an abnormal α chain ($α^G$) and an abnormal β chain ($β^S$). Because both are present in the heterozygous state, the abnormal chains also coexist with the normal α and β chains ($α^A$ and $β^A$) from the unaffected alleles. This allows for the production of four major hemoglobin species: Hb A ($α^A_2 β^A_2$), Hb S ($α^A_2 β^S_2$), Hb G ($α^G_2 β^A_2$), and Hb S/G ($α^G_2 α^S_2$). Hb S and Hb G-Philadelphia both migrate in the same position on alkaline gels, producing a large "S" band, and Hb S/G migrates in the Hb A_2/C position. The faint band seen near carbonic anhydrase is known as Hb G_2. Hb G_2 is composed of two abnormal α chains and two normal δ chains; it is the abnormal counterpart of Hb A_2. On acid gels, only two major bands are present: Hb G-Philadelphia migrates with Hb A, and Hb S/G migrates with Hb S. Isoelectric focusing and HPLC are capable of resolving Hb S and Hb G-Philadelphia, and reveals four major hemoglobin bands: A, S, G-Philadelphia, and S/G. Note that Hb A_2 can be quantified in this case by HPLC. (See Figures 19.1 and 19.2.)

The most likely misdiagnosis in this case is S/β-thalassemia, given that the "S" band is larger than the A band, and that there is an increase in what appears to be Hb A_2. The key to avoiding this pitfall is the recognition that Hb A_2 never comprises greater than 10% of the total hemoglobin (and only very rarely exceeds 8%). The recognition of the Hb G_2 band is also an important clue, but this faint, slow-moving band may be easily missed, especially when obscured by carbonic anhydrase. Hb G_2 may be distinguished from carbonic anhydrase by application of a heme-specific stain to the membrane. The presence of three major bands (each comprising greater than 10% of the total hemoglobin) in the A, S, and C positions is nearly diagnostic of S/G-Philadelphia, barring transfusion or accidental mixing of specimens. Such a pattern should prompt a search for a faint Hb G_2 band and/or additional testing, such as isoelectric focusing. Globin chain electrophoresis can be helpful in these cases, as the presence of both an alpha and beta chain variant (Figure 19.3) is clearly demonstrated.

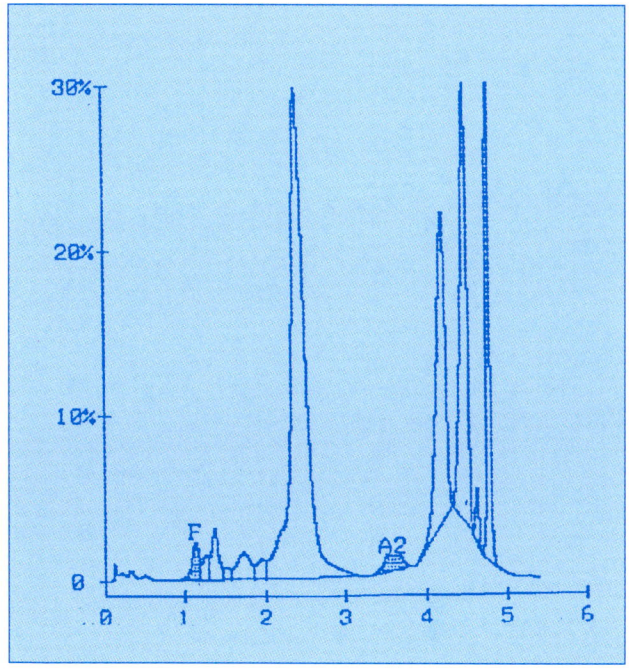

Figure 19.1
An example of Hb S/Hb G-Philadelphia by HPLC. There are three major peaks seen that have a retention time between four to five minutes. The earliest of these, just after four minutes, represents Hb G-Philadelphia. The second peak represents Hb S in the S window. The third peak at just under five minutes represents the S/G hybrid ($α^G_2 β^S_2$).

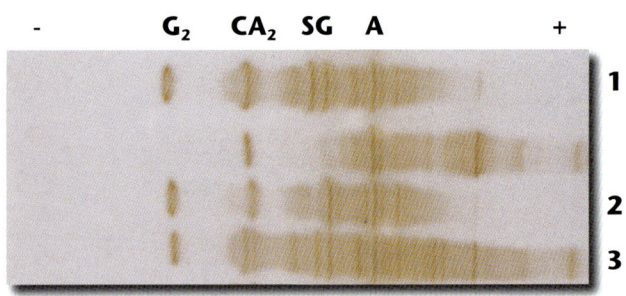

Figure 19.2
An example of Hb S/Hb G-Philadelphia by isoelectric focusing (lane 1). Although they appear together on alkaline electrophoresis, Hb S and Hb G-Philadelphia appear as separate bands on isoelectric focusing. The G-Philadelphia band is the more anodal band (closer to Hb A). Also seen are the S/G hybrid ($\alpha^G_2\beta^S_2$) in the A_2 position and the G_2 band ($\alpha^G_2\delta_2$). 2-Hb G-Philadelphia trait, 3-control.

Figure 19.3
Alkaline globin chain electrophoresis. The presence of both an α chain variant and a β chain variant are clearly demonstrated.

References

Baglioni C, Ingram VM. Abnormal human hemoglobins, V: chemical investigation of haemoglobins A, G, C, X from one individual. *Biochim Biophys Acta.* 1961;48:253-265.

Ballas SK, Walker BK, Atwater J. Globin synthesis studies in a person heterozygous for alpha-thalassemia-2, Hb S, and Hb G-Philadelphia. *Clin Chim Acta.* 1980;100:1-6.

Lawrence C, Hirsch RE, Fataliev NA, Patel S, Fabry ME, Nagel RL. Molecular interactions between Hb alpha-G Philadelphia, Hb C, and Hb S: phenotypic implications for SC alpha-G Philadelphia disease. *Blood.* 1997;90:2819-2825.

Rising JA, Sautter RL, Spicer SJ. Hemoglobin G-Philadelphia-S: a family study of an inherited hybrid hemoglobin. *Am J Clin Pathol.* 1974;61:92-102.

Sancar GB, Tatsis B, Cedeno MM, Rieder RF. Proportion of hemoglobin G Philadelphia (alpha 268 Asn→Lys beta 2) in heterozygotes is determined by alpha-globin gene deletions. *Proc Natl Acad Sci USA.* 1980;77:6874-6878.

Surrey S, Ohene-Frempong K, Rappaport E, Atwater J, Schwartz E. Linkage of alpha G-Philadelphia to alpha-thalassemia in African-Americans. *Proc Natl Acad Sci USA.* 1980;77:4885-4889.

Case 20

HISTORY
The patient is an asymptomatic 33-year-old African-American male who was told that he has sickle cell anemia when he was younger. No abnormalities noted on the physical examination.

BLOOD COUNT DATA
RBC.................................4.94 x 10^{12}/L
Hb...................................14.8 g/dL
MCV................................89.0 fL
WBC................................10.2 x 10^9/L
Plt....................................196 x 10^9/L

PERIPHERAL BLOOD SMEAR
No abnormalities.

OTHER LABORATORY TESTS
The solubility test for sickling hemoglobin is positive.

Alkaline Electrophoresis (pH 8.6)

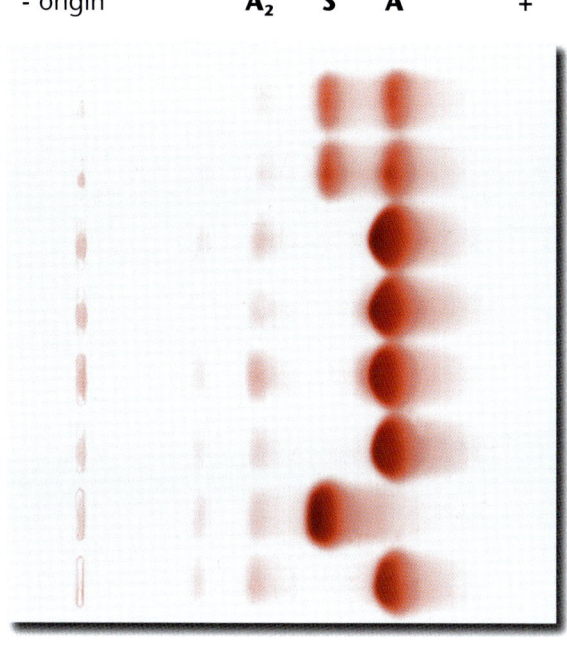

- origin   A₂   S   A   +

Acid Electrophoresis (pH 6.2)

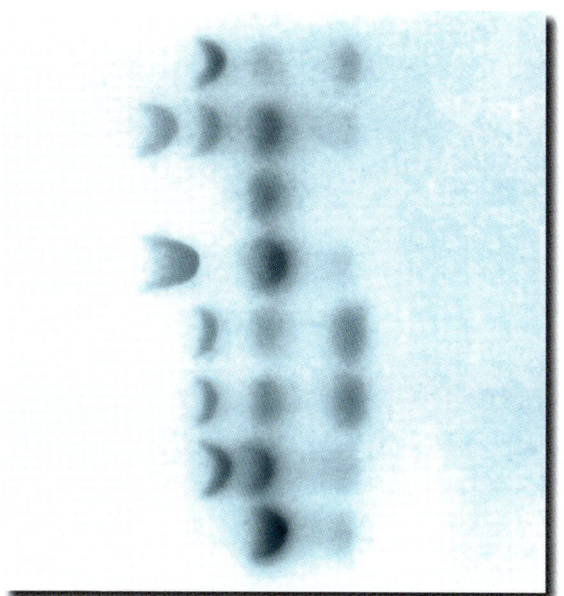

+   C   S   A   F   -

Case 20 Discussion

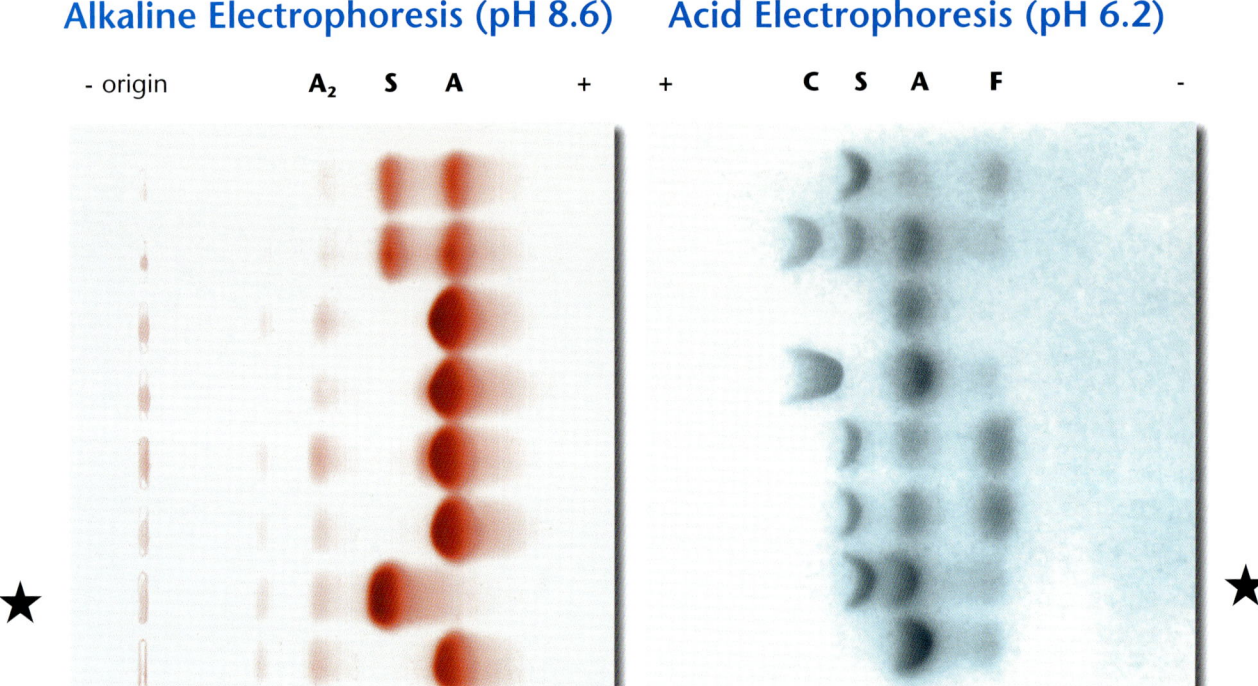

Interpretation

On alkaline electrophoresis, there is no Hb A present. There is a major band in the S position. Acid electrophoresis shows a band in the S position, confirming the presence of Hb S. Additionally, there is a second band which is just slightly anodic to the Hb A position. Further testing including high performance liquid chromatography, isoelectric focusing, and globin chain electrophoresis identified this second variant as Hb Korle-Bu.

Diagnosis

Hb S/Hb Korle-Bu.

Performance

This combination has appeared only once in the survey. This was a difficult specimen, with only 41% of laboratories reporting a combination of Hb S plus a D or G β trait. The D or G variant was identified as Hb D-Punjab by 7% of laboratories and Hb Korle-Bu by 2% of laboratories. 28% of laboratories identified this combination as Hb S/G-Philadelphia. This combination was erroneously reported as homozygous Hb S by 3% of laboratories.

Discussion

Hb Korle-Bu results from a substitution of aspartic acid by asparagine at the 73rd position of the β chain [β73 (E17) Asp→Asn]. This variant is found predominantly in African-Americans who trace their ancestry back to western Africa, where it is found in the Ghana and Ivory Coast areas. This variant has no clinical or hematologic effects. Similarly, the combination of Hb S with Hb Korle-Bu is equivalent to Hb S trait.

Hb Korle-Bu is interesting from a historical standpoint. It was first described in 1954 in a survey of blood samples from the Gold Coast in a west-African male. Hb Korle-Bu is the original Hb G. As other hemoglobin variants with the same electrophoretic mobility were discovered, it was redesignated Hb G-Accra (for the city in Ghana). In 1968, it was renamed Hb Korle-Bu (for Korle-Bu Hospital in Ghana). Hb Korle-Bu is also related to Hb C-Harlem (C-Georgetown), a doubly substituted hemoglobin variant. In addition to the Hb S mutation at the 6th position, the other mutation is the Hb Korle-Bu mutation at the 73rd position. Hb C-Harlem also traces back to western Africa; it is likely that a crossover event occurred in the distant past to place both mutations on the same chromosome.

This case illustrates the utility of acid electrophoresis. By alkaline electrophoresis, the electrophoretic pattern is identical to homozygous Hb S with a single band in the S position. However, on acid electrophoresis, Hb Korle-Bu migrates with Hb A, and thus two hemoglobin variants are evident. It is always important to further evaluate a single band in the S position by another method to ensure that this band is due solely to Hb S or to two co-migrating variants. This method does not need to be acid electrophoresis; other methods such as HPLC or isoelectric focusing could also serve as a confirmatory method. The patient's history may indicate that such a confirmation was not performed.

Hb S/Hb Korle-Bu is electrophoretically similar to the combination of Hb S with other D or G hemoglobins. The most important of these is Hb D-Los Angeles (D-Punjab). By most electrophoretic methods, these two variants are very difficult to separate. The difference is clinically important as Hb S/Hb D-Los Angeles is a sickling disorder, whereas Hb S/Hb Korle-Bu is not. As discussed in Case 11, HPLC is very helpful in distinguishing these two variants (see Figure 20.1).

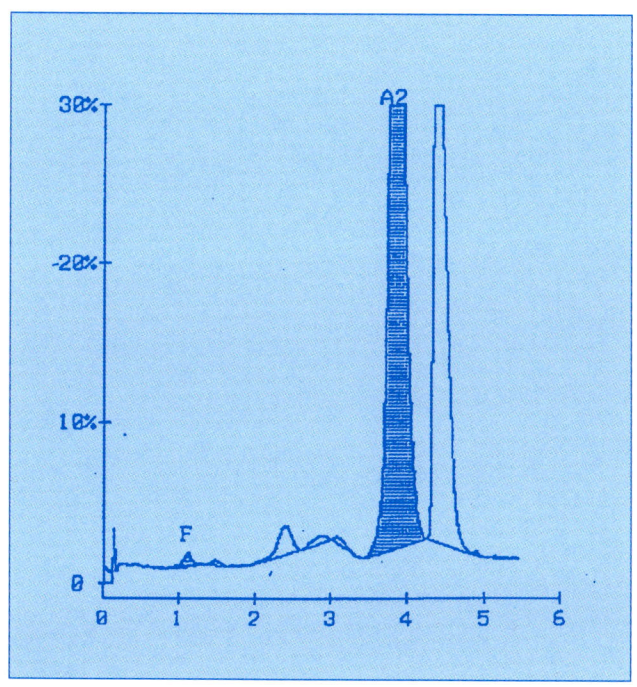

Figure 20.1
An example of Hb S/Hb Korle Bu by HPLC. There is no Hb A present. There is a large peak in the S window, corresponding to Hb S, and a large peak in the A_2 window, corresponding to Hb Korle-Bu.

References

Bookchin RM, Nagel RL, Ranney HM. Structure and properties of hemoglobin C-Harlem: a human hemoglobin variant with amino acid substitutions in two residues of the β-polypeptide chain. *J Biol Chem.* 1967;242:248-255.

Edington GM, Lehmann H. Haemoglobin G: a new haemoglobin found in West Africa (preliminary communication). *Lancet.* 1954;2:173-174.

Edington GM, Lehman H, Schneider RG. Characterization and genetics of Haemoglobin G (letter-to-editor). *Nature.* 1955;175:850-851.

Konotey-Ahulu FID, Gallo E, Lehmann H, Ringelhann B. Hemoglobin Korle-Bu (β73 aspartic acid→ asparagine). *J Med Genet.* 1968;5:107-111.

Lehmann H, Beale D, Boi-Doku FS. Hemoglobin G-Accra. *Nature.* 1964;203:363-365.

Case 21

HISTORY
The patient is a 34-year-old African-American male who has had recurrent myalgias for many years, particularly after sports or when at high altitude.

BLOOD COUNT DATA
- RBC .... 6.17×10^{12}/L
- Hb .... 15.0 g/dL
- MCV .... 77.4 fl
- WBC .... 4.2×10^9/L
- Plt .... 320×10^9/L

PERIPHERAL BLOOD SMEAR
The red blood cells showed hypochromia, microcytosis, and occasional target cells.

OTHER LABORATORY TESTS
Test for unstable hemoglobin is positive.

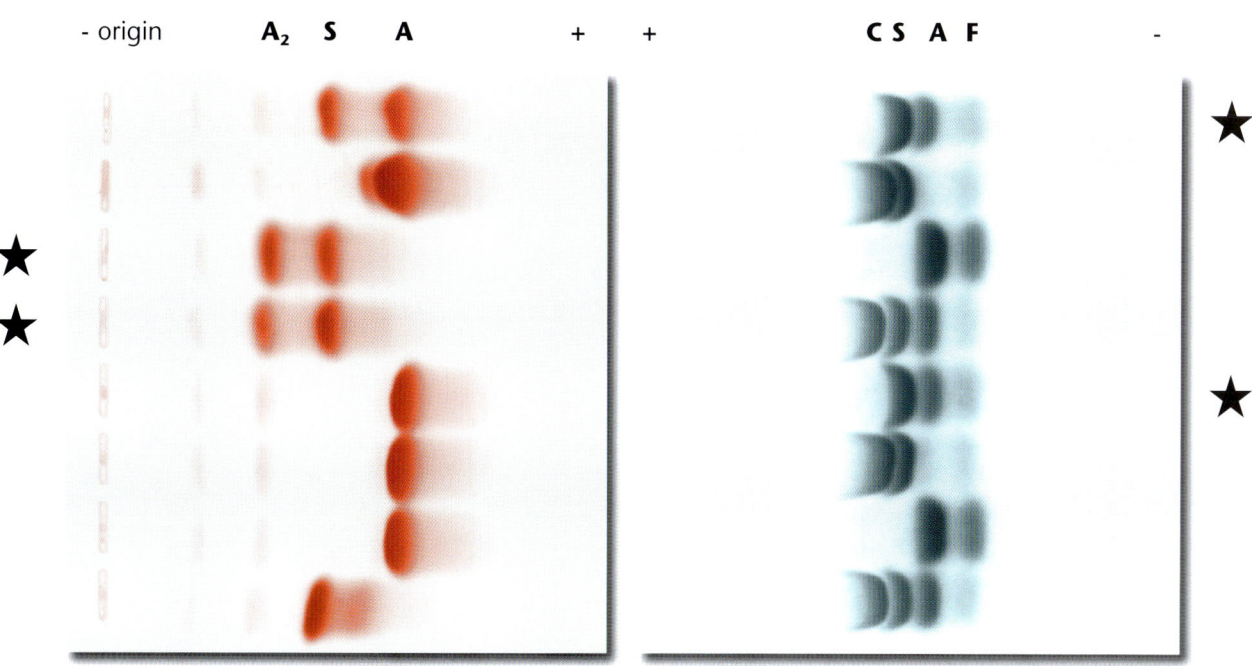

Alkaline Electrophoresis (pH 8.6)   Acid Electrophoresis (pH 6.2)

Case 21 Discussion

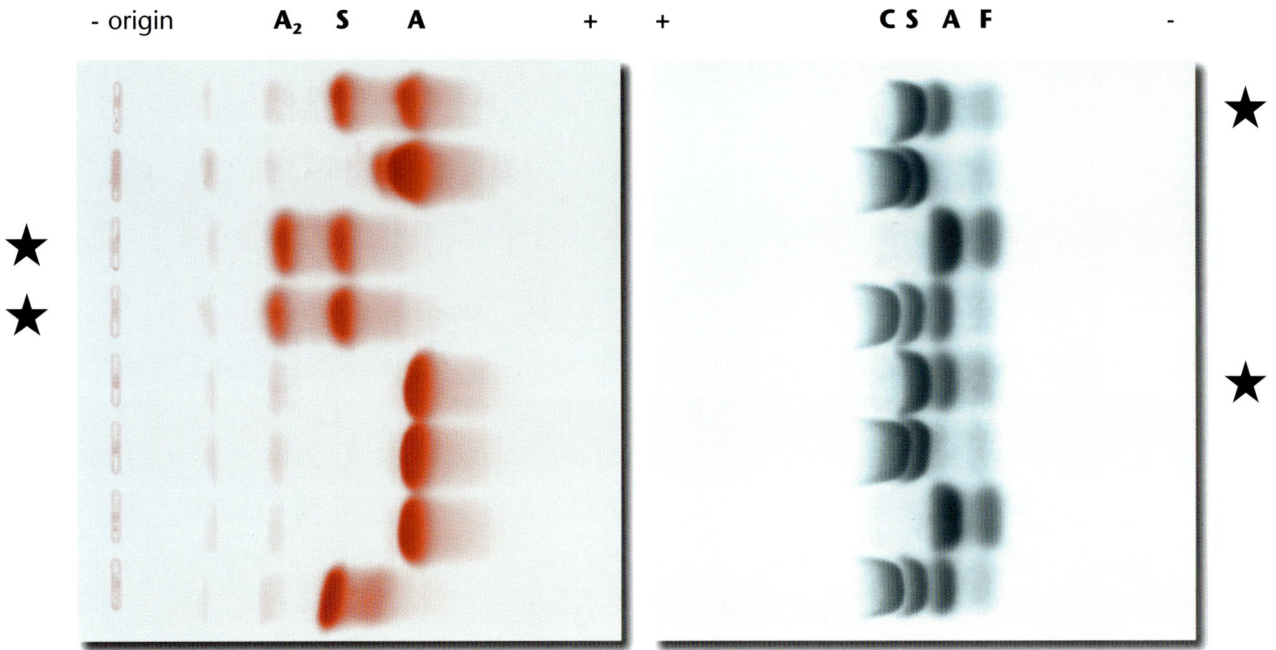

Interpretation

Alkaline electrophoresis shows a band in the S position and a band in the A_2 position. There is no Hb A present. Acid electrophoresis shows bands in the A and S positions.

Diagnosis

Hb S/Hb E combination.

Performance

Hb S/Hb E has appeared in the survey once as a wet specimen, with 70.5% of laboratories correctly identifying this combination. This has also appeared as a dry lab challenge, with 78.2% of laboratories giving a correct response.

Discussion

Hb S and Hb E are the most common hemoglobin variants worldwide, yet compound heterozygosity for Hb S and Hb E is extremely rare due to different ethnic distributions. Hb S is the most common variant in African Americans, with a gene frequency of approximately 0.04 (corresponding to about 8% of African Americans with Hb S trait). Hb E is the most prevalent β globin chain variant in Southeast Asia, with the highest prevalence in Thailand, Cambodia, and northeast India. Both hemoglobin variants offer a protective advantage against malaria, and their ethnic and geographic gene frequency distributions are influenced by the regional prevalence of malaria. The gene frequency of Hb E in Thailand and Burma ranges from 0.05 to 0.10; in Cambodia it is 0.20; and in a tribe of Assam, in northeast India, it is 0.5. Approximately 32% of Cambodians have Hb E trait, and 3% are homozygous. These gene frequencies result in approximately 30 million people in Southeast Asia who are heterozygous for Hb E and one million who are homozygous. Hb E has been detected in about 1 in 50,000 African Americans, and several cases of Hb S/E have now been described in African Americans. Hb S/E has also been observed in Saudi Arabia, India, and Pakistan, and in persons of Filipino, Creole, and Turkish origin.

In most hemoglobinopathy conditions in which there is compound heterozygosity for two β globin chain variants, the two variants are present in roughly equal proportion, although the more anodic variant is usually present in slightly greater amounts. The reason for this is that the more anodic variants have β chains that are more negatively charged and have a greater binding affinity for the α globin chains. In Hb S/E, the percentage of Hb S is consistently greater than the percentage of Hb E, with relative proportions ranging from 60-70% Hb S and 30-40% Hb E (plus Hb A_2). The explanation for this is that Hb E, in addition to being a structural variant of the β globin chain, is also underproduced and thus mimics β-thalassemia (see Case 9). Molecular studies have shown that there is a deficiency of $β^E$ mRNA due to abnormal splicing, which results in a decrease in $β^E$ globin chain production. Therefore, there are fewer $β^E$ globin chains than $β^S$ chains to bind with normal α globin chains, resulting in a relative excess of Hb S.

Hb S/E appears to be a generally benign condition with few clinical manifestations. The majority of patients described, although few in number, have mild to absent anemia, microcytic indices, some target cells, and slight splenomegaly. The microcytosis and target cells may be attributed to the Hb E. Although severe sickling manifestations have not been documented, a few patients have been described who appear to have had episodes of splenic sequestration and transient hyposplenism. The high percentage of Hb S, which is typically greater than 50%, may contribute to complications in pregnancy.

Under alkaline electrophoresis conditions, compound heterozygosity for Hb S and Hb E produces a band in the Hb S region and another in the Hb A_2 position. On acid electrophoresis, the identity of Hb S is confirmed and Hb E migrates in the Hb A position. As noted earlier, the percentage of Hb S is greater than that of Hb E (approximately 60% and 40%, respectively). Hb A_2 does not separate from Hb E by these electrophoresis methods, and therefore the band in the Hb A_2 position represents the sum of Hb E and Hb A_2. It is essential to distinguish Hb S/E from Hb S/C, Hb S/C-Harlem and Hb S/O-Arab, because the latter three conditions are often severe sickling disorders. However, these disorders are excluded by the acid electrophoresis, since Hb C, Hb C-Harlem, and Hb O-Arab have mobilities that are distinct from Hb A under acid conditions. Examples of Hb S/Hb E are shown on HPLC (Figure 21.1) and isoelectric focusing (Figure 21.2).

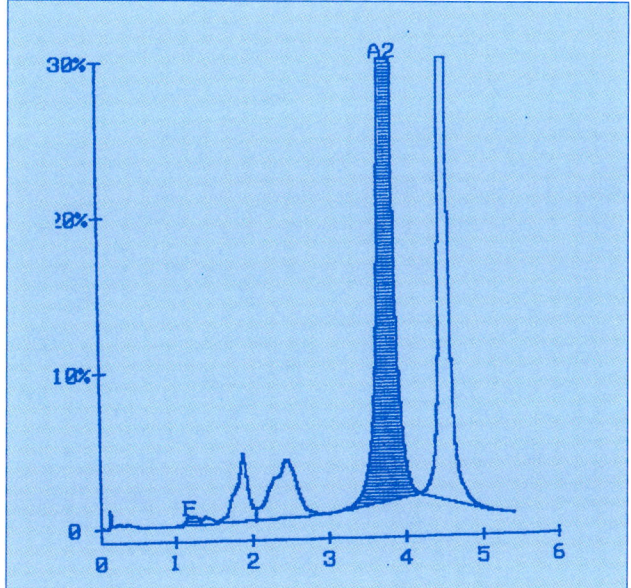

Figure 21.1
An example of Hb S/Hb E by HPLC. In addition to a major peak in the S window, there is a major A_2 peak representing Hb E. By HPLC, this case has an identical chromatogram to Case 20.

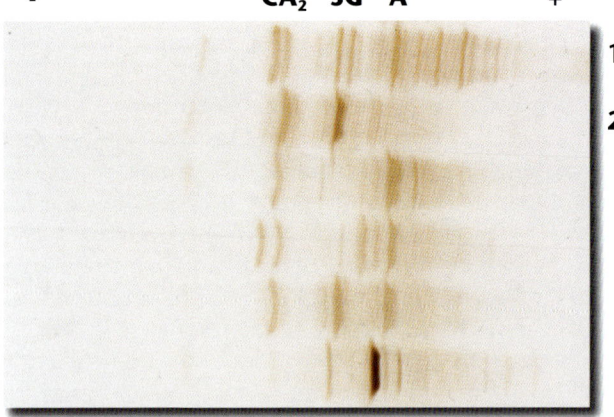

Figure 21.2
An example of Hb S/Hb E by isoelectric focusing. The control (lane 1) contains hemoglobins S, C, G-Philadelphia, J-Baltimore, and I. In Lane 2, there is no Hb A present, but only a major band in the S position and in the A_2 position.

References

Aksoy M, Lehmann H. The first observation of sickle-cell haemoglobin E disease. *Nature.* 1957;179:1248-1249.

Aksoy M. The hemoglobin E syndromes, II: sickle-cell hemoglobin E disease. *Blood.* 1960;15:610-613.

Altay G, Niazi GA, Huisman THJ. The combination of Hb S and Hb E in a black female. *Hemoglobin.* 1977;1:100-102.

Anderson HM, Ranney HM. Southeast Asian immigrants: the new thalassemias in Americans. *Semin Hematol.* 1990;27:239-246.

Englestad BL. Functional asplenia in hemoglobin SE disease. *Clin Nucl Med.* 1982;7:100-102.

Hardy MJ, Ragbeer MS. Homozygous HbE and HbSE disease in a Saudi family. *Hemoglobin.* 1995;9:47-52.

Monzon CM, Fairbanks VF, Burgert O Jr, et al. Hematologic genetic disorders among Southeast Asian refugees. *Am J Hematol.* 1985;19:27-36.

Ramahi AJ, Lewkow LM, Dombrowski MP, Bottoms SF. Sickle cell E hemoglobinopathy and pregnancy. *Obstet Gynecol.* 1988;71:493-495.

Rey SK, Unger CA, Sreedhar R, Miller ST. Sickle cell-hemoglobin E disease: clinical findings and implications. *J Pediatr.* 1991;119:949-951.

Sandhaus LM, Smith CM, Peterson L. Hb E disorders in a Minnesota Southeast Asian immigrant population: morphology, indices, electrophoretic patterns and clinical manifestations. *Minn Med.* 1983;66:163-166.

Schneider RG, Hightower B, Hosty TS, et al. Abnormal hemoglobins in a quarter million people. *Blood.* 1976;48:629-637.

Shroeder WA, Powars D, Reynolds RD, Fisher JI. Hb-E in combination with Hb-S and Hb-C in a black family. *Hemoglobin.* 1977;1:287-289.

Case 22

HISTORY
The patient is a 51-year-old African-American female. She has been healthy her entire life and has never needed a blood transfusion.

BLOOD COUNT DATA
RBC .... 4.36 x 10^{12}/L
Hb .... 12.2 g/dL
MCV .... 86.3 fL
WBC .... 7.6 x 10^9/L
PLT .... 202 x 10^9/L

PERIPHERAL BLOOD SMEAR
No abnormalities.

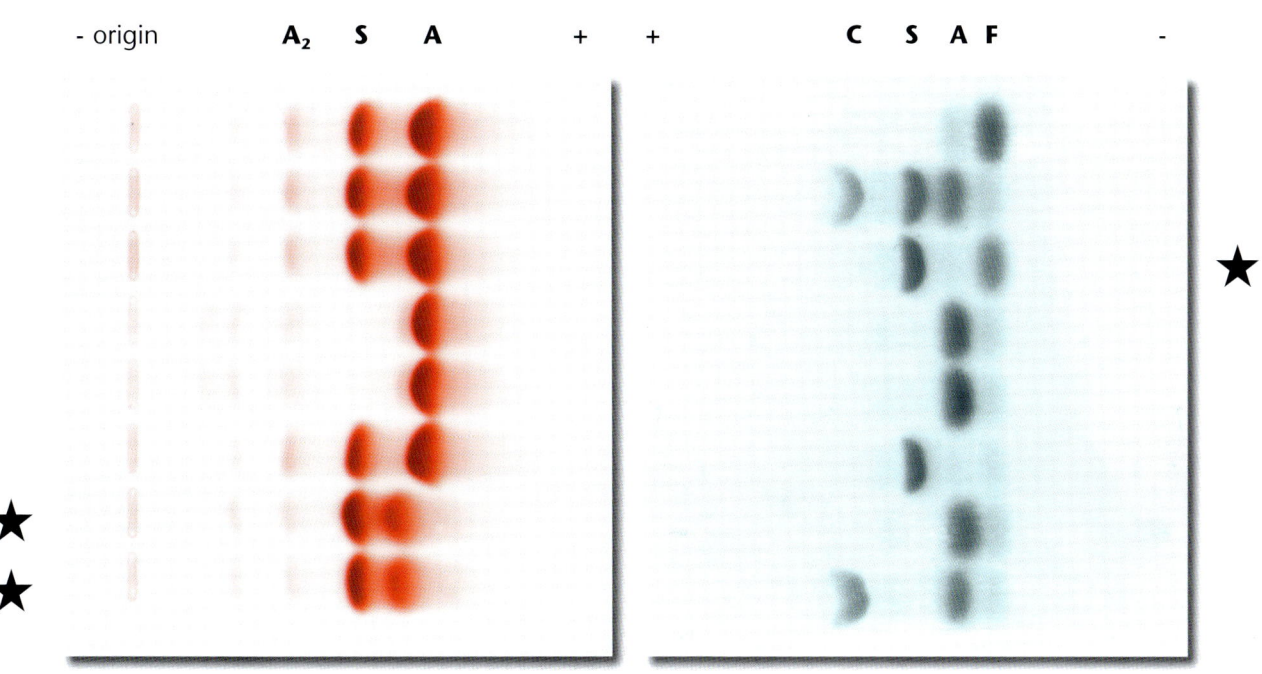

Alkaline Electrophoresis (pH 8.6)   **Acid Electrophoresis (pH 6.2)**

- origin A_2 S   A   +   +   C   S   A   F   -

Case 22 Discussion

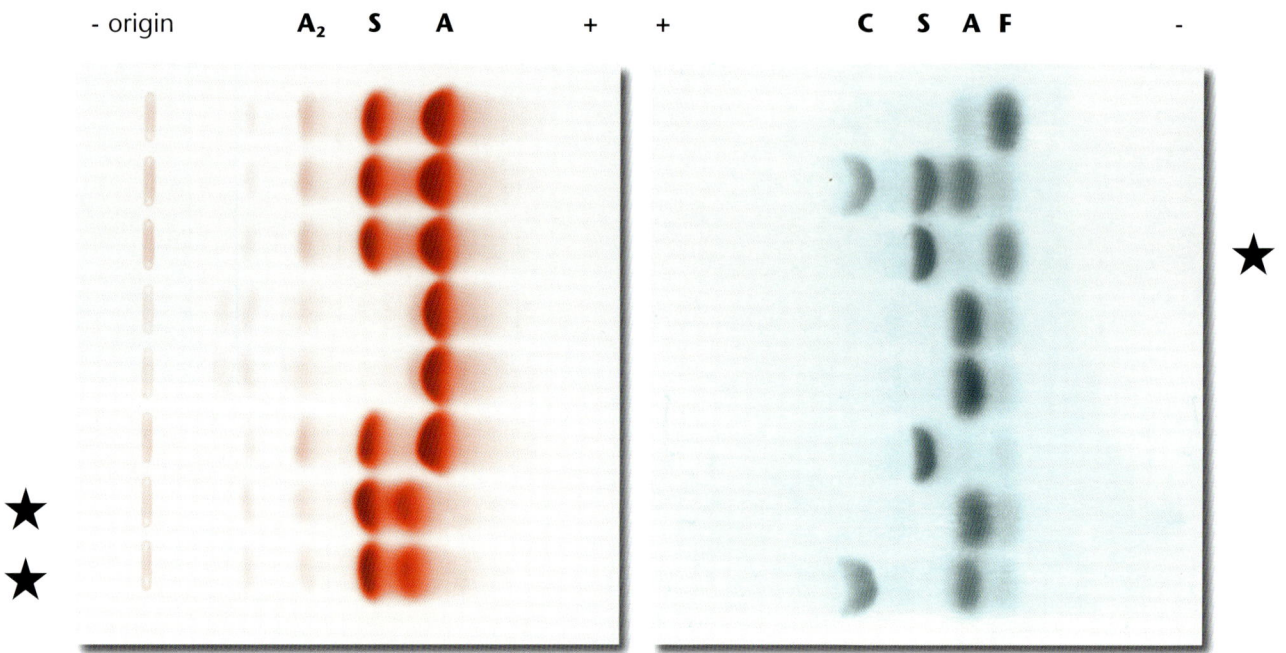

Interpretation

On alkaline electrophoresis, there are two bands present, one in the S position and one in the position of Hb F. There is no Hb A present. Similarly, on acid electrophoresis, there are bands seen in the S and F positions.

Diagnosis

Hb S trait/Hereditary persistence of fetal hemoglobin trait (Hb S/HPFH).

Performance

Hb S/HPFH has been included in the survey twice, with correct responses of 93% and 91%.

Discussion

This represents a case of Hb S trait in combination with hereditary persistence of fetal hemoglobin (HPFH trait). Hereditary persistence of fetal hemoglobin is heterogeneous at the molecular level and is found in multiple ethnic groups (see Case 4). In African Americans, there are three mutations that are most commonly seen. Two of these involve large deletions (105-106 kb) that involve both the δ and β genes. There is no production of Hb A from the affected chromosome, and Hb F levels range from 25-35% in patients with HPFH trait. The third type of mutation is non-deletional and is due to a C to G substitution at position 202 (upstream) from the beginning of the $^G\gamma$ gene (in the promoter region). This appears to cause a change in the binding site of two proteins, which causes persistent overexpression of the $^G\gamma$ chains. Because this is not a deletional mutation, there is still some production of normal β chains from the affected chromosome. An interesting feature is that almost all of the Hb F produced is of the $^G\gamma$ type; thus this mutation has been termed "$^G\gamma\beta^+$ HPFH." When this mutation is present in combination with Hb S, the following percentages are obtained: Hb A, 25-35%; Hb S, 40-45%; Hb F, 20%; Hb A_2, 2-2.5%.

All three of the common African-American forms of HPFH show a pancellular distribution of Hb F by the Kleihauer-Betke acid elution test. With the development of a monoclonal antibody against the γ chain, it is now possible to analyze the cellular distribution of Hb F by flow cytometry. A pretreatment step is used to permeabilize the red cells without lysing them, and fluorescence labeled anti-Hb F is added. The red cells are then analyzed by single color flow cytometry. In a normal person, a single peak with minimal fluorescence is seen, corresponding to Hb A. In neonates, there is a single peak with bright fluorescence, corresponding to Hb F. In young infants, there are typically two peaks present, representing both Hb A and Hb F. In patients with HPFH trait of one of the above types, a single peak with intermediate fluorescence is seen. This corresponds to the pancellular pattern seen with the Kleihauer-Betke test. Other conditions with elevated levels of Hb F, such as β-thalassemia trait or δβ-thalassemia trait, will give two peaks, corresponding to the heterocellular pattern by the Kleihauer-Betke test.

In the current case, alkaline electrophoresis demonstrates only Hb S, Hb F, and Hb A_2; there is no Hb

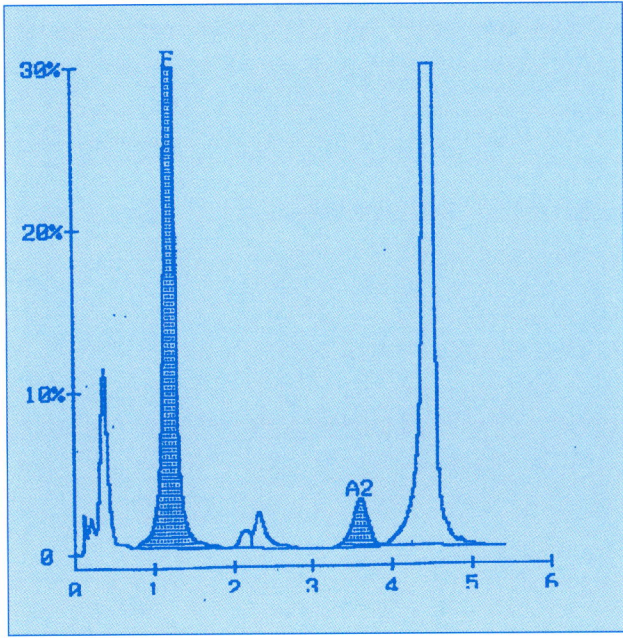

Figure 22.1
An example of Hb S/HPFH by HPLC. In addition to a major peak in the S window, there is also an increased amount of Hb F.

A. The Hb F accounts for approximately 25-35% of the hemoglobin present. The main differential with Hb S/HPFH in this case is either homozygous Hb S or Hb S/β^0-thalassemia. The Hb F level seen in this case would be unusual for homozygous S (unless being treated with hydroxyurea; see below). Both the CBC and clinical course are also key discriminators between these possibilities. Patients with Hb S/HPFH are usually not anemic and do not have any of the sickling manifestations of sickle cell anemia. This is because the high levels of Hb F inhibit the polymerization of Hb S within the red cells. Because of the inhibitory effect of Hb F on the polymerization of Hb S, many patients with sickle cell anemia are now treated with hydroxyurea, which will elevate their level of Hb F. This level of Hb F can sometimes be so high as to cause confusion with Hb S/HPFH. This is particularly true when no clinical information is known. In confusing situations, flow cytometry studies can be valuable. Patients with sickle cell anemia will give two peaks (Hb S and Hb F), whereas, patients with Hb S/HPFH will give a peak with intermediate fluorescence similar to patients with HPFH trait.

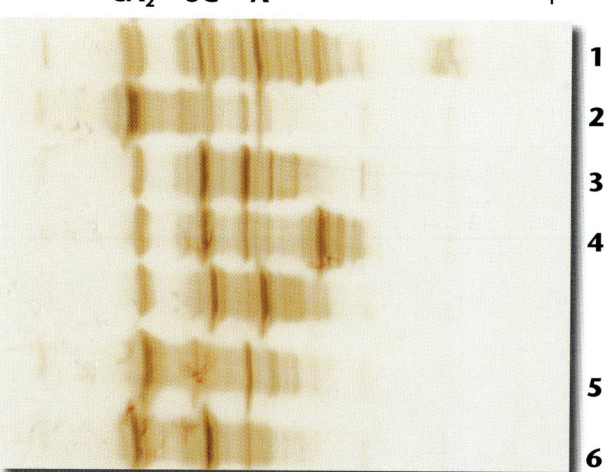

Figure 22.2
An example of Hb S/hereditary persistence of fetal hemoglobin by isoelectric focusing (lane 3). In addition to the Hb S and Hb A_2 bands, there is an increased amount of Hb F. The band seen just anodal to the Hb A position represents acetylated Hb F. Lane 1-control, 2-homozygous C, 4-Hb S/Hb N-Baltimore, 5-Hb E/β^0-thalassemia, 6-Hb S/C disease.

References

Bollekens JA, Forget BG. Delta beta thalassemia and hereditary persistence of fetal hemoglobin. *Hematol Oncol Clin North Am.* 1991;5:399-422.

Charache S, Clegg JB, Weatherall DJ. The Negro variety of hereditary persistence of fetal haemoglobin is a mild form of thalassemia. *Br J Haemtol.* 1976;34:527-533.

Conley CC, Weatherall DJ, Richardson SN, et al. Hereditary persistence of fetal hemoglobin: a study of 79 affected persons in 15 Negro families in Baltimore. *Blood.* 1963;21:261-279.

Davis BH, Bigelow NC, Chen JC. Detection of fetal red cells in fetomaternal hemorrhage using a fetal hemoglobin monoclonal antibody by flow cytometry. *Immunohematology.* 1998;38:749-756.

Hoyer JD, Penz CS, Fairbanks VF, et al. Flow cytometric measurement of hemoglobin F in RBCs: diagnostic usefulness in the distinction of hereditery persistence of fetal hemoglobin (HPFH) and hemoglobin S-HPFH from other conditions with elevated levels of hemoglobin F. *Am J Clin Pathol.* 2002;117:857-863.

Jacob GF, Raper AB. Hereditary persistence of foetal haemoglobin production and its interaction with the sickle cell trait. *Br J Haematol.* 1958;4:138-149.

Murray N, Serjeant BE, Serjeant GR. Sickle cell-hereditary persistence of fetal haemoglobin and its differentiation from other sickle cell syndromes. *Br J Haemotol.* 1988;6:89-92.

Rubin EM, Rowley PT. Sickle cell trait/hereditary persistence of fetal hemoglobin trait: misdiagnosis as sickle cell anemia by newborn screening. *Am J Dis Child.* 1979;133:1248-1250.

Case 23

HISTORY

A 61-year-old diabetic male of African-American heritage was found to have a Hb A_{1c} value of 70%. This extraordinary high value of Hb A_{1c} led to further testing. Except for diabetes mellitus, requiring insulin therapy, he was well and asymptomatic (#1). A specimen was also received from the 32-year-old healthy asymptomatic daughter of the gentleman above (#2).

Note: In order to provide participants with a sufficient volume of sample to measure Hb F, the father's blood was diluted 2:1 with washed, packed normal erythrocytes. Thus, the level of Hb A is higher and the level of Hb F is lower than in the original specimen. The original hemoglobin percentages in the father were as follows: Hb A=28.7%; Hb F=67.7%; Hb A_2=3.6%.

BLOOD COUNT DATA

	Father (#1)	Daughter (#2)
RBC	6.98	$5.35 \times 10^{12}/L$
Hgb	15.2	13.1 g/dL
MCV	69	74 fL
WBC	7.0	$9.4 \times 10^9/L$
Plt	175	$281 \times 10^9/L$

PERIPHERAL BLOOD SMEAR
No abnormalities.

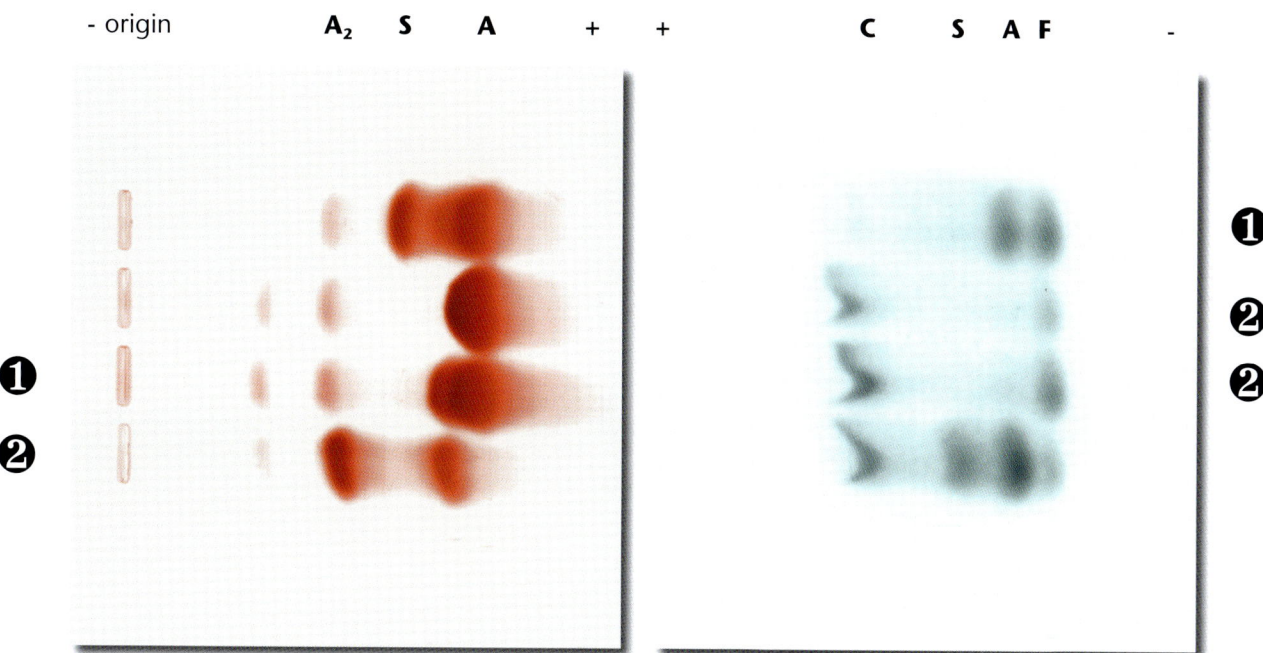

Alkaline Electrophoresis (pH 8.6)

Acid Electrophoresis (pH 6.2)

Case Studies

Case 23 Discussion

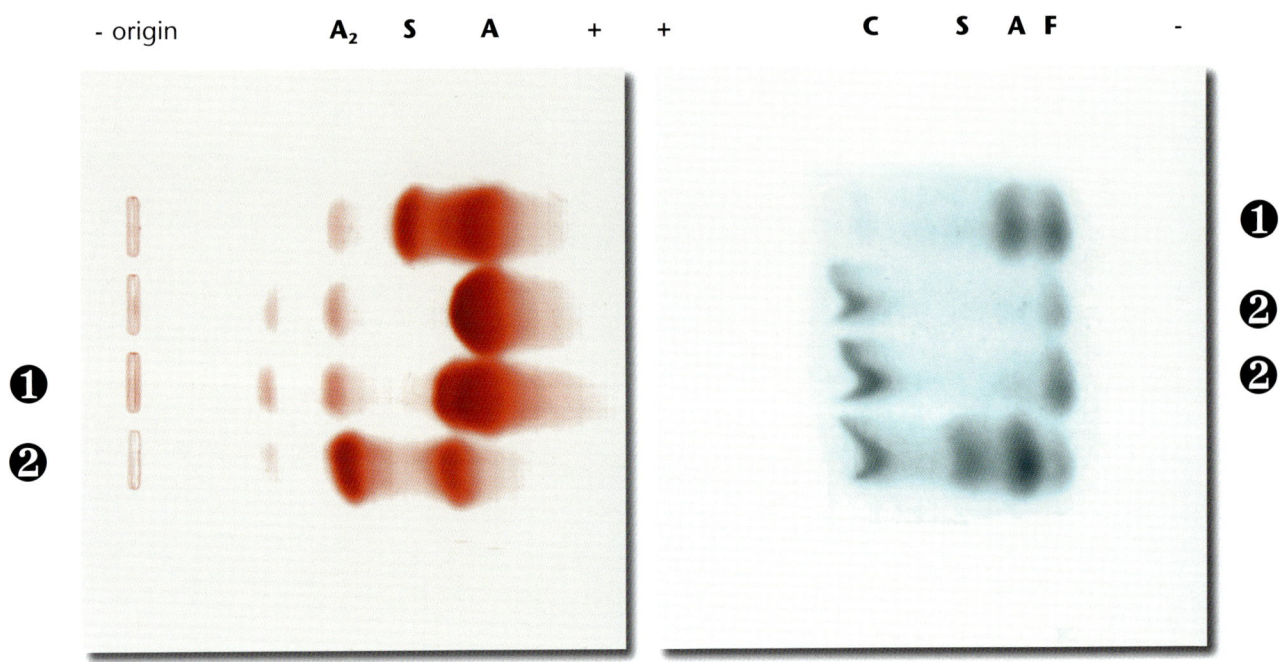

Interpretation

Both alkaline and acid electrophoresis of the father (#1) shows Hb A and increased Hb F level. Alkaline electrophoresis of the daughter's sample shows a band in the C position and an elevated level of Hb F. Acid electrophoresis confirms the presence of Hb C and Hb F.

Diagnosis

Father – HPFH trait/β-thalassemia trait.
Daughter – Hb C trait/HPFH trait.

Performance

The dilution of the father's sample with normal erythrocytes caused some confusion in its interpretation. Although 87.2% of laboratories recognized the presence of HPFH trait, only 48.5% of laboratories recognized concurrent β-thalassemia trait. For the daughter's specimen, approximately 64% recognized the combination of Hb C with HPFH; 26% interpreted this as Hb C/β-thalassemia; and 9.5% as homozygous Hb C.

Discussion

These two samples illustrate the value of family studies in puzzling cases. The Hb F value obtained in the father is too low for homozygous HPFH and yet too high for HPFH trait. Thus, the results obtained represent either HPFH trait in combination with a β-thalassemia mutation or, alternatively, two mild β⁺-thalassemia mutations. The MCV seen in the father could be compatible with either possibility. However, examination of the results of the daughter shows an elevation of Hb F of around 40%, consistent with HPFH trait. The daughter then inherited HPFH trait from her father; the Hb C trait is inherited from her mother. Had the daughter inherited β-thalassemia trait from her father, she would have a Hb C/β⁺-thalassemia combination, with 20-30% Hb A and 60-70% Hb C (see Case 29). Thus, the findings seen in the father are due to HPFH trait in combination with β-thalassemia trait.

The type of HPFH trait present in this family is likely one of the deletional forms seen in African Americans as discussed in Case 22. The extremely high values for Hb A_{1c} that were originally obtained in the father are the result of the high Hb F being interpreted as Hb A_{1c} on ion-exchange chromatography. This has long been known to be a limitation of this technique and is remedied by using affinity chromatography.

References

Bollekens JA, Forget BG. Delta beta thalassemia and the hereditary persistence of fetal hemoglobin. *Hematol Oncol Clin North Am.* 1991;5:399-423.

Fairbanks VF. *Hemoglobinopathies and Thalassemias.* New York, NY: Brian C. Decker; 1980:22-25.

Fairbanks VF. Measurement of glycosylated hemoglobin by affinity chromatography. *Mayo Clin Proc.* 1987;58:770-773.

Case 24

HISTORY
The patient is a 34-year-old, asymptomatic Native-American woman. The physical examination was unremarkable.

BLOOD COUNT DATA
RBC..............................4.7 x 10^{12}/L
Hb................................12.8 g/dL
MCV..............................84 fL
WBC..............................6.8 x 10^9/L
Plt.................................229 x 10^9/L

PERIPHERAL BLOOD SMEAR
No abnormalities.

OTHER LABORATORY TESTS
A test for unstable hemoglobin was negative.

Alkaline Electrophoresis (pH 8.6)   Acid Electrophoresis (pH 6.2)

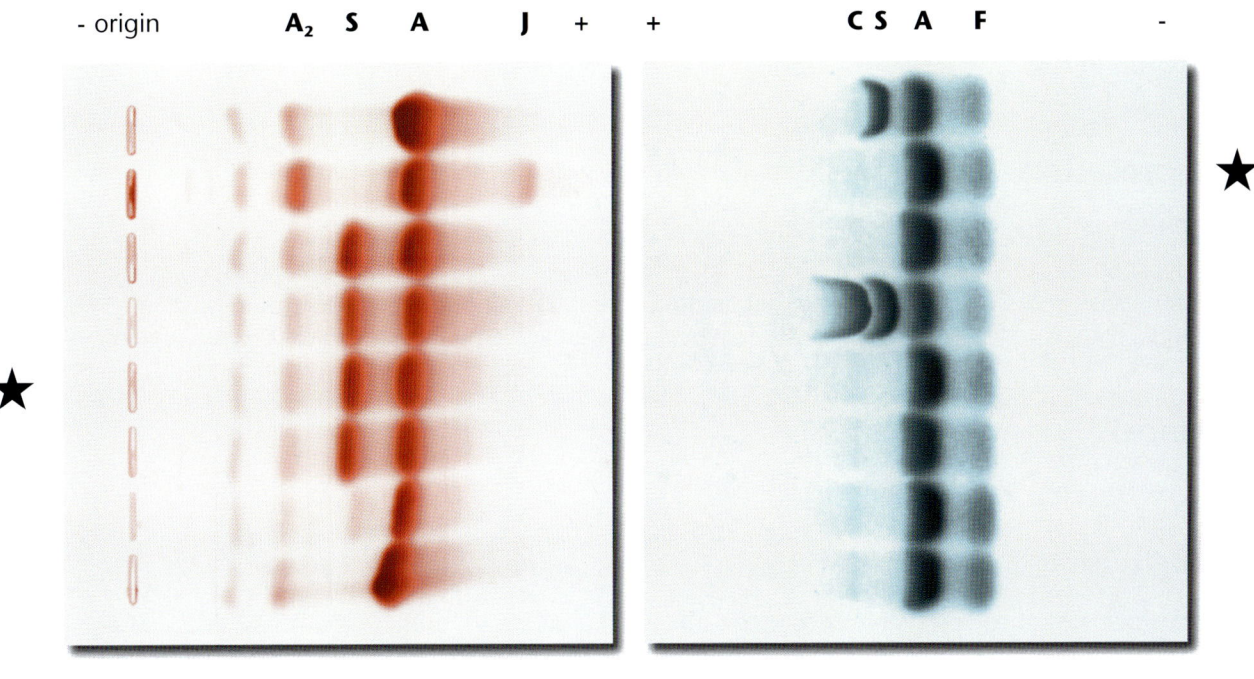

Case Studies

Case 24 Discussion

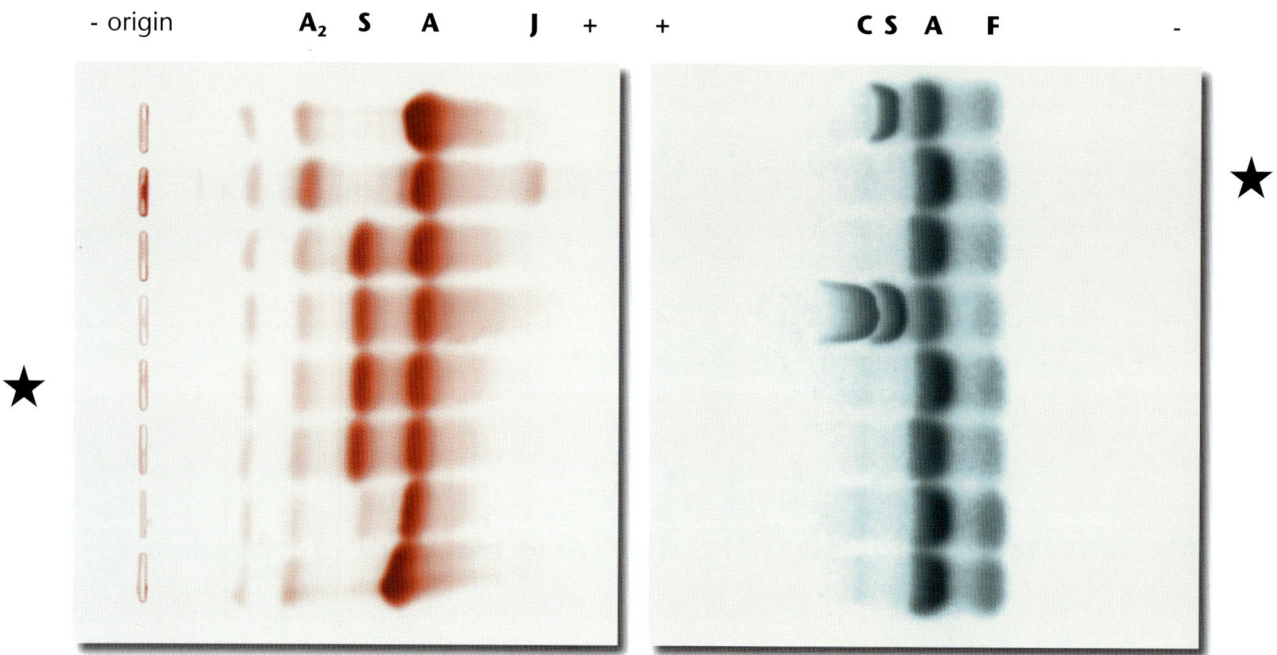

Interpretation

The alkaline electrophoresis gel demonstrates two similarly-sized major bands at the A and S/D/G/Lepore positions; densitometry revealed 55% hemoglobin A and 42% of the variant. The hemoglobin A_2 band appears to be the same size as in the other lanes on this gel, and no additional minor slow-moving band is evident. Acid electrophoresis demonstrates a single major band in the A position and a minor band in the F position. Other studies, such as HPLC, globin chain electrophoresis, and isoelectric focusing, identified the variant as Hb G-Coushatta.

Diagnosis

Hb G-Coushatta trait.

Performance

Hb G-Coushatta has been used only once in the survey. Of laboratories using both alkaline and acid electrophoresis, 94% of participants correctly identified the presence of a variant migrating in the S/D/G/Lepore position. Of participants, 57% correctly chose Hb G beta trait in the interpretive portion of the survey; 42% and 41% chose Hb D-Punjab trait and Hb D-other trait (many participants registered more than one response in this section). All three answers were considered correct for the purposes of grading.

Discussion

Hb G-Coushatta is a structural hemoglobin variant resulting from a glutamic acid to alanine substitution at the 22nd amino acid of the beta globin chain (β22 Glu→Ala). It has also been referred to as G-Saskatoon, G-Taegu, and G-Hsin-Chu. This variant was originally described in Native Americans of the Alabama-Coushatta tribe in eastern Texas but has since been described in Chinese, Korean, Japanese, Thai, Turkish, and Algerian individuals. The incidence of this abnormal hemoglobin in these populations is unknown. Genetic studies suggest that the mutation originated independently in Asia and North America. In the heterozygous state, Hb G-Coushatta represents 38-45% of total hemoglobin. Homozygotes are very rare.

Hb G-Coushatta is a stable hemoglobin with no known functional abnormalities. In most reports, patients have had no hematologic abnormalities, although a single report from China described anemia in both heterozygotes and homozygotes. The anemia in that particular cohort may have been due to other coexistent states, such as iron deficiency.

The identification of an abnormal hemoglobin in the S position was relatively straightforward in this case, and the presence of a single major band in the A position on acid electrophoresis rules out hemoglobin S and several other rare variants (Hasharon, Q-Thailand, Tarrant, and Sogn). Thus, the task largely becomes the differentiation of G, D, and Lepore hemoglobins. These all migrate similarly on alkaline and acid electrophoresis, but examination of the densitometry, blood count, and historical data allow a reasonably confident identification of the abnormal hemoglobin as G-Coushatta. Hemoglobin Lepore is a δβ fusion hemoglobin that is under-produced relative to normal β chains. (See Case 10.) Because it is under-produced, it represents only around 8% of the total hemoglobin and produces a thalassemic picture including microcytosis. In addition, the Hb A$_2$ band is typically reduced in heterozygous Hb Lepore. Thus, based on the absence of these features, Hb Lepore may be ruled out in this case. The most common type of hemoglobin G is G-Philadelphia. (See Case 13.) This is an α chain variant, so in addition to the major band migrating in the S position, a second minor band is present representing α$^G_2$/δ$_2$. This represents the abnormal counterpart of Hb A$_2$, often referred to as Hb G$_2$. The absence of this band rules out G-Philadelphia as well as other G α variants. The final distinction between a G beta trait and a D beta trait [the most common of which is Hb D-Los Angeles (Punjab)] (see Case 11) is impossible based on the hematologic and electrophoretic data provided. However, the fact that the patient is Native American is an important clue, as Hb G-Coushatta is seen almost exclusively in Native Americans and East Asians. Hb D-Los Angeles is seen primarily in Caucasians. Examples of Hb G-Coushatta on HPLC and isoelectric focusing are shown in Figures 24.1 and 24.2. Differentiating clinical and electrophoretic features for hemoglobins at or near the S position are provided in the accompanying table and figures.

Table 24.1 Some Hb S-like Variants With Characteristic Ethnic Distribution

Variants	Ethnic Distribution	Frequency	Stability (Isopropanol)	Hematologic Effect
Alpha Chain Variants				
G-Philadelphia	Afro-Americavn	Common	Stable	None or mild microcytosis (often linked to α-thal-2)
Hasharon	Ashkenazic Jewish, Italian	Uncommon	Unstable (stable by heat test)	Drug-inducible hemolysis
Q-Thailand (Mahidol)	Chinese, SE Asian	Uncommon	Stable	None or mild microcytosis (linked to α-thal-2)
Tarrant	Mexican	Rare	Stable	High O$_2$ affinity; erythrocytosis (mild)
Beta Chain Variants				
S	African, Mediterranean, Indian*	Common	Stable	Sickling
D-Punjab (Los Angeles)	British, Afro-American, Indian*	Common	Stable	None (interacts with Hb S)
G-Coushatta	Native American, Chinese, Taiwanese, Korean, Aglerian, Iranian	Unknown	Stable	None (except in 1 case report)
Sogn	Norwegian	Rare	Unstable	None
Fusion Gene				
Lepore	Mediterranean	Common	Stable	Microcytosis

*Ancestry from Indian subcontinent, i.e., India or Pakistan

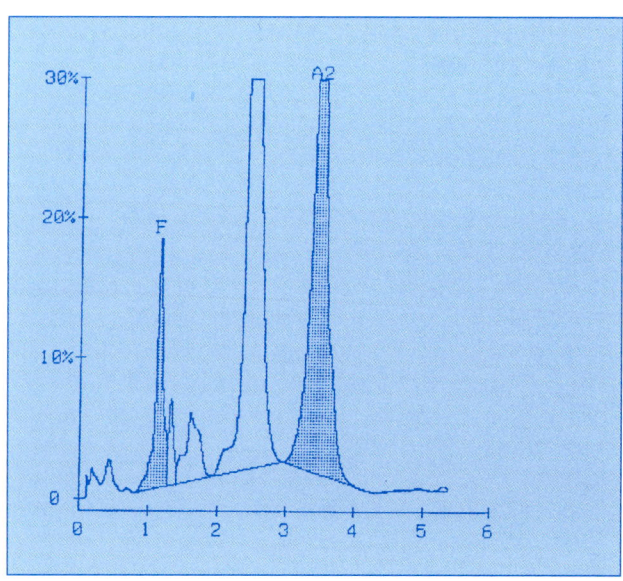

Figure 24.1
An example of Hb G Coushatta by HPLC. Hb G Coushatta elutes in the A_2 position, with a retention time of approximately 3.5 minutes.

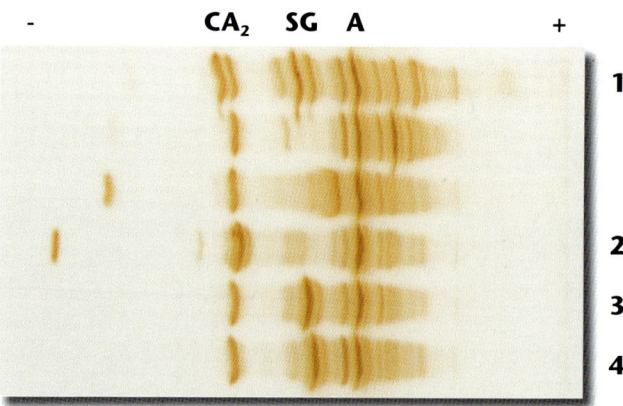

Figure 24.2
An example of Hb G Coushatta trait by isoelectric focusing. Lane 1-control specimen, consisting of a mixture of Hb C, Hb G-Philadelphia, Hb S, Hb J-Baltimore, and Hb I. Lane 2-Hb O-Indonesia, 3-Hb D-Punjab, 4-Hb G-Coushatta.

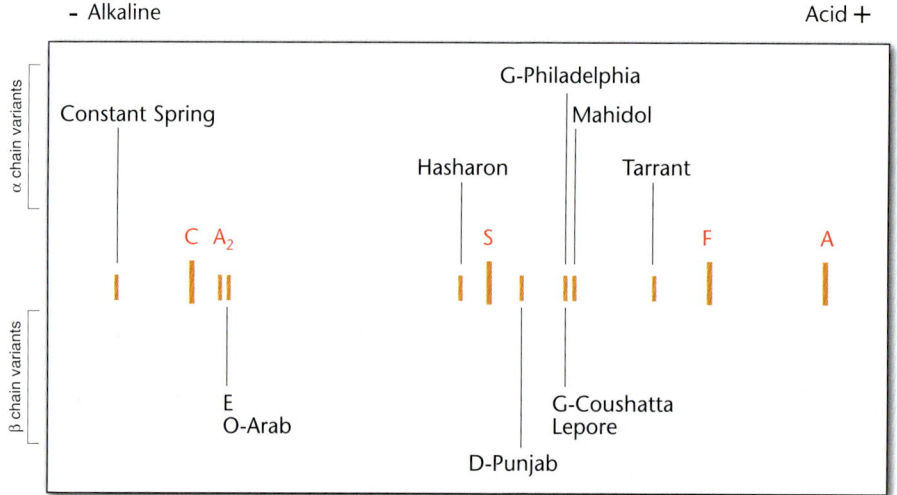

Figure 24.3
Position of S-like hemoglobin on isoelectric focusing. (Relative positions based on data of Galacteros; α chain variants are labeled above, β chain variants below the path of focusing.)

Alkaline Electrophoresis, pH 8.6

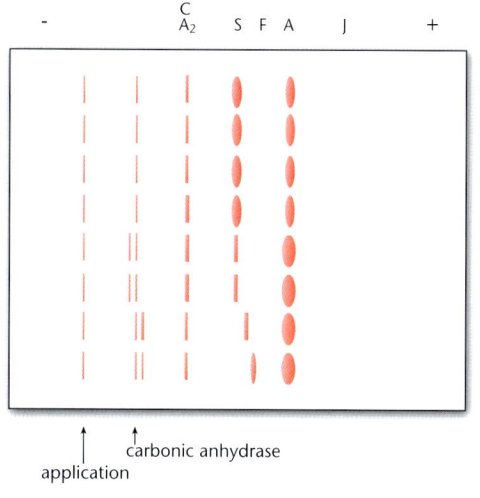

Acid Electrophoresis, pH 8.6

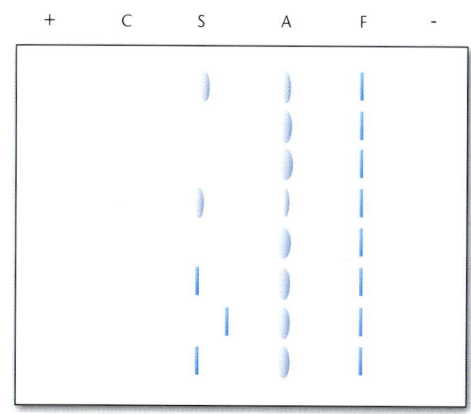

Globin Chain Electrophoresis, pH 8.9

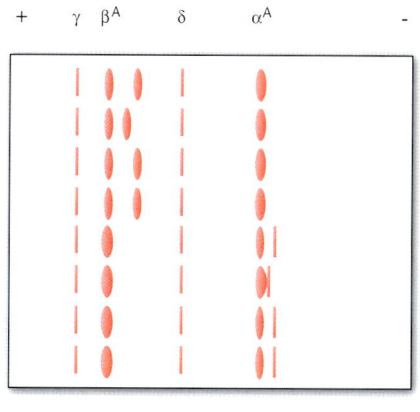

Globin Chain Electrophoresis, pH 6.2

Figure 24.4
Electrophoretic mobilities of many Hb S-like hemoblobins.

References

Blackwell RQ, Huang JT, Ro IH. Hemoglobin variants in Koreans: hemoglobin G Taegu. *Science.* 1967;158: 1056-1057.

Blackwell RQ, Liu CS, Yang HJ, Wang CC, Huang JT. Hemoglobin variant common to Chinese and North American Indians: alpha-2-beta-22 Glu-Ala. *Science.* 1968;161:381-382.

Blackwell RQ, Ro IH, Liu CS, Yang HJ, Wang CC, Huang JT. Hemoglobin variant found in Koreans, Chinese, and North American Indians: alpha-2 beta-2 22 Glu Ala. *Am J Phys Anthropol.* 1969;30:389-391.

Boissel JP, Wajcman H, Labie D, Dahmane M, Benabadji M. [Hemoglobin G Coushatta (beta 22 (β4) glu leads to ala) in Algeria: an homozygous case]. *Nouv Rev Fr Hematol.* 1979;21: 225-230. French.

Bowman BH, Barnett DR, Hite R. Hemoglobin G-Coushatta: a beta variant with a delta-like substitution. *Biochem Biophys Res Commun.* 1967;26:466-470.

Dincol G, Dincol K, Erdem S. Hb G-Coushatta or alpha 2 beta 2 22(B4)Glu→Ala in a Turkish male. *Hemoglobin.* 1989;13:75-77.

Itchayanan D, Svasti J, Srisomsap C, Winichagoon P, Fucharoen S. Hb G-Coushatta [beta22 (β4) Glu→Ala] in Thailand. *Hemoglobin.* 1999;23:69-72.

Case 25

HISTORY
The patient is a 27-year-old African-American woman who was thought to have poorly controlled diabetes mellitus because of elevated levels of glycosylated hemoglobin, sometimes exceeding 40%. Her insulin dosage was repeatedly increased, but the percentage of glycosylated Hb remained persistently elevated. She began to have recurrent spells of faintness, palpitations, shakes, and sweats.

BLOOD COUNT DATA
RBC .... 4.5×10^{12}/L
Hb .... 12.3 g/dL
MCV .... 84 fL
WBC .... 8.6×10^9/L
Plt .... 207×10^9/L

PERIPHERAL BLOOD SMEAR
Normal erythrocyte morphology.

OTHER LABORATORY TESTS
Blood glucose = 40 mg/dL

Alkaline Electrophoresis (pH 8.6)

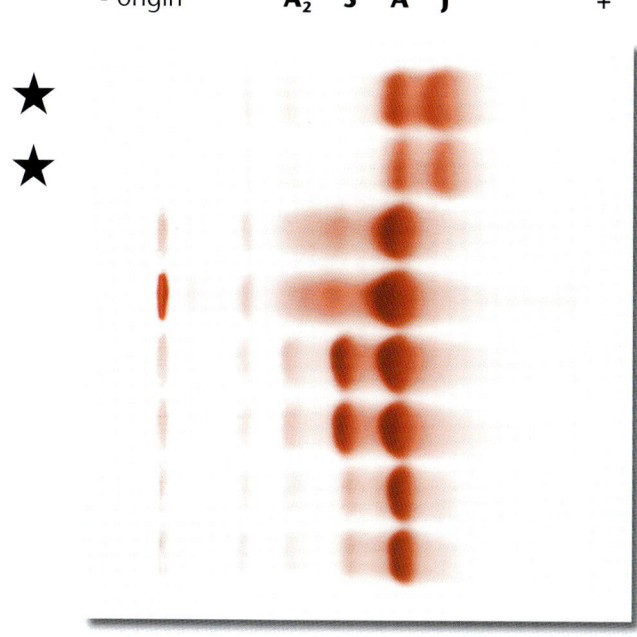

Acid Electrophoresis (pH 6.2)

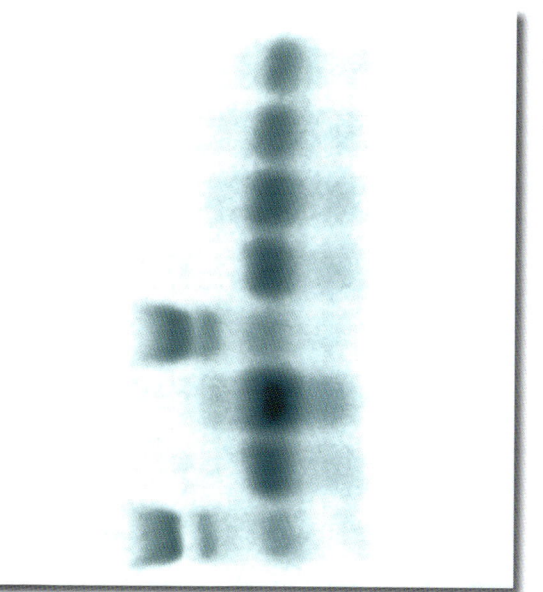

Case 25 Discussion

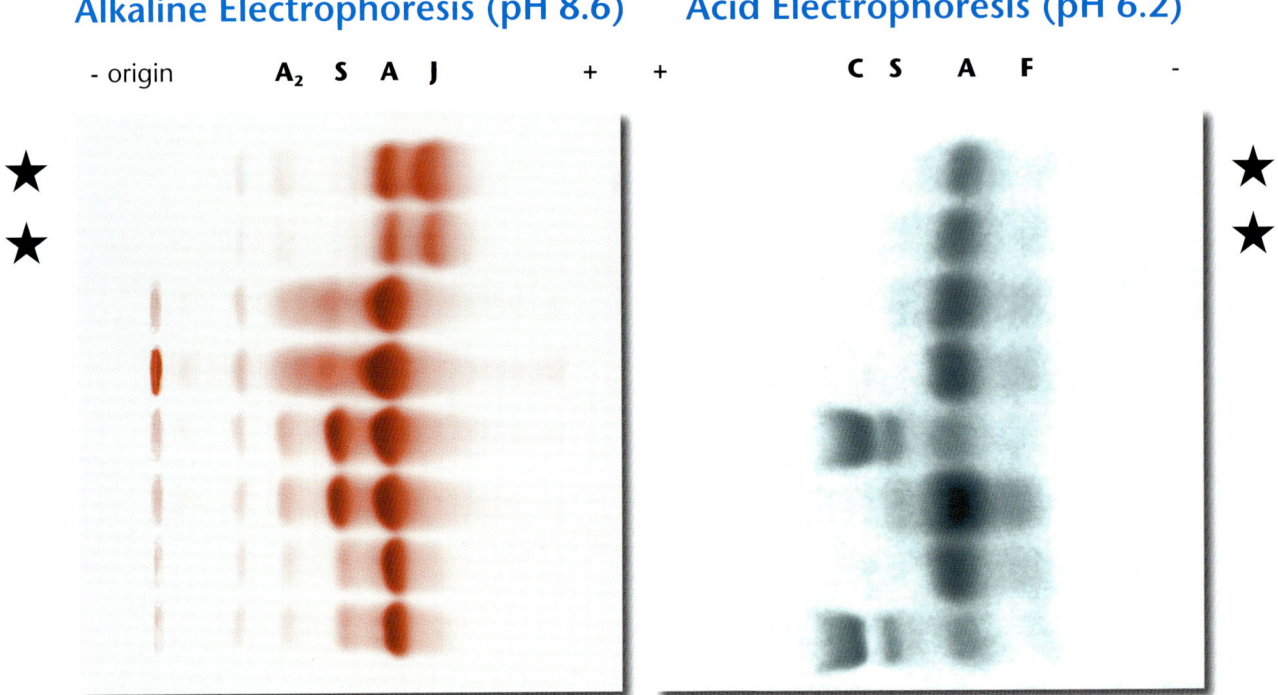

Interpretation

On alkaline electrophoresis, there is a fast moving hemoglobin band that is as far in front (anodal) of Hb A as Hb S is behind (cathodal) Hb A. The abnormal variant is present in approximately equal proportion to Hb A. On acid electrophoresis, the hemoglobin variant migrates with Hb A.

Diagnosis

Hb J-Baltimore trait.

Performance

Nearly 50% of laboratories correctly identified this variant as Hb Jβ trait. Other responses included Hb N trait and Hb I trait.

Discussion

Hb J-Baltimore is a β globin chain variant that arises from a mutation in codon 16, resulting in the replacement of glycine by aspartic acid (β16 Gly→Asp). This variant has no hematological consequences. The major clinical significance is that in persons with diabetes mellitus, Hb J may result in spuriously elevated levels of glycosylated Hb A (Hb A_{1c}). These spurious results depend upon the assay method used. When an ion exchange resin method is used, the presence of a fast hemoglobin, such as Hb J, I, or N, will cause falsely elevated results. Affinity chromatography with aminoboronic acid columns circumvents this problem. The specimen in this case yielded 50% Hb A_{1c} by ion exchange chromatography and 7% by affinity chromatography. The patient's diabetes had actually been under excellent control before the insulin dosage was increased, which resulted in her repeated attacks of hypoglycemia. Hb J-Baltimore is present in low frequency in blacks and is very rarely encountered in other ethnic groups such as English, Dutch, French, Swedish, or Spanish.

Hb J-Baltimore migrates anodal to Hb A under alkaline conditions and is present in approximately equal proportion to Hb A. Hbs H and I are considerably faster moving hemoglobins and migrate anodal to Hb J (see Case 27). Hb N is slightly faster than Hb J-Baltimore. There are also several α chain variants (Hb Jα) with similar electrophoretic mobility as Hb J-Baltimore. These α chain variants are usually present in a proportion of 1:3 relative to Hb A, because only one of the 4 α globin gene loci carries the Jα mutation.

Increased levels of Hb F can also cause falsely elevated levels of Hb A_{1c}. In contrast, the presence of Hbs S, D, G, C, E, or other electrophoretically slow hemoglobin variants will result in falsely low levels of HbA_{1c} by ion exchange chromatography. Examples of HB J-Baltimore trait by HPLC and isoelectric focusing are shown in Figures 25.1 and 25.2.

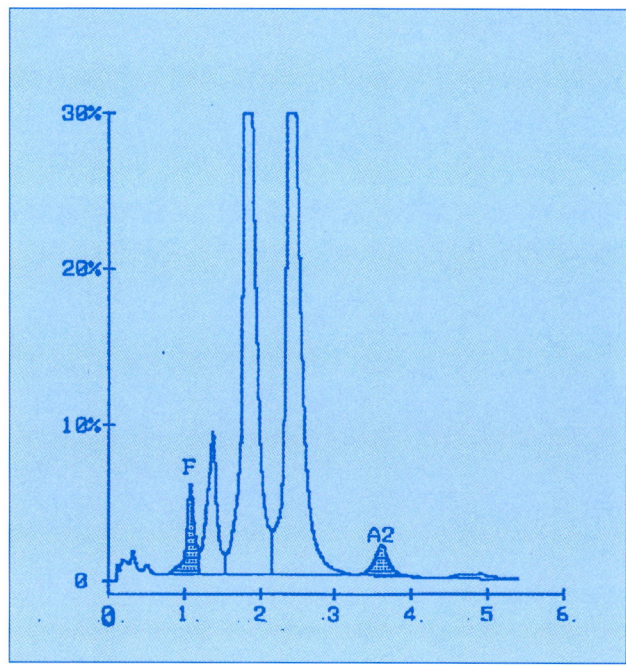

Figure 25.1
An example of Hb J-Baltimore trait by HPLC. Hb J-Baltimore elutes ahead of Hb A in the P3 position, with a retention time of approximately 1.8-1.9 minutes.

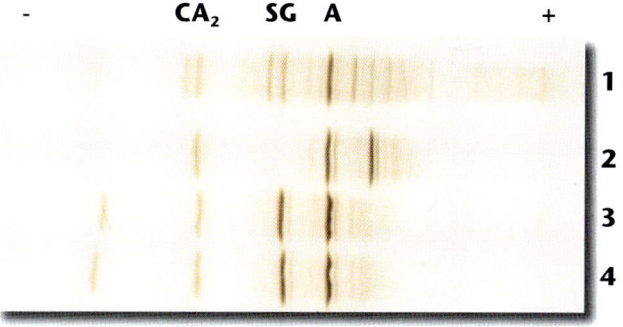

Figure 25.2
An example of Hb J-Baltimore trait by isoelectric focusing. Lane 1-control, 2-Hb J-Baltimore trait, 3-Hb Q-Thailand, 4-Hb G-Philadelphia.

References

Arribalzaga K, Ricard MP, Carreno DC, et al. Hb J-Baltimore [β 16 (A13) Gly→Asp] associated with β+ thalassemia in a Spanish family. *Hemoglobin.* 1996;20:79-84.

Baglioni C, Weatherall DJ. Abnormal human hemoglobins, IX: chemistry of Hb J Baltimore. *Biochim Biophys Acta.* 1963;87:637-643.

Fairbanks VF, Zimmerman BR. Measurement of glycosylated hemoglobins by affinity chromatography. *Mayo Clin Proc.* 1983;58:770-773.

Landis B, Jeppsson JO. Rare beta globin variants found in Swedish patients during Hb A_{1c} analysis. *Hemoglobin.* 1993;17:303-318.

Syndenstrycker JP. Studies on a fast hemoglobin variant found in a Negro family in association with thalassemia. *Clin Chim Acta.* 1961;6:677-685.

Case 26

HISTORY
The patient is a 43-year-old woman of Italian ancestry, who is diabetic and believed to be well controlled with insulin. There has been a problem measuring her Hb A_{1c} due to interference by a hemoglobin variant. There are no abnormalities on the physical examination.

BLOOD COUNT DATA
RBC .... 4.4 x 10^{12}/L
Hb .... 12.8 g/dL
MCV .... 89 fL
WBC .... 7.8 x 10^9/L
Plt .... 289 x 10^9/L

PERIPHERAL BLOOD SMEAR
No abnormalities noted.

OTHER LABORATORY TESTS
Test for unstable hemoglobin is negative.

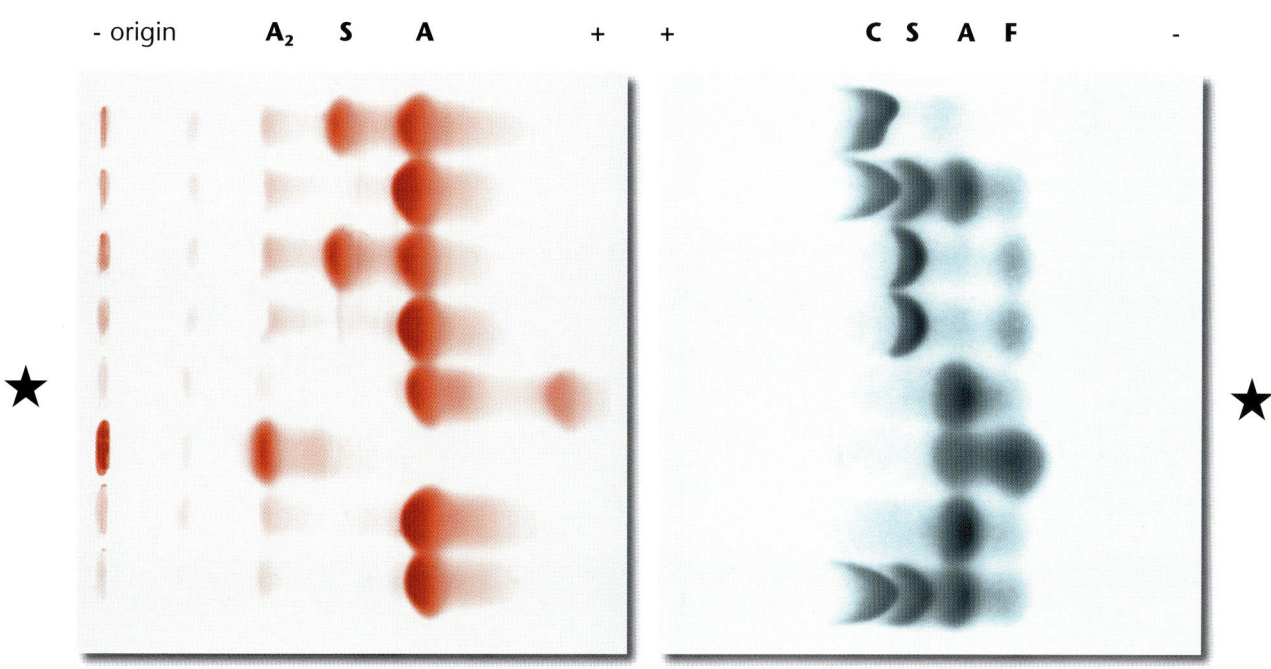

Alkaline Electrophoresis (pH 8.6)
- origin A_2 S   A   +

Acid Electrophoresis (pH 6.2)
+   C   S   A   F   -

Case 26 Discussion

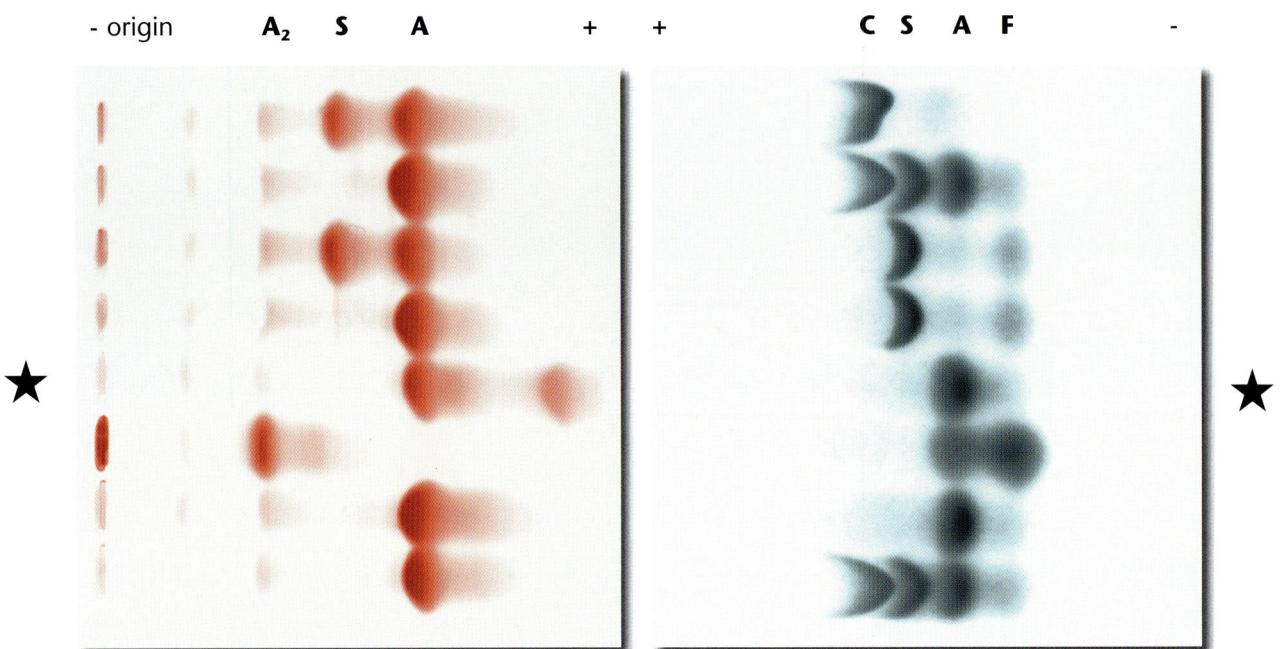

Alkaline Electrophoresis (pH 8.6) — origin A₂ S A +
Acid Electrophoresis (pH 6.2) + C S A F −

Interpretation

On alkaline electrophoresis, there is a fast band present which accounts for approximately 25% of the total hemoglobin. This band is as anodal to Hb A as Hb C is cathodal to Hb A. Acid electrophoresis shows only a band in the A position.

Diagnosis

Hb I trait.

Performance

Hb I has been used in the survey three times, with correct identifications ranging from 35.8–56%.

Discussion

Hb I (α16 Lys→Glu) is a fast α chain variant that was one of the first hemoglobin variants described (1955). It has been given a number of different names, such as I-Burlington, I-Philadelphia, I-Texas, and I-Skamania. It is stable, has a normal oxygen affinity, and has no clinical or hematologic effect. Hb I is found in persons of Northern European, Mediterranean, African, and Native American heritage.

The electrophoretic findings seen in this case are typical. Hb I must be differentiated from other fast hemoglobin variants, particularly Hb H, which has an almost identical electrophoretic mobility on alkaline electrophoresis. However, at electrophoresis at pH 6.2, Hb I migrates in the A position, but Hb H migrates between the A and S positions. Unlike other α variants, the δ chain variant (I_2 or $\alpha^I_2 \delta_2$) is not seen because it co-migrates with Hb A. Other pertinent findings that serve to distinguish between these two variants are (1) Hb I will usually be a greater percentage of the total hemoglobin than Hb H, (2) Hb H is an unstable hemoglobin, and (3) Hb I is not associated with clinical or hematologic manifestations, whereas patients with Hb H are moderately to severely anemic. Because both Hb H and Hb I are very fast variants, there is a danger of running this band off the alkaline electrophoresis gel if the length of the electrophoresis is too long or the voltage is too high.

Like other fast variants, such as Hb J or Hb N, Hb I will give falsely elevated Hb A_{1c} levels on ion-exchange chromatography methods. The use of affinity chromatography methods will remedy this interference. Examples of Hb I trait by HPLC and isoelectric focusing are shown in Figures 26.1 and 26.2.

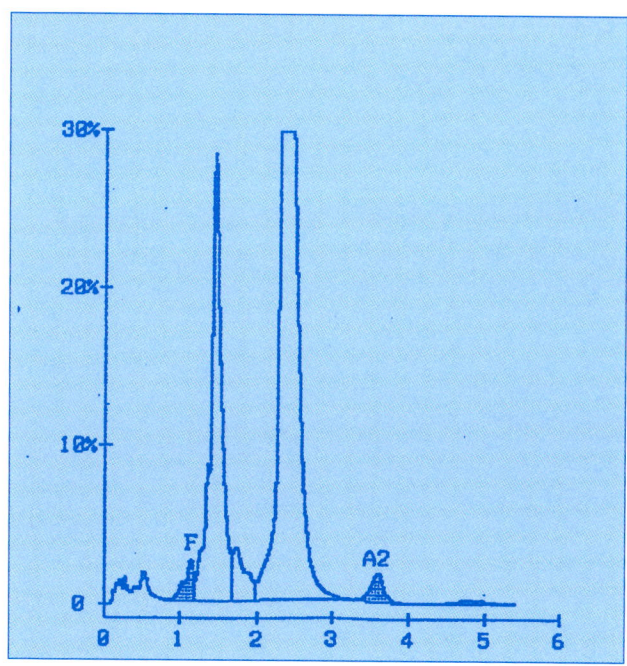

Figure 26.1
An example of Hb I trait by HPLC. The Hb I elutes ahead of the Hb A peak. It can appear in either the P2 or P3 position at approximately 1.45-1.50 minutes.

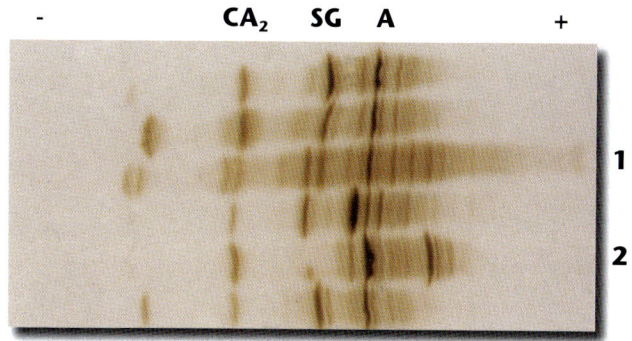

Figure 26.2
An example of Hb I trait by isoelectric focusing. Lane 1-control, 2-Hb I trait.

References

Bowman BH, Barnett DR. Amino acid substitution in hemoglobin I (Texas variant). *Nature*. 1967;214: 494.

Fairbanks VF, Zimmerman BR. Measurement of glycosylated hemoglobin by affinity chromatography. *Mayo Clin Proc*. 1983;58:770-773.

Rucknagel DL, Page EB, Jensen WN. Hemoglobin I: an inherited hemoglobin anomaly. *Blood*. 1955;10: 999-1009.

Schneider RG, Alperin JB, Beale D, Lehman H. Hemoglobin I in an American Negro family: structural and hematologic studies. *J Lab Clin Med*. 1966;68: 940-946.

Case 27

HISTORY
The patient is a 29-year-old asymptomatic male of African-American ancestry. The physical examination revealed no abnormalities.

BLOOD COUNT DATA
RBC .... 5.1×10^{12}/L
Hb .... 12.2 g/dL
MCV .... 77.0 fL
WBC .... 7.9×10^{9}/L
Plt .... 288×10^{9}/L

PERIPHERAL BLOOD SMEAR
No abnormalities.

OTHER LABORATORY TESTS
Test for unstable hemoglobin was negative.

Alkaline Electrophoresis (pH 8.6)   Acid Electrophoresis (pH 6.2)

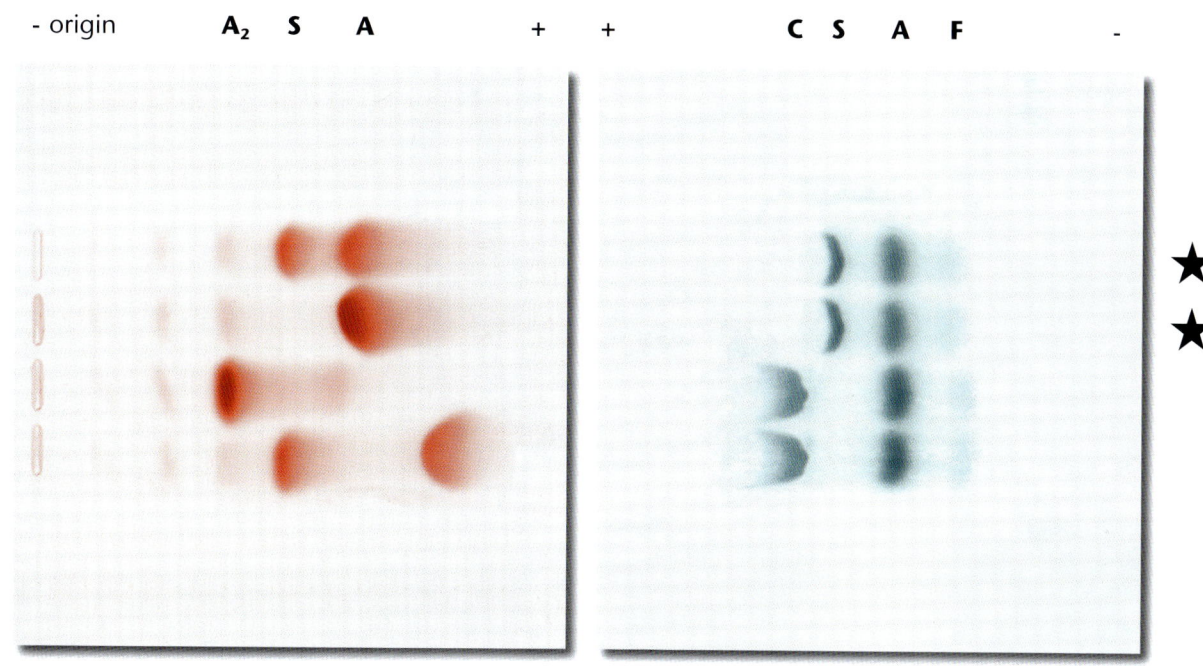

Case 27 Discussion

Alkaline Electrophoresis (pH 8.6)   Acid Electrophoresis (pH 6.2)

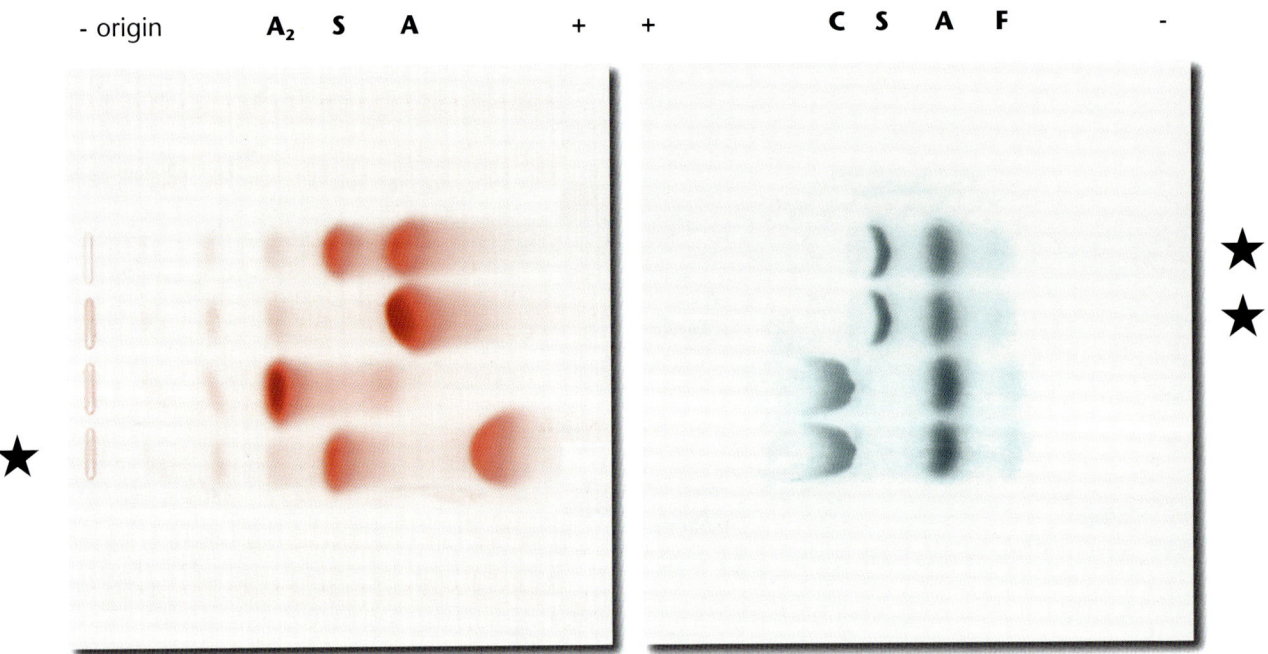

Interpretation

On alkaline electrophoresis, there is no Hb A present. There is a major band in the S position, as well as a fast band. On acid electrophoresis, there is a band in the A position and one in the S position.

Diagnosis

Hb S/Hb N-Baltimore.

Performance

This combination has been included in the survey only once. Approximately 95% of laboratories correctly identified Hb S, and 83% identified Hb N-Baltimore.

Discussion

Hb N-Baltimore results from a lysine to glutamic acid substitution at the 95th position of the beta chain (β95 Lys→Glu). Hb N-Baltimore was one of the earlier hemoglobin variants described and has been found to be of primary west African origin. Hb N-Baltimore trait has no clinical or hematologic effects. Because it is found in African Americans, it can sometimes be seen with other β chain variants such as Hb S (as in this case) or Hb C. The combination of Hb S with Hb N-Baltimore is equivalent to Hb S trait alone. The fast mobility of Hb N-Baltimore is due to an additional two negative charges on the β chain as compared with Hb A. Thus, it moves faster towards the anode. One interesting aspect of this variant is that when it is present in the simple heterozygote, it usually comprises more of the total hemoglobin than does Hb A (55-60%), as opposed to Hb S, which comprises less (30-40%). McDonald and colleagues have demonstrated that β chain variants that are more negatively charged than Hb A bind more avidly to α chains. This may help to explain the empirical observation that in heterozygotes "fast" β chain variants (more negatively charged) are usually in greater proportion than Hb A, whereas "slow" β chain variants (more positively charged) are usually in lesser proportion than Hb A. This also explains why in Hb S/C disease there is slightly more Hb S than Hb C (see Case 17).

Hb N-Baltimore must be differentiated from other fast hemoglobins, such as Hb J, Hb I, or Hb H. The J hemoglobins migrate as far in the anodal direction from Hb A as Hb S is in the cathodal direction. Hb I and Hb H, on the other hand, are as far in the anodal direction from Hb A as Hb C is in the cathodal direction. Hb N-Baltimore (and the other N-hemoglobins such as N-Seattle) has an electrophoretic mobility between Hb J and Hb I on alkaline electrophoresis, but it is closer to Hb I. Acid electrophoresis is not helpful in distinguishing these hemoglobins, as they all (except Hb H) migrate with Hb A. Other features that are helpful in distinguishing Hb N from Hb I and Hb H are that Hb I is an α chain variant (and so comprises only 25% of the total hemoglobin rather than 50-60%), and that Hb H gives a positive unstable hemoglobin test. Examples of Hb S/Hb N-Baltimore on HPLC and isoelectric focusing are shown in Figures 27.1 and 27.2.

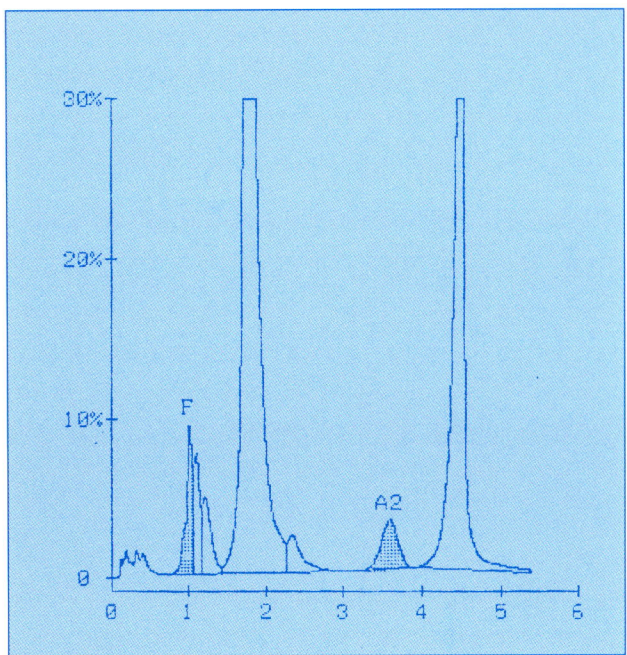

Figure 27.1
An example of Hb S/Hb N-Baltimore by HPLC. In addition to a major peak which elutes in the S window, there is also a peak that elutes in the P3 position at approximately 1.7-1.75 minutes, which represents Hb N-Baltimore.

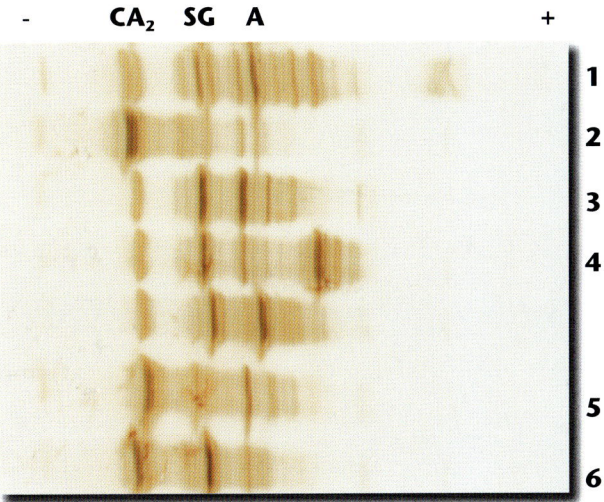

Figure 27.2
An example of Hb S/Hb N-Baltimore by isoelectric focusing (lane 4). The slight increase in Hb F seen is due to the young age of this patient. Lane 1-control, 2-homozygous C, 3-Hb S/HPFH, 5-Hb E/β⁰-thalassemia, 6-Hb S/C disease.

References

Clegg JB, Naughton MA, Weatherhall DJ. An improved method for the characterization of human haemoglobin mutants: identification of $\alpha_2\beta_2$ 95 glu haemoglobin N (Baltimore). *Nature.* 1965;207: 945-947.

Dobbs NB, Jr, Simmons JW, Wilson JB, Huisman THJ. Hemoglobin Jenkins on hemoglobin N-Baltimore or $\alpha_2\beta_2$ 95 glu. *Biochim Biophys Acta.* 1966;117: 492-494.

Johnson C, Powars D, Schroeder WA. A case with both hemoglobins C and N-Baltimore. *Acta Haematol.* 1976;56:183-188.

McDonald MJ, Turci SM, Mrabet NT, et al. The kinetics of assembly of normal and variant human oxyhemoglobins. *J Bio Chem.* 1987;262:5951-5956.

Case 28

HISTORY
A specimen was received from a 39-year-old African-American woman who was asymptomatic and without abnormalities on physical examination. She had been found to have an unusual Hb electrophoresis pattern.

BLOOD COUNT DATA
RBC .... 4.0×10^{12}/L
Hgb .... 10.0 g/dL
Hct 32%
MCV .... 80.0 fL

PERIPHERAL BLOOD SMEAR
Unremarkable.

OTHER LABORATORY TESTS
The solubility test for sickling hemoglobin is positive.

Alkaline Electrophoresis (pH 8.6)

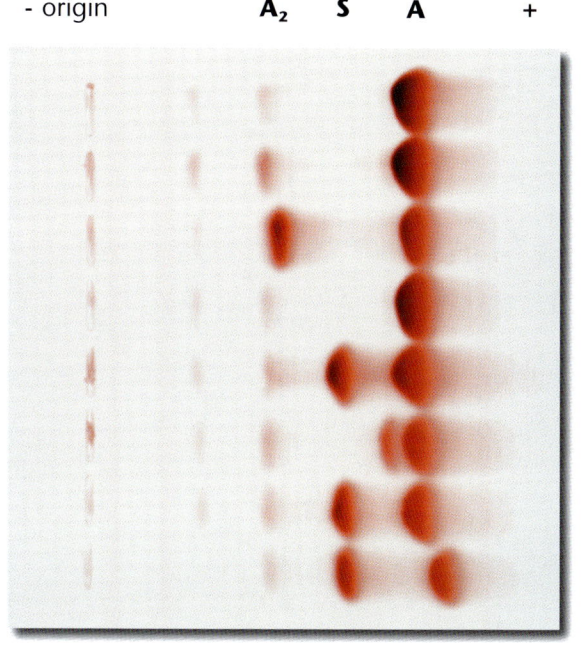

Acid Electrophoresis (pH 6.2)

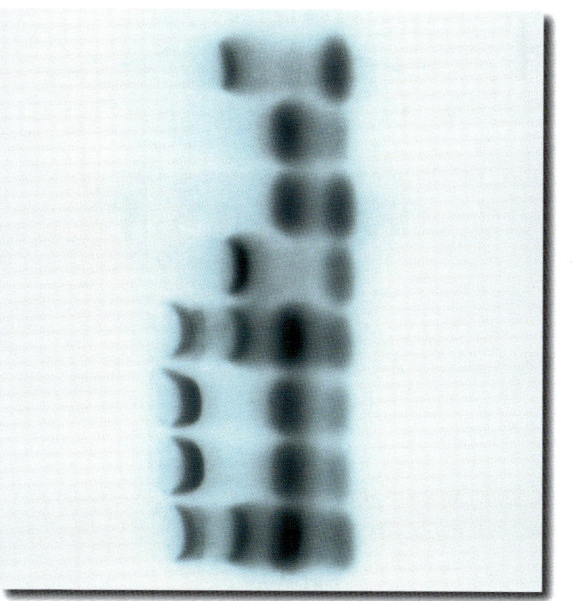

Case 28 Discussion

Alkaline Electrophoresis (pH 8.6)   Acid Electrophoresis (pH 6.2)

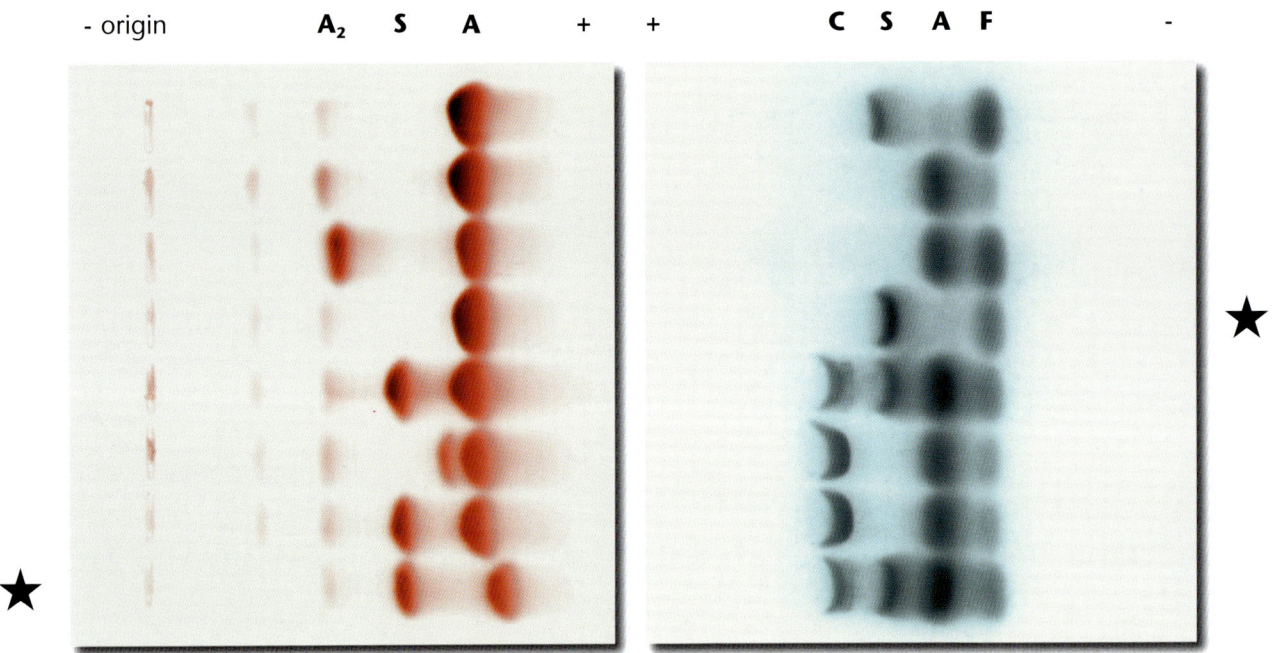

Interpretation

On alkaline electrophoresis, there are two major bands present, one in the S position and one slightly faster than Hb A. There is no Hb A present. On acid electrophoresis, there is a band in the S position and a band in the F position.

Diagnosis

Hb S/Hb Hope.

Performance

The Hb S/Hope combination has been used twice in the survey, with 46.0% and 41.6% of laboratories correctly identifying both variants.

Discussion

Hemoglobin Hope results from substitution of aspartate for glycine at the 136th position of the β chain [β 136 (H14) Gly→Asp]. Hb Hope has slightly reduced oxygen affinity, and for this reason it delivers oxygen to tissues more readily than does normal Hb A. Hb Hope has also been reported as being mildly unstable. However, tests for unstable hemoglobin are nearly always negative. It is usually harmless, and the combination Hb S/Hb Hope is believed to be equivalent to Hb S trait. In this country, it is usually encountered incidentally in African Americans. Hemoglobin Hope has also been reported from France in people of west African origin, and in Japanese, Laotian, and Thai individuals.

Because Hb Hope has decreased oxygen affinity, less hemoglobin is needed for oxygen transport. Thus, while many Hb Hope heterozygotes are hematologically normal, some have a mild "physiological anemia." This appears to be the explanation for the slight anemia in Case 28. A case has been reported of Hb Hope trait together with α-thalassemia-2 trait in which there was a marked microcytic anemia.

Hemoglobin Hope comprises 40-50% of total hemoglobin in the heterozygous state. It is a fast hemoglobin that migrates between J and A on alkaline electrophoresis. Several other abnormal hemoglobins migrate in this position, including several rare types of Hb K, Hb Camden, Hb Osler, and Hb Andrew-Minneapolis (see Case 42). The latter two abnormal hemoglobins are high oxygen affinity hemoglobins that are associated with erythrocytosis. The location of Hb Hope on acid electrophoresis (identical migration as Hb F) helps to establish a diagnosis. Note that Hemoglobin Hope is one of many hemoglobin variants that co-elute with Hb A_{1c} from ion exchange columns, and may lead to the erroneous interpretation of very poorly controlled diabetes mellitus.

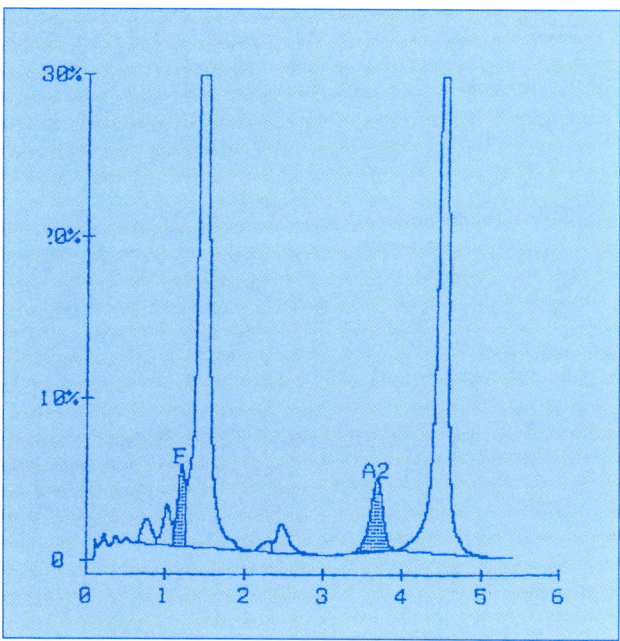

Figure 28.1

An example of Hb S/Hb Hope by HPLC. In addition to a major peak in the S window, there is a major peak that elutes at approximately 1.4-1.5 minutes (P2 position), representing Hb Hope.

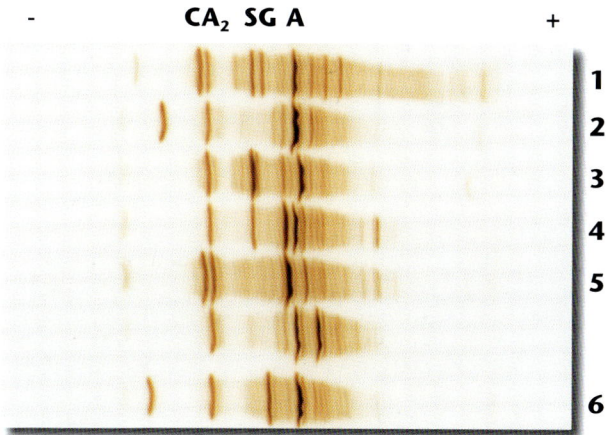

Figure 28.2

An example of Hb S/Hb Hope by isoelectric focusing (lane 3). Hb Hope migrates slightly anodal to the Hb A position. Lane 1-control, 2-Hb A_2', 4-Hb S trait in a neonate showing the presence of Hb Bart's, indicating concurrent α-thalassemia, 5-Hb C/Hb O-Arab in a young child, 6-Hb Q-Thailand.

References

Araki E, Wada Y, Ishihara K, et al. Hemoglobin Hope found in a patient with basal cell carcinoma of the genial region. *Nippon Ketsueki Gakkai Zasshi.* 1989;52(6):972-976. Japanese. (Note: "genial region" (sic, as listed by MedLine) may have been an error in translation.)

Charache S, Achuff S, Winslow R, Kazazian H. Oxygen transport in a woman with hemoglobin Hope/β+-thalassemia. *J Lab Clin Med.* 1976; 93:316-320.

Endoki Y, Ohga Y, Furukawa K, et al. Hb Hope, beta 136 (H14) Gly→Asp, in a diabetic Japanese female and its functional characterization. *Hemoglobin.* 1989;13(l):17-32.

Hubbard M, Wilson JB, Wrightstone RN, et al. Hb Camden and Hb Hope found during routine testing. *Acta Haematol.* 1975;54:53-58.

King ME, Rifai N, Malekpour A. Hemoglobin "Hope" interferes with measurement of glycated hemoglobin by ion-exchange chromatography and electrophoresis [letter]. *Clin Chem.* 1984;30(6):1106-1107.

Minnich V, Hill RJ, Khuri PD, et al. Hemoglobin Hope: a beta chain variant. *Blood.* 1965;25:830-838.

Moo-Penn W, Jue D, George B, et al. Hemoglobin Hope β136 (H13) (Gly→Asp) in Georgia. *Am J Clin Pathol.* 1975;63:87-90.

Pillers DM, Jones M, Head C, Jones RT. Hb Hope [beta 136(H14) Gly→Asp] and Hb E [beta 26 (B8) Glu→Lys], compound heterozygosity in a Thai Mien family. *Hemoglobin.* 1992;16:81-84.

Rahbar S, Nozari G, Asmerom Y, et al. Association of Hb Hope [beta 136 (H14) Gly→Asp] and alpha-thalassemia-2 (3.7 Kb deletion) causing severe microcytic anemia. *Hemoglobin.* 1992;16:421-425.

Steinberg MH, Adams JG, Thigpen JT, et al. Hemoglobin Hope ($\alpha_2\beta_2$136 gly→asp) S disease: clinical and biochemical studies. *J Lab Clin Med.* 1974;84: 632-642.

Steinberg MH, Lovell WJ, Wells S, et al. Hemoglobin Hope: studies of oxygen equilibrium in heterozygotes, hemoglobin S-Hope disease, and isolated hemoglobin. *J Lab Clin Med.* 1976;88:125-131.

Case 29

HISTORY
The patient is a 58-year-old African-American woman with a history of high blood pressure and anemia. Previous iron administration for presumed iron deficiency was without effect. She has never received blood transfusions. The physical examination was normal.

BLOOD COUNT DATA
RBC.................................5.6 x 10^{12}/L
Hb...................................11.9 g/dL
MCV.................................63.4 fL
WBC.................................5.0 x 10^9/L
Plt....................................323.0 x 10^9/L

PERIPHERAL BLOOD SMEAR
Numerous target cells, occasional microcytes, rare spherocytes.

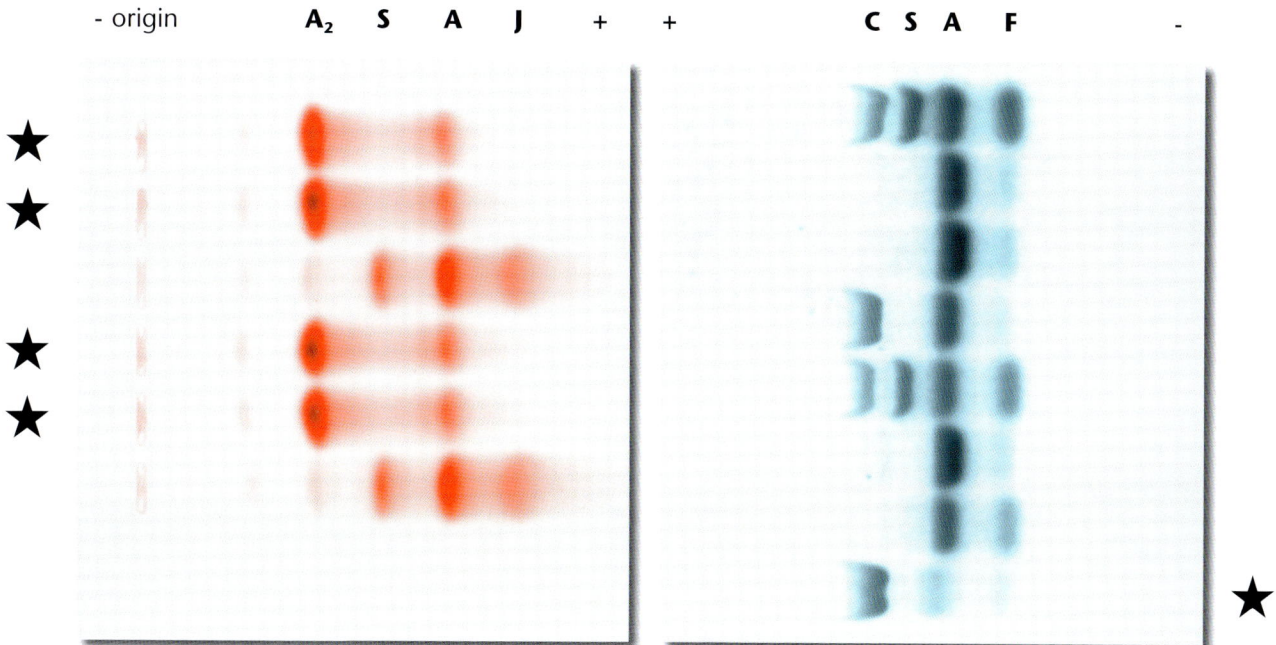

Alkaline Electrophoresis (pH 8.6)   Acid Electrophoresis (pH 6.2)

Case Studies

Case 29 Discussion

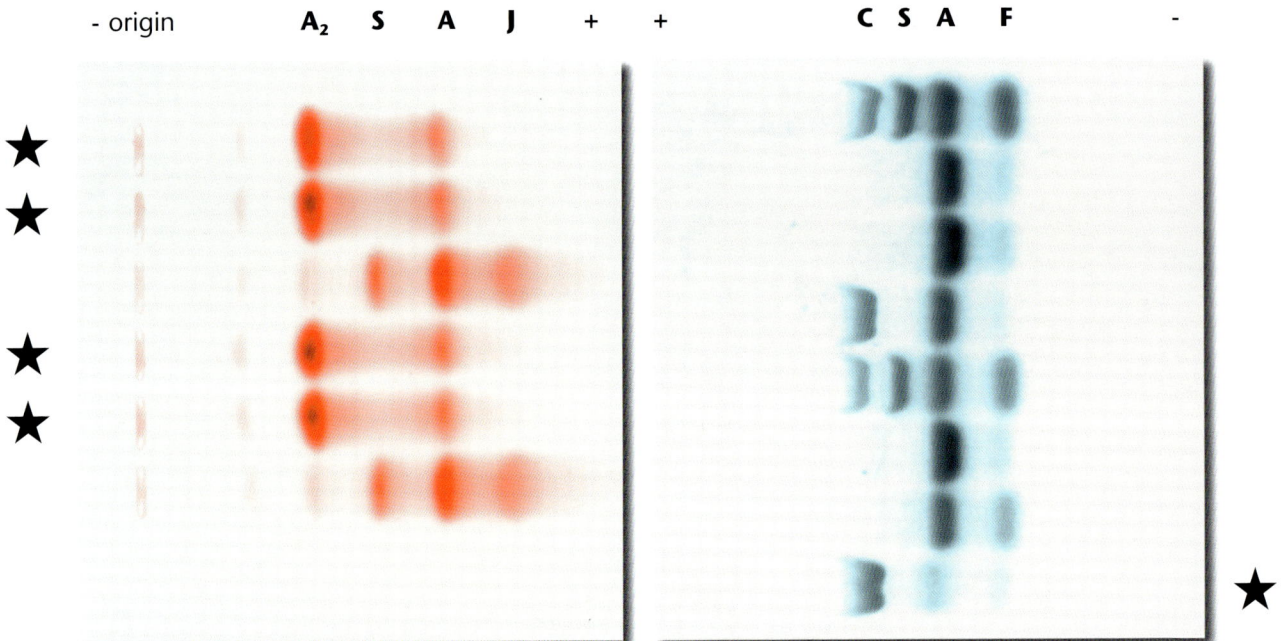

Interpretation

Both alkaline and acid electrophoresis gels demonstrate two major bands in the C and A positions, with the former being considerably larger than the latter.

Diagnosis

Hb C/β⁺-thalassemia.

Performance

One previous case in the survey was intended to illustrate Hb C/β⁺-thalassemia. However, this case had 22% HbF and no microcytosis. It was subsequently determined that this in fact represented Hb C and a form of hereditary persistence of fetal hemoglobin (HPFH). Therefore another case has been substituted for discussion in this text. Nevertheless, for that challenge, of laboratories using both alkaline and acid electrophoresis, 68% correctly identified the presence of Hb A, and 99% correctly identified the presence of Hb C; 70% of labs correctly reported that Hb A_2 was not measurable, and 47% percent of labs provided the interpretation of Hb C/β⁺-thalassemia. The remainder provided a variety of interpretations, including Hb C trait, homozygous Hb C disease, HPFH, and "other."

Discussion

Hb C/β⁺-thalassemia has been described in both black and Mediterranean populations. In the African-American population, β-thalassemia mutations have a prevalence of approximately 1%. In this patient group, a variety of β gene mutations are seen, but these are most commonly of the β⁺ variety in which β chain production is decreased but not absent (see Case 18, page 89; and *A Closer Look At...Beta-Thalassemia*, page 24). In uncomplicated Hb C trait, the level of Hb C is less than Hb A, in part because of decreased affinity of the β^C chains for α chains compared to normal β chains. When a β⁺ thalassemia gene is located in trans to a Hb C gene, the output of normal β chains is reduced. Thus, the amount of Hb C is greater than Hb A in these patients. The relative proportions will vary depending on the amount of normal β chain output, which in turn depends on the type of mutation present. Hb C/β⁺-thalassemia is a mild hemolytic anemia that is generally asymptomatic. In the African-American population, this disorder is hematologically most similar to the common β-thalassemia minor. The hemoglobin level is only mildly reduced (11-13 g/dL), although the anemia may be exacerbated during pregnancy. The MCV is also reduced to levels similar to those seen in β-thalassemia minor (50-70 fL). Splenomegaly is usually not present. As in β-thalassemia minor, the blood smear in Hb C/β⁺-thalassemia demonstrates microcytosis and hypochromia; however, target cells are much more prominent than in uncomplicated thalassemia. Electrophoresis typically reveals 65-80% Hb C, 20-30% Hb A, and 2-5% Hb F. These patients usually suffer no complications and have a normal life span.

The identification of the presence of hemoglobins A and C in this sample provides little difficulty given their characteristic electrophoretic mobilities in both alkaline and acid gels. What is important to observe in this case is that the Hb C band is larger than the Hb A band. In uncomplicated Hb C trait, the A band is always larger than the C band (approximately a 60:40 ratio). Furthermore, patients with Hb C trait will not be anemic or microcytic; at most they will have increased target cells on their blood smears. Other than Hb C/β⁺-thalassemia, the only scenario that could produce the pattern seen in this case would be a patient with homozygous Hb C disease who had recently received blood transfusions; patients with homozygous C disease produce no Hb A. This possibility is ruled out by the history. Note that the Hb A_2 in this case is unmeasurable by alkaline electrophoresis and by routine micro-column chromatography methods due to interference from Hb C. In a case such as this, isoelectric focusing or HPLC would likely demonstrate an increase in Hb A_2 resulting from the presence of a β-thalassemia gene, as these methods separate Hb A_2 from Hb C.

References

Bunn HF, Forget BG. *Hemoglobin: Molecular, Genetic, and Clinical Aspects.* Philadelphia, PA: WB Saunders Co;1986:422.

Nagel RL, Steinberg MH. Hb S/C disease and Hb C disorders. In: Steinberg MH, Forget BJ, Higgs DR, Nagle RL. *Disorders of Hemoglobin: Genetics, Pathophysiology and Clinical Management.* Cambridge, England: Cambridge University Press; 2001:756-785.

Singer K, Josephson AM, Singer L, Heller P, Zimmerman HJ. Studies on abnormal hemoglobins, XIII: hemoglobin S-thalassemia disease and hemoglobin C-thalassemia. *Blood.* 1957;12:593-602.

Singer K, Kraus AP, Singer L, Rubenstein HM, Goldberg SR. Studies on abnormal hemoglobins, X: a new syndrome: hemoglobin C-thalassemia disease. *Blood.* 1954; 9:1032-1046.

Smith EW, Krevans JR. Clinical manifestations of haemoglobin C disorders. *Bull Johns Hopkins Hosp.* 1959;104:17-43.

Weatherall DJ, Clegg JB. *The Thalassemia Syndromes.* 4th ed. Oxford, England: Blackwell Science Ltd; 2001:415-419.

Case 30

HISTORY
The patient is a 29-year-old African-American woman who is asymptomatic except that she perhaps tires more easily than do some of her friends. The physical examination revealed no icterus, but her spleen was palpable.

BLOOD COUNT DATA
RBC ....5.6×10^{12}/L
Hb ....11.1 g/dL
MCV ....60.7 fL
WBC..............................7.2×10^9/L
Plt..................................167.0×10^9/L

PERIPHERAL BLOOD SMEAR
Hypochromia, microcytosis, abundant target cells, occasional coarse basophilic stippling.

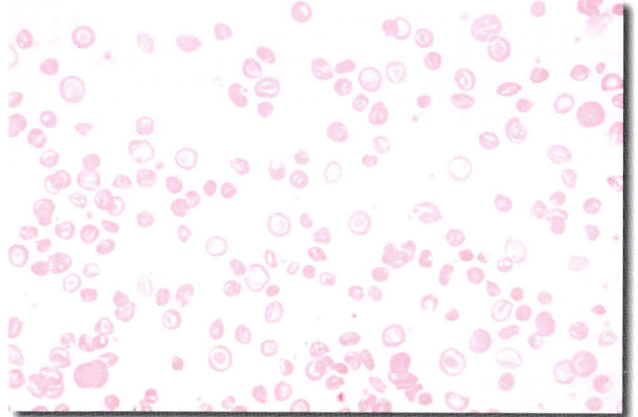

Alkaline Electrophoresis (pH 8.6) Acid Electrophoresis (pH 6.2)

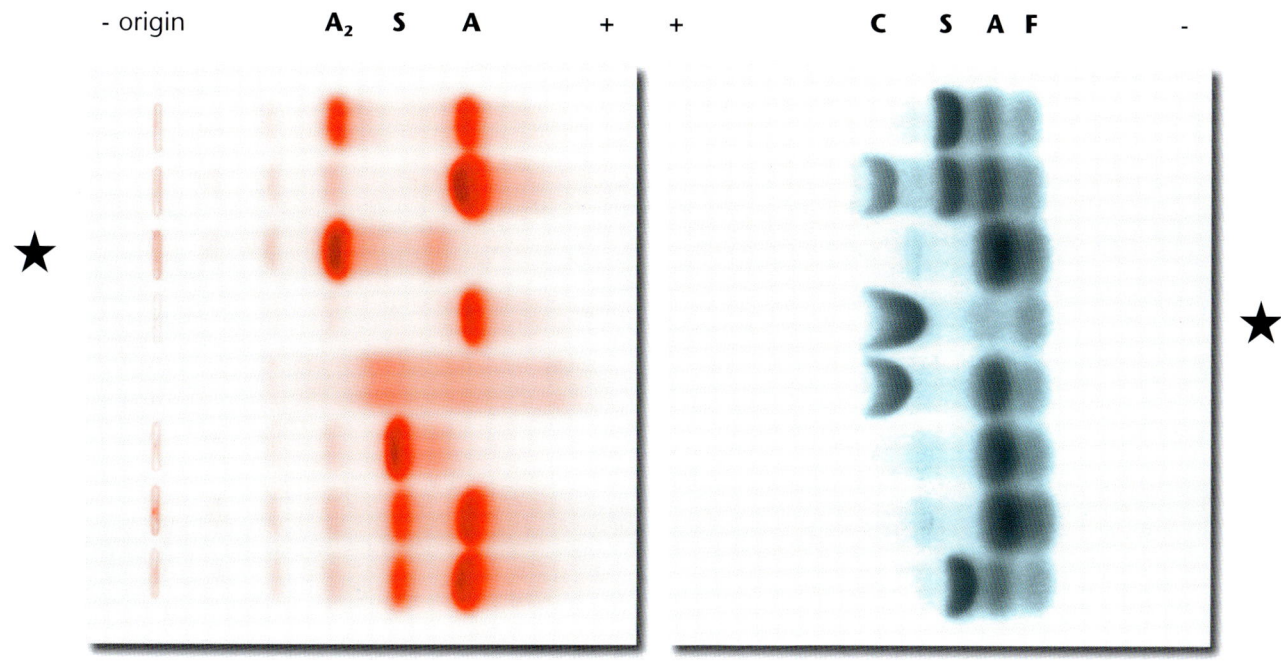

Case Studies

Case 30 Discussion

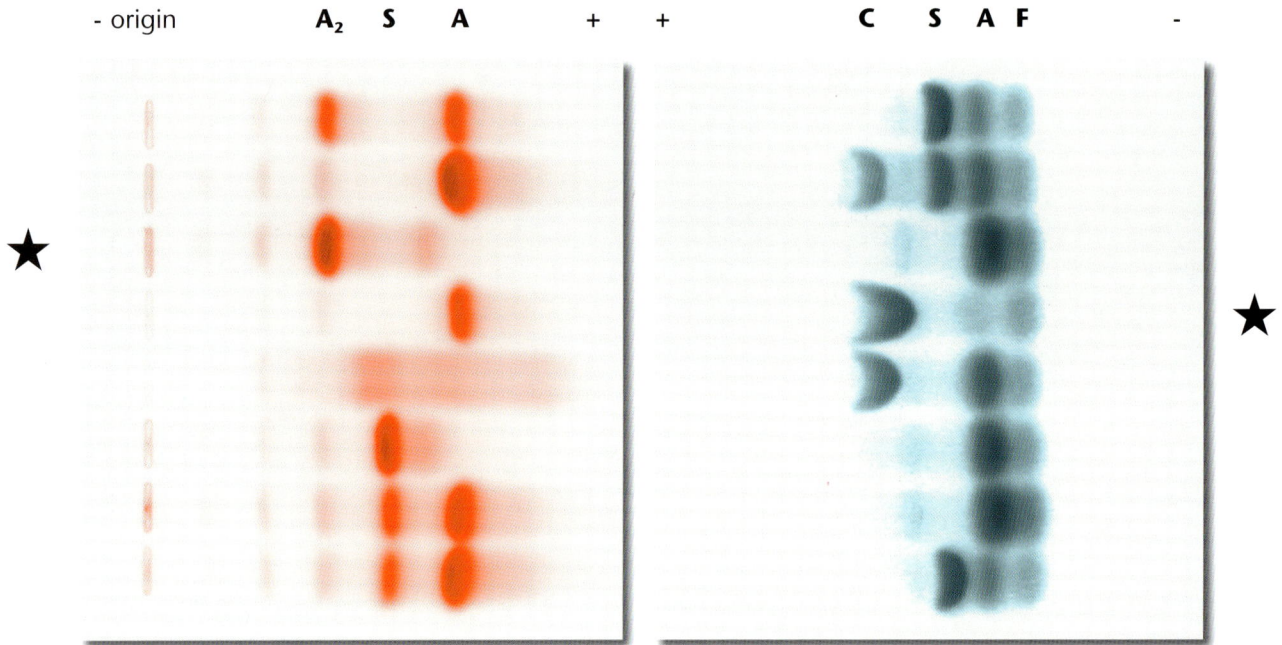

Interpretation

The alkaline electrophoresis gel demonstrates a single major band at the C position and a small band in the F position. The acid electrophoresis demonstrates a single major band in the C position and minor bands in the F and A positions.

Diagnosis

Hb C/β^0-thalassemia.

Performance

Hb C/β^0-thalassemia has been used only once in the survey. Of laboratories using both alkaline and acid electrophoresis, 99% of participants correctly identified the presence of a variant migrating in the C, E, or O position. Nearly all laboratories reported that hemoglobin A was not measurable. Roughly 60% favored a diagnosis of homozygous hemoglobin C disease, whereas 40% favored hemoglobin C/β^0-thalassemia. Both answers were considered correct for the purposes of grading.

Discussion

Like Hb C/β^+-thalassemia, Hb C/β^0-thalassemia has been described in both black and Mediterranean populations. As discussed in Case 29, β^0 mutations, in which there is no β chain output from the affected allele, are quite uncommon in the African-American population. When such a mutation is inherited in trans to a β^C mutation, the result is an absence of normal β chain production, and thus an absence of hemoglobin A. Red cells in patients with Hb C/β^0-thalassemia therefore have predominantly Hb C with elevated Hb A_2 in most cases. Hemoglobin F may be mildly elevated as well. The consequences of this disorder for the red cells appear to be similar to those in homozygous Hb C disease (see Case 15). In addition, however, the thalassemic component will lead to enhanced microcytosis and hypochromia. The precise mechanisms of hemolysis in these patients have not been specifically investigated but presumably involve a combination of the cellular dehydration resulting from hemoglobin C and the excess α chains associated with the β-thalassemia. Interestingly, crystal formation does not appear to be a feature of Hb C/β^0-thalassemia, perhaps because of the decreased intra-cellular hemoglobin concentration resulting from the thalassemia.

The clinical features of Hb C/β^0-thalassemia appear to be similar to homozygous hemoglobin C disease in that patients have a mild to moderate chronic hemolytic anemia, with hemoglobin levels in the range of 8-12 g/dL, accompanied by prominent splenomegaly. The blood smear demonstrates large numbers of target cells, folded cells, scattered spherocytes, hypochromia, microcytosis, and polychromasia (Figure 30.1). The MCV in Hb C/β^0-thalassemia ranges from 55-70 fL, in contrast to homozygous C disease in which the average MCV is 72 fL. This disorder is compatible with a normal life span, although, as in homozygous Hb C disease, complications of chronic hemolysis may be seen. Patients may be asymptomatic, however.

As the performance data for this case indicate, the identification of the presence of Hb C without the presence of Hb A was a straightforward task. Specifically, other hemoglobin species migrating with Hb C on alkaline electrophoresis (such as Hb E and Hb O) are ruled out by the migration pattern in the acid gel. However, the distinction of Hb C/β^0-thalassemia from homozygous Hb C disease is problematic using routine electrophoretic methods. The reason for this is that the quantification of Hb A_2 from the alkaline electrophoretic gel or with microcolumn chromatography is impossible because Hb A_2 is obscured by Hb C. While a small Hb A_2 band is evident in the A position of the acid gel, quantification is generally not performed from that analysis. However, based on the MCV of 60.7 fL, it is a reasonable assumption that this represents Hb C/β^0-thalassemia. This may be confirmed by either isoelectric focusing or HPLC, as both of these methods separate Hb A_2 from Hb C. In this case, the Hb A_2 level measured by HPLC was 7.1%, confirming the diagnosis of the double heterozygous state for both Hb C and β^0-thalassemia. Note that the absence of any Hb A rules out Hb C/β^+-thalassemia (see Case 29, page 135).

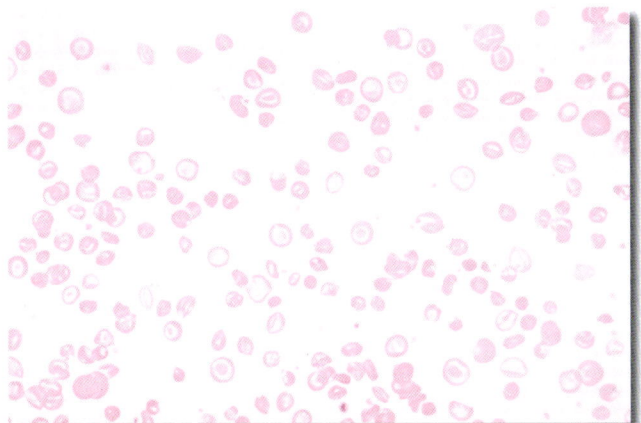
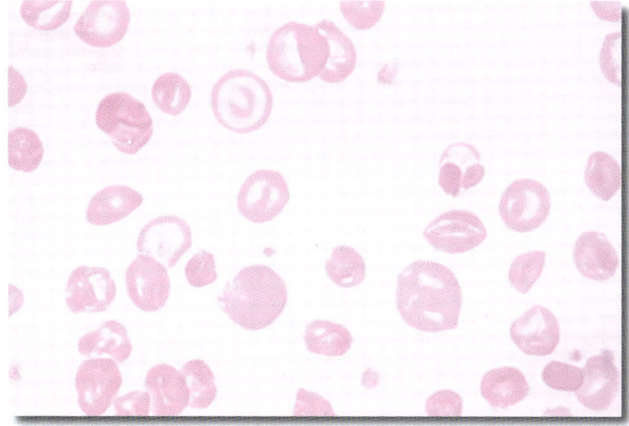

Figure 30.1 (Wright-Giemsa, 160x and 400x)
Low- and high-power views of the peripheral blood smear from a patient with Hb C/β^0-thalassemia. In contrast with homozygous Hb C, there is a greater degree of anisopoikilocytosis.

References

Bunn HF, Forget BG. *Hemoglobin: Molecular, Genetic, and Clinical Aspects.* Philadelphia, PA: WB Saunders Co;1986:422.

Casado A, Pellicer A, Olmeda F, et al. Double heterozygosis for hemoglobin C-beta thalassemia: description of a Spanish family. Hemoglobin C-beta thalassemia in a Spanish family. *Clin Genet.* 1978;13:265-270.

Fairbanks VF. *Hemoglobinopathies and Thalassemias. Laboratory Methods and Case Studies.* New York, NY: Brian C. Decker; 1980:154-156.

Nagel RL, Steinberg MH. Hb S/C disease and Hb C disorders. In: Steinberg MH, Forget BJ, Higgs DR, Nagle RL. *Disorders of Hemoglobin: Genetics, Pathophysiology and Clinical Management.* Cambridge, England: Cambridge University Press; 2001:756-785.

Ozsoylu S, Sipahioglu H, Altay F. Hemoglobin C-beta (0) thalassemia. *Isr J Med Sci.* 1989;25:410-412.

Weatherall DJ, Clegg JB. *The Thalassemia Syndromes.* 4th ed. Oxford, England: Blackwell Scientific Ltd; 2001:415-419.

Case 31

HISTORY
The patient is a 42-year-old black woman who had a myocardial infarction in October 1989. Subsequently, coronary angiography revealed no obstructions. The physical examination at that time revealed mild splenomegaly, which has persisted. She does not smoke. There was no family history of polycythemia.

BLOOD COUNT DATA
RBC .... 6.4 x 10^{12}/L
Hb .... 14.1 g/dL
MCV .... 65.0 fL
WBC .... 17.0 x 10^9/L
Plt .... 1200 x 10^9/L

PERIPHERAL BLOOD SMEAR
The peripheral blood smear confirmed leukocytosis, neutrophilia, hypochromia, microcytic erythrocytes, and marked thrombocytosis.

OTHER LABORATORY TESTS
Serum ferritin concentration was 6 µg/L.
Initial therapy included oral iron to correct iron deficiency. However, the patient's hemoglobin concentration then rose to 17.5 g/dL, RBC 7.6 x 10^{12}/L, MCV 68 fL, and HCT 52%. Leukocytosis, neutrophilia, and thrombocytosis persisted. Because of the persistent microcytosis, hemoglobin studies were obtained.

Alkaline Electrophoresis (pH 8.6)

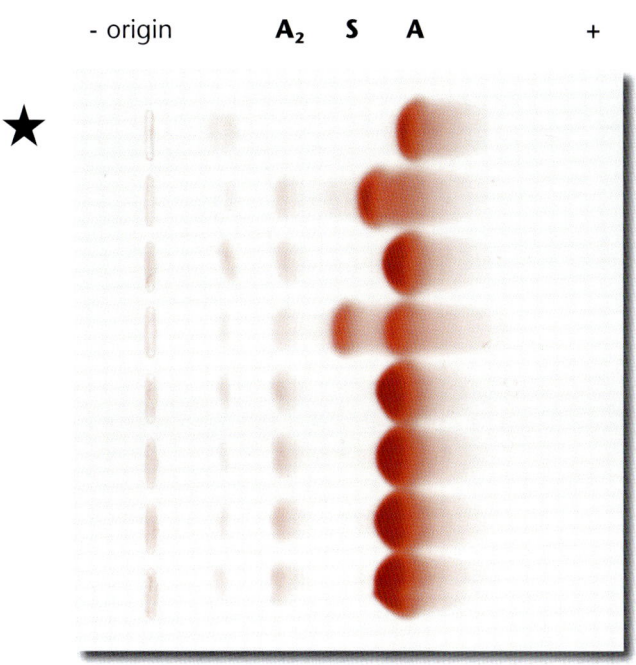

Case 31 Discussion

Alkaline Electrophoresis (pH 8.6)

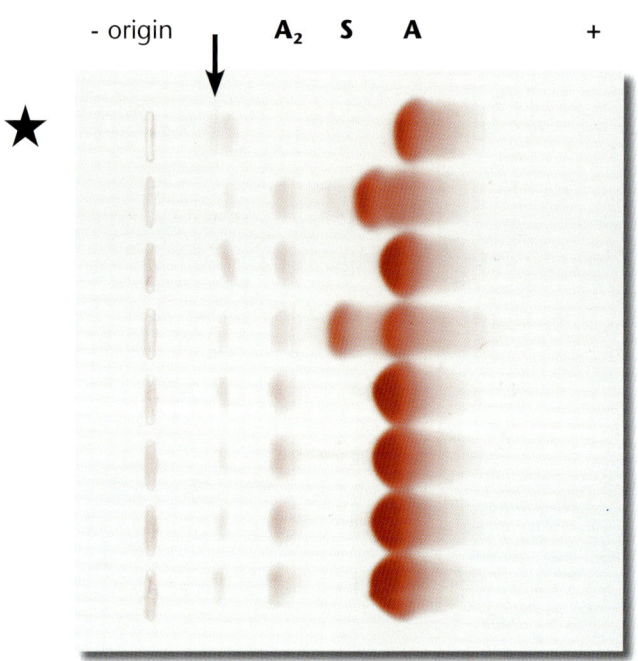

Interpretation

Examination of alkaline electrophoresis shows no band in the A_2 position. However, there is a distinct band seen just cathodal to the carbonic anhydrase position (arrow). Acid electrophoresis (not shown) showed no abnormal bands.

Diagnosis

Homozygous Hb A_2'.

Performance

This variant is usually a difficult one for laboratories to identify due to its low percentage. On this specimen, 18.9% correctly identified homozygous Hb A_2', with an additional 13.2% of laboratories being partially correct, identifying Hb A_2' trait.

Discussion

Hb A_2' is a δ chain variant that is due to a glycine to arginine substitution at the 16th position of the delta globin chain (δ 16 Gly→Arg). It has also been called Hb B_2. This is the commonest δ chain variant seen and occurs in 1-2% of African Americans. The homozygous state (as in this case) is much less common but may be predicted to occur in 1/20,000 African Americans. Hb A_2' has no clinical or hematological manifestations. However, because this variant migrates separately from normal Hb A_2', the amount of Hb A_2 will be underestimated by quantitative measurements. The history in this case shows leukocytosis, thrombocytosis, and microcytosis with iron deficiency (but with a normal hemoglobin level). These findings are all suggestive of a chronic myeloproliferative disorder, and the patient carries a diagnosis of polycythemia vera. Examples of homozygous Hb A_2' on HPLC and isoelectric focusing are shown in Figures 31.1 and 31.2.

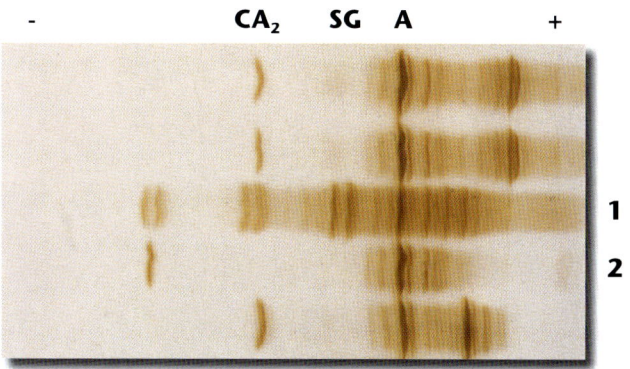

Figure 31.2
An example of homozygous Hb A_2 by isoelectric focusing (lane 2). A band in the A_2 position is not seen. Rather, there is a single band seen cathodal to the A_2 position. Lane 1-control.

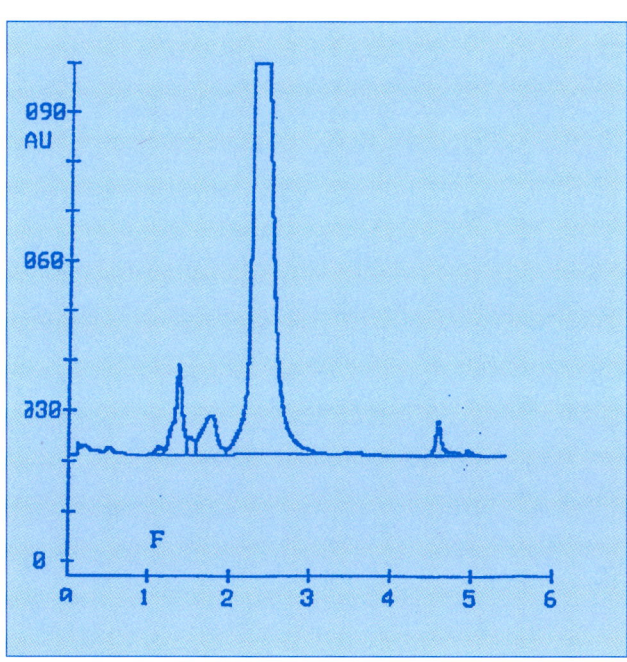

Figure 31.1
An example of homozygous Hb A_2' by HPLC. A peak in the A_2 position (3.3-3.9 minutes) is not seen. Instead, there is a slower peak corresponding to Hb A_2' which is seen in the S window at approximately 4.5-4.6 minutes.

References

Ball EW, Mynell MJ, Beal D, et al. Haemoglobin $A_2':\alpha_2\delta_2 16$ glycine→argine. *Nature.* 1966;209:1217-1218.

Huisman THJ, Lee RC. Two δ-chain abnormal hemoglobins in one individual. *Blood.* 1965;26:677-681.

Jones RT, Brimhall B, Huisman THJ. Structural characterization of two δ-chain variants: hemoglobin A_2' (B_2) and hemoglobin Flatbush. *J Biol Chem.* 1967;242:4141-4145.

Case 32

HISTORY
The patient is an asymptomatic 29-year-old woman who was examined because she had recently given birth to a child who, on neonatal screening for hemoglobinopathy, was found to have 14% Hb S, 86% Hb F, and no demonstrable Hb A. During a three-month postnatal period, her infant exhibited no clinical manifestations of sickle cell disease. Hemoglobin electrophoresis has not yet been repeated. She has an older child with sickle cell trait. The physical examination revealed an alert, healthy-appearing, young black woman with no abnormalities.

BLOOD COUNT DATA
RBC.................5.6 x 10^{12}/L
Hb...................12.8 g/dL
MCV.................68 fL
WBC.................5.4 x 10^9/L
Plt....................373 x 10^9/L

PERIPHERAL BLOOD SMEAR
Erythrocytic microcytosis, hypochromia, target cells, and coarse basophilic stippling.

OTHER LABORATORY TESTS
Quantitation of Hb F was within normal limits. A test for unstable hemoglobin was negative. Serum ferritin concentration was 44 µg/L.

Alkaline Electrophoresis (pH 8.6)

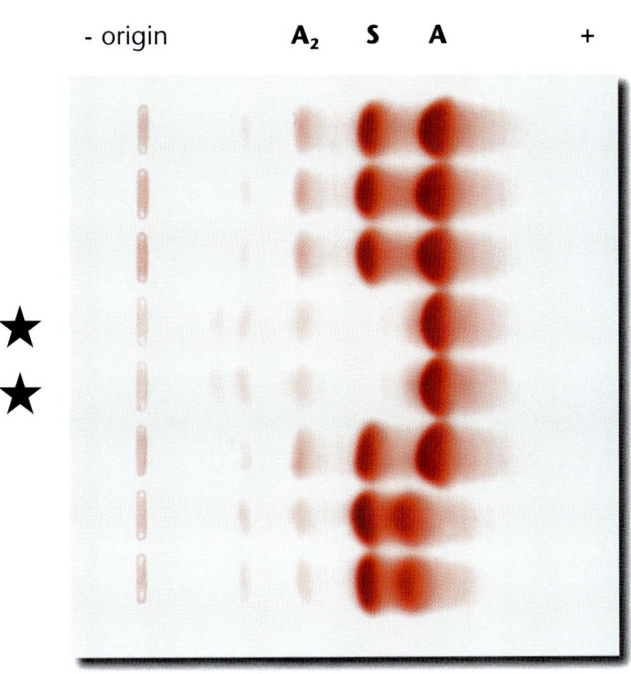

Case 32 Discussion

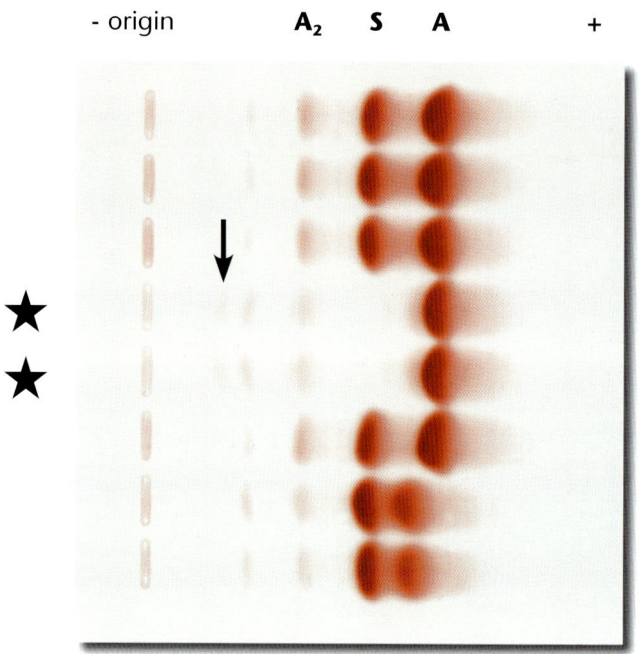

Interpretation

On alkaline electrophoresis, there is a band in the A position and a minor band in the A_2 position. Additionally, there is a minor band just cathodal to the carbonic anhydrase position (arrow). Laboratories that measured Hb A_2 by column chromatography obtained a mean value of Hb A_2 of 5.50%, whereas those laboratories who estimated Hb A_2 by densitometry obtained a mean value of only 3.05%.

Diagnosis

β-thalassemia trait with Hb A_2' trait.

Performance

73.3% of laboratories correctly identified β-thalassemia trait, whereas only 21.5% of laboratories recognized Hb A_2' trait.

Discussion

Hb A_2' was discussed in Case 31. It is important to remember that the total Hb A_2 is the sum of the Hb A_2 plus Hb A_2'. In this case, the total Hb A_2 is elevated, indicating β-thalassemia trait. If Hb A_2' is not recognized, it may result in underestimation of the total Hb A_2. This is true of laboratories that estimate Hb A_2 by densitometry, but also true of laboratories that quantitate Hb A_2 by high performance liquid chromatography (Figure 32.1). An example of Hb A_2' on isoelectric focusing is shown in Figure 32.2.

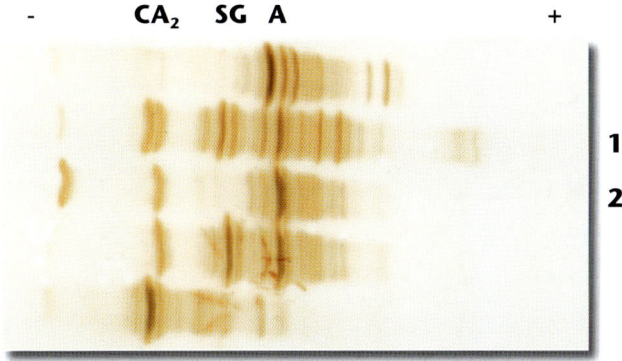

Figure 32.2
The same case illustrated in Figure 32.1 by isoelectric focusing (lane 2). Both the normal A_2 band as well as the Hb A_2' band are seen. Lane 1-control.

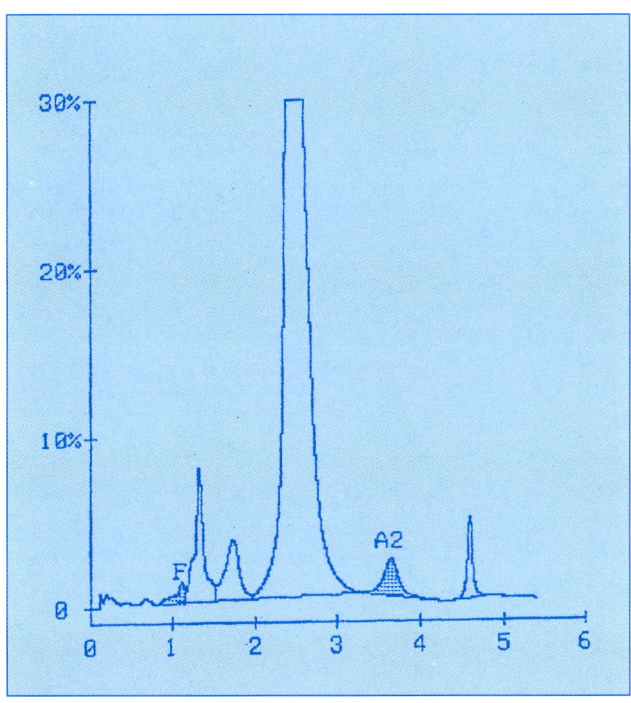

Figure 32.1
An example of Hb A_2' in combination with β–thalassemia trait by HPLC. In addition to a peak in the A_2 position, there is a peak at approximately 4.5-4.6 minutes (S window) representing Hb A_2'. The sum of Hb A_2 and A_2' in this example is 5.8%, consistent with β-thalassemia trait.

References

Ball EW, Mynell MJ, Beal D, et al. Haemoglobin A_2':$α_2δ_2$16 glycine→argine. *Nature.* 1966;209: 1217-1218.

Huisman THJ, Lee RC. Two δ-chain abnormal hemoglobins in one individual. *Blood.* 1965;26: 677-681.

Jones RT, Brimhall B, Huisman THJ. Structural characterization of two δ-chain variants: hemoglobin A_2' (B_2) and hemoglobin Flatbush. *J Biol Chem.* 1967; 242:4141-4145.

Case 33

HISTORY
A 26-year-old black woman was seen for a chief complaint of headaches. She was otherwise asymptomatic. Many years previously she had been told that she had sickle cell trait. The physical examination showed no abnormalities.

BLOOD COUNT DATA
RBC..............................4.33×10^{12}/L
Hb................................12.0 g/dL
MCV..............................82.4 fL
WBC..............................7.4×10^9/L
Plt................................284×10^9/L

PERIPHERAL BLOOD SMEAR
No abnormalities.

OTHER LABORATORY TESTS
The solubility test for sickling hemoglobin is positive.

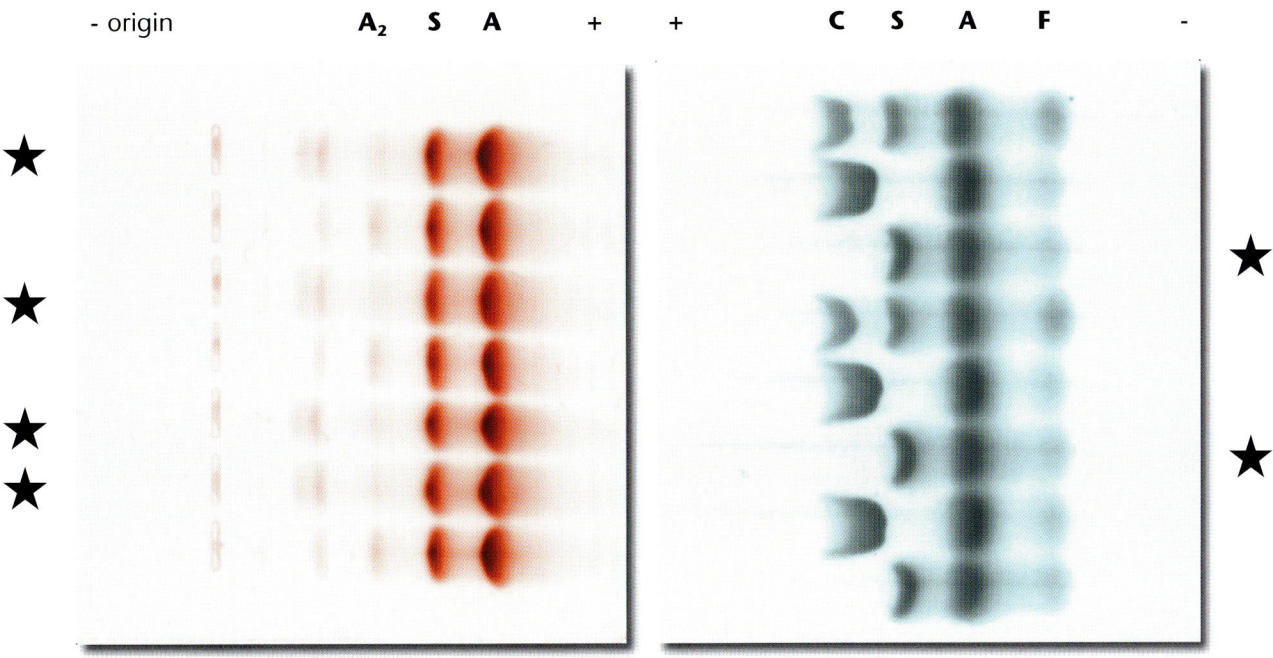

Alkaline Electrophoresis (pH 8.6) **Acid Electrophoresis (pH 6.2)**

Case 33 Discussion

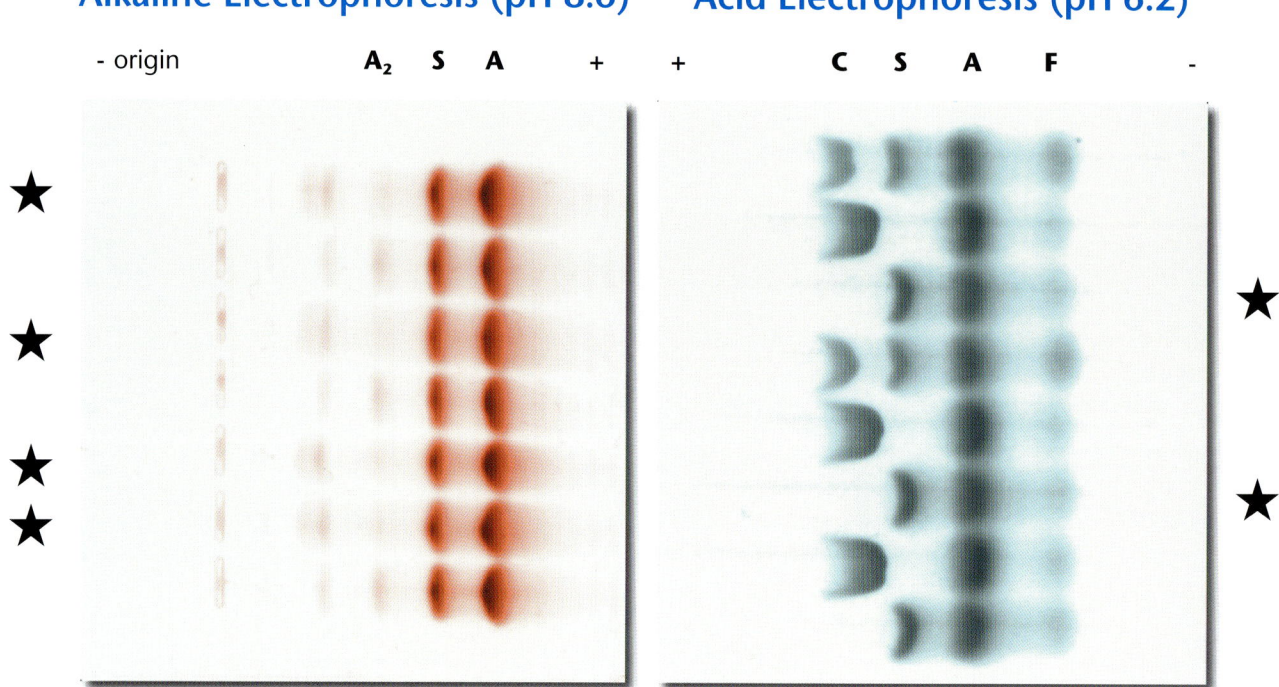

Interpretation

On alkaline electrophoresis, there are two major bands present, one in the A position and one in the S position. The band in the S position accounts for 30% of the total hemoglobin. Additionally, there is a minor band seen cathodal to the carbonic anhydrase position. On acid electrophoresis, there are major bands seen in the A and S positions.

Diagnosis

Hb S trait/Hb A_2' trait/α-thalassemia-2 trait.

Performance

This combination appeared in the survey once. Although 86.5% of laboratories correctly identified Hb S trait, only 15.4% of laboratories recognized concurrent α-thalassemia, and 7.1% of laboratories the presence of Hb A_2'.

Discussion

This case represents the combination of three separate abnormalities that can be seen in African Americans. This patient is a heterozygote for two different and unrelated hemoglobin variants as well as a single gene deletion α-thalassemia. This combination is not rare; with the prevalence of these traits as given in previous cases, it may be expected that approximately 1/3000 African Americans would have this combination. The differential diagnosis of Hb S/Hb A_2' is discussed more fully in dry lab challenge DL-20, page 293.

References

Ball EW, Mynell MJ, Beal D, et al. Haemoglobin A_2': $\alpha_2\delta_2$16 glycine→argine. *Nature.* 1966;209:1217-1218.

Huisman THJ, Lee RC. Two δ-chain abnormal hemoglobins in one individual. *Blood.* 1965;26:677-681.

Jones RT, Brimhall B, Huisman THJ. Structural characterization of two δ-chain variants: hemoglobin A_2'(B_2) and hemoglobin Flatbush. *J Biol Chem.* 1967;242: 4141-4145.

Case 34

HISTORY
The patient is a 30-year-old Cambodian man evaluated for mild anemia. The physical examination showed no splenomegaly.

BLOOD COUNT DATA
RBC .... 6.35 x 10^{12}/L
Hb .... 12.2 g/dL
MCV .... 64.1 fL
WBC .... 7.3 x 10^9/L
Plt .... 323 x 10^9/L

PERIPHERAL BLOOD SMEAR
RBC hypochromia and microcytosis with many target cells.

OTHER LABORATORY TESTS
Serum bilirubin 0.7 mg/dL.
Serum ferritin 154 µg/L.
Test for unstable hemoglobin was positive.

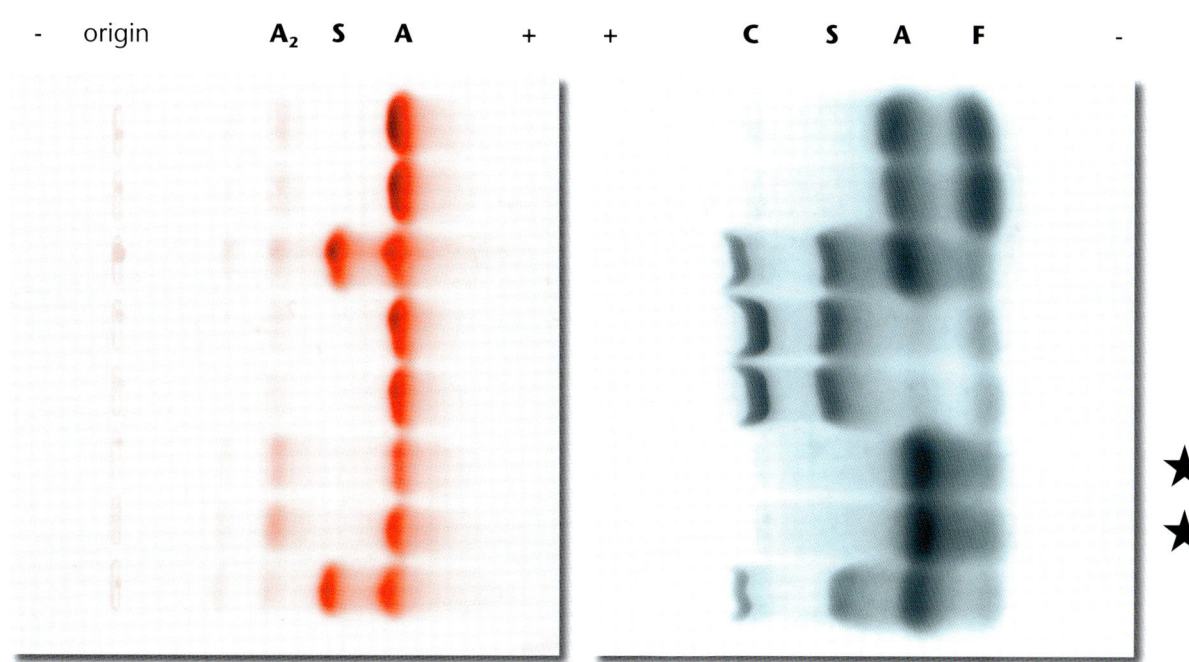

Alkaline Electrophoresis (pH 8.6)   Acid Electrophoresis (pH 6.2)

Case 34 Discussion

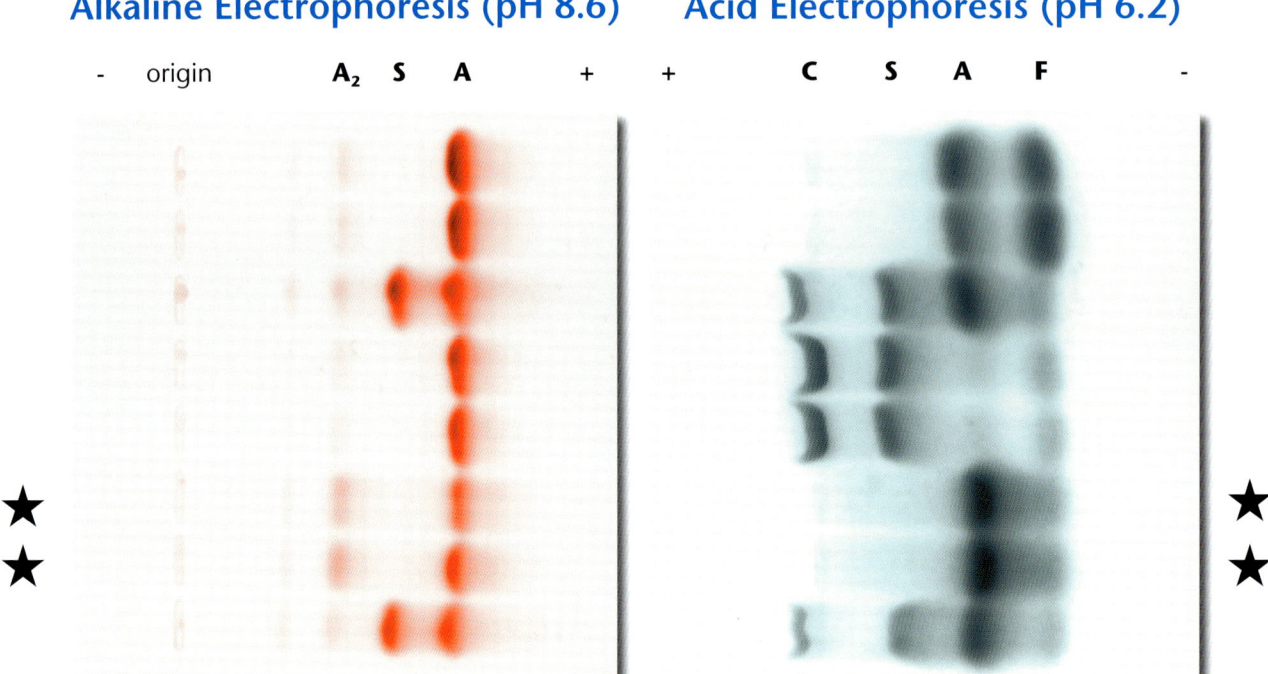

Interpretation

Alkaline electrophoresis shows two major bands, one in the A position and one in the A_2 position. This second band accounts for approximately 20-25% of the total hemoglobin. On acid electrophoresis, only a band in the A position is seen.

Diagnosis

Hb E trait in combination with α-thalassemia.

Performance

Virtually all laboratories identified Hb E trait, with 44.0% of laboratories correctly identifying Hb E trait with concurrent α-thalassemia.

Discussion

Hb E has been previously discussed in detail in Cases 9, 14, and *A Closer Look At…Hb E-Associated Disorders* (page 72). The identification of Hb E in this case is relatively straightforward. However, the percentage of the variant and the MCV in this case are too low for uncomplicated Hb E trait, in which Hb E is 30-35% of the total hemoglobin, and the MCV is 70-75 fL. Both concurrent α-thalassemia or iron deficiency will serve to lower both the percentages of the hemoglobin variant as well as the MCV. However, as the history indicates, the serum ferritin is normal. The Hb E percentage of 20-25% is also too low for Hb E/α-thalassemia-2 trait (i.e., one α-chain deletion). With that combination, the percentage of Hb E would be 25-30% and the MCV approximately 70 fL. Therefore, the patient must have a two α chain deletion, either α-thalassemia-1 trait (--/αα) or homozygous α-thalassemia-2 (-α/-α). A 3 α-chain deletion would result in a form of Hb H disease which has been termed "Hb AE Bart's syndrome," and is illustrated in a subsequent dry lab challenge (case DL-4, page 229; also see *A Closer Look At…Hb E-Associated Disorders,* page 72).

Iron deficiency and α-thalassemia can easily co-exist in the same patient. In this situation, the percentage of Hb E will be 10-15% or possibly even <10%, and one must be careful not to interpret the band in the A_2 position as simply Hb A_2 (i.e., β-thalassemia trait). A good rule of thumb is that Hb A_2 almost is never elevated above 10% in β-thalassemia trait.

References

Fairbanks VF, Gilchrist GS, Brimhall B, et al. Hemoglobin E trait re-examined: a cause of microcytosis and erythrocytosis. *Blood.* 1979;53:109-115.

Tuchinda S, Rucknagel DL, Minnich V, et al. The co-existence of the genes for hemoglobin E and α-thalassemia in traits with resultant suppression of Hb E synthesis. *Am J Hum Genet.* 1964;10:311-335.

Case 35

HISTORY
This specimen was obtained from a recently postpartum 29-year-old woman of Chinese ancestry because on neonatal hemoglobinopathy screening of a specimen from her baby, several hemoglobin bands were seen. She was asymptomatic and had no history of anemia. The physical examination was normal.

BLOOD COUNT DATA
RBC .... 6.3×10^{12}/L
Hb .... 14.1 g/dL
MCV .... 68.0 fL
WBC .... 7.4×10^9/L
Plt .... 287×10^9/L

PERIPHERAL BLOOD SMEAR
Slight microcytosis only.

OTHER LABORATORY TESTS
Reticulocytes 1.3%.
Serum ferritin 47.0 µg/L.
The solubility test for sickling hemoglobin is negative.

Alkaline Electrophoresis (pH 8.6)

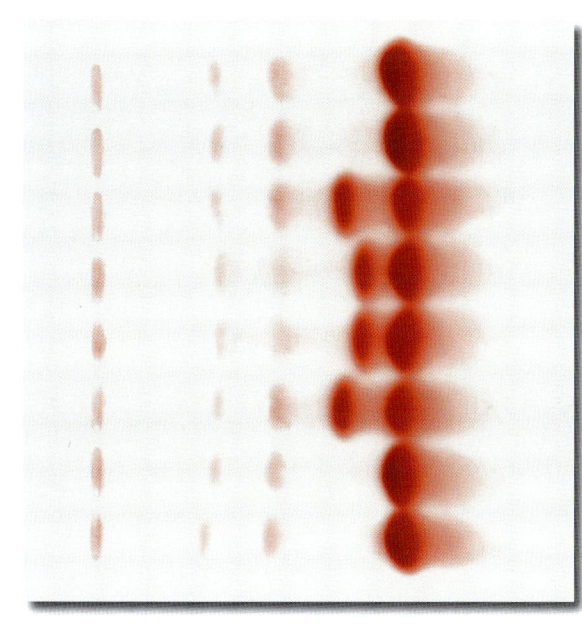

Acid Electrophoresis (pH 6.2)

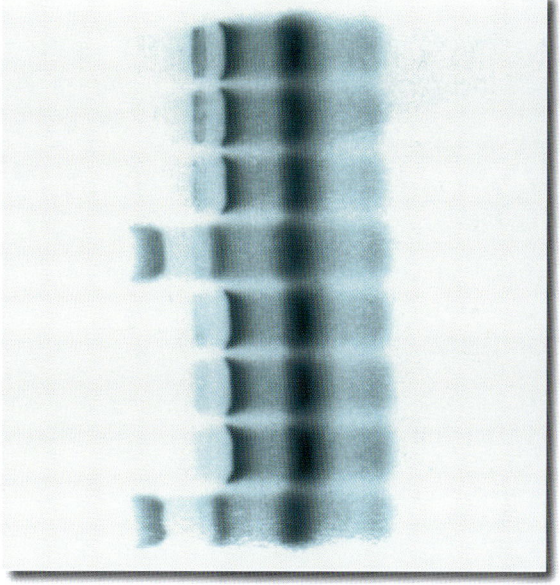

Case 35 Discussion

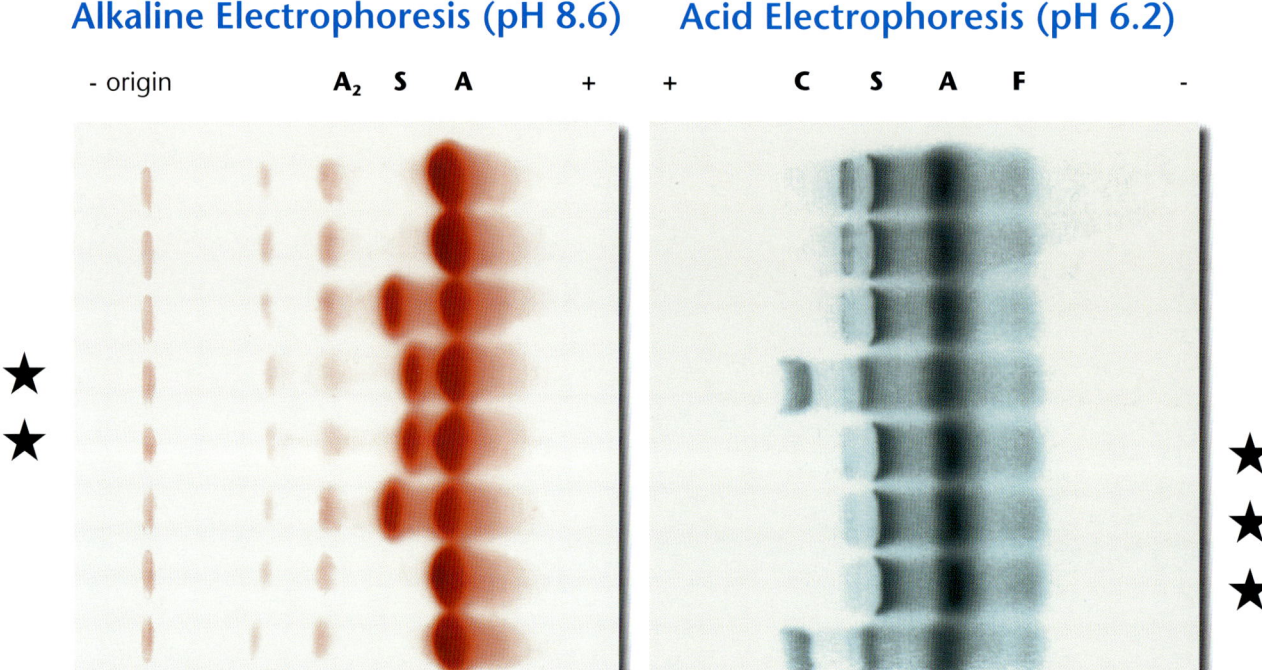

Interpretation

On alkaline electrophoresis, there are two bands seen, one in the A position and a band that is slightly anodal to the Hb S position. This band accounts for approximately 30% of the total hemoglobin. On acid electrophoresis, in addition to a band in the A position, there is a band that is slightly cathodal to the S position. Other methods identified the variant as Hb Q-Thailand.

Diagnosis

Hb Q-Thailand trait with α-thalassemia-2 trait.

Performance

Hb Q-Thailand has been included in the survey once. 25.8% of laboratories correctly identified Hb Qα trait, with 22.7% of laboratories also recognizing co-existent α-thalassemia.

Discussion

Hb Q-Thailand results from a substitution of aspartic acid to histidine at the 74th position of the α globin chain (α 74 Asp→His). This variant has many synonyms and has also been called Hb Mahidol, Q-Chinese, G-Taichung, Kurashiki, and Asabara. Hb Q-Thailand has no clinical or hematologic effects but is always associated with a deletion of the contiguous upstream α 2 globin gene. When Hb Q-Thailand is seen in trans with α-thalassemia-1 trait (-α^Q/--), a form of Hb H disease (Hb Q/H) is produced. This is the subject of a subsequent dry lab challenge (see case DL-10, page 253). Hb Q-Thailand is found only in persons of Asian ancestry, particularly in Chinese individuals.

Hb Q-Thailand represents 30-35% of total hemoglobin in the heterozygous state (rather than 25%) because of the concurrent α gene deletion that always accompanies it. Although it migrates with Hb S on alkaline electrophoresis, it should not be confused with Hb S because of a negative sickle solubility test. The slightly anodal position should also differentiate Hb Q-Thailand from other D or G hemoglobins. Hb Q-Thailand migrates in the S window on HPLC (Figure 35.1). Isoelectric focusing is very helpful because it clearly shows the presence of the δ chain variant ($α^Q_2δ_2$) (Figure 35.2). Differentiation from other α variants is difficult and requires ancillary tests, possibly including amino acid or DNA sequencing.

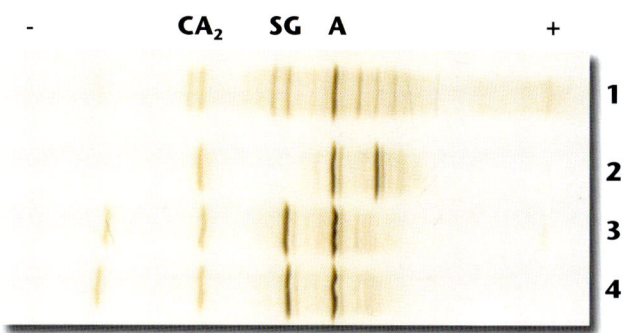

Figure 35.2
An example of Hb Q-Thailand by isoelectric focusing (lane 3). In lane 4 is Hb G-Philadelphia trait, another α chain variant. Lane 1-Control, Lane 2-Hb J-Baltimore trait.

References

Beris P, Huber P, Miescher PA, et al. Hb Q-Thailand-Hb H disease in a Chinese living in Geneva, Switzerland: characterization of the variant and identifications of the two α-thalassemic chromosomes. *Am J Hematol.* 1987;24:395-400.

Blackwell RQ, Liu CS. Hemoglobin G Taichung: α 74 Asp→His. *Biochim Biophys Acta.* 1970;200:70-75.

Jen PC. Abnormal hemoglobins found in Guangdong, P.R. China. *Hemoglobin.* 1987;11:573-579.

Lie-Injo LE, Dozy AM, Kam YW, et al. The α-globin gene adjacent to the gene for Hb Q-α 74 Asp→His is deleted, but not that adjacent to the gene for Hb G-α 30 Glu→Gln; three fourths of the α-globin genes are deleted in Hb Q-α-thalassemia. *Blood.* 1979;54:1407-1416.

Liu JF, Lu YQ, Liu XQ, et al. Hb G-Taichung [α 74(EF3)Asp→His] in a Hunanese family in China. *Hemoglobin.* 1989;13:163-167.

Lorkin PA, Charlesworth D, Lehmann H, Rahbar S, et al. Two hemoglobins Q, α 74 (EF3) and α 75 (EF4) aspartic acid-histidine. *Br J Haematol.* 1970;19:117-125.

Pootrakui S, Dixon GH. Hemoglobin Mahidol: a new hemoglobin α-chain mutant. *Can J Biochem.* 1970;48:1066-1078.

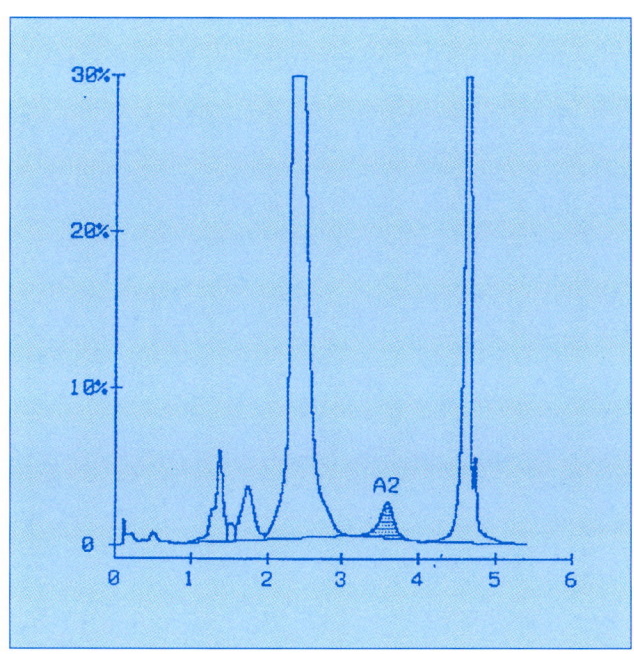

Figure 35.1
An example of Hb Q-Thailand trait by HPLC. Hb Q-Thailand elutes in the S window at approximately 4.6-4.7 minutes.

Case 36

HISTORY
The patient is a 34-year-old diabetic male of Polish-Jewish ancestry who was tested for a hemoglobinopathy because an endocrinologist thought that his diabetes was not as well-controlled as implied by nearly normal glycated hemoglobin assay results (ion-exchange method). No abnormalities were noted on the physical examination.

BLOOD COUNT DATA
RBC .... $4.51 \times 10^{12}/L$
Hb .... 13.4 g/dL
MCV .... 91 fL
WBC .... $8.9 \times 10^9/L$
Plt .... $301 \times 10^9/L$

PERIPHERAL BLOOD SMEAR
Normal erythrocyte morphology.

OTHER LABORATORY TESTS
Isopropanol test: positive; heat stability test: negative
Solubility test for sickling hemoglobin: negative
Plasma glucose (fasting) 150 mg/dL
Glycated Hb by affinity column, 9.9% (normal: 4-6%)

Alkaline Electrophoresis (pH 8.6)

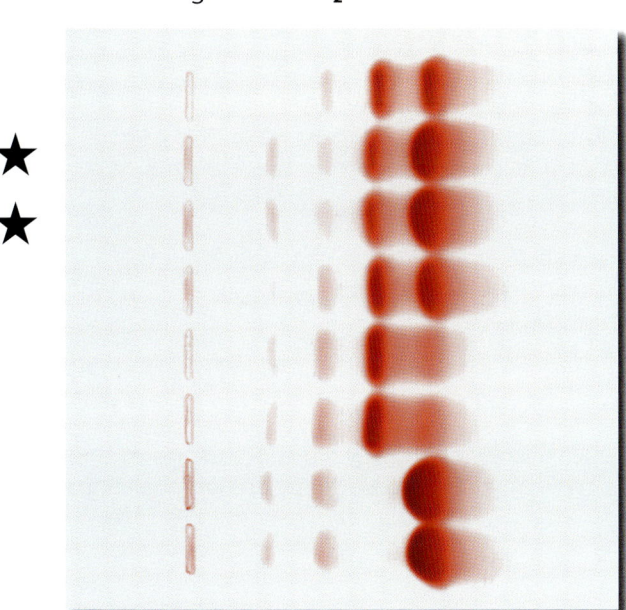

Acid Electrophoresis (pH 6.2)

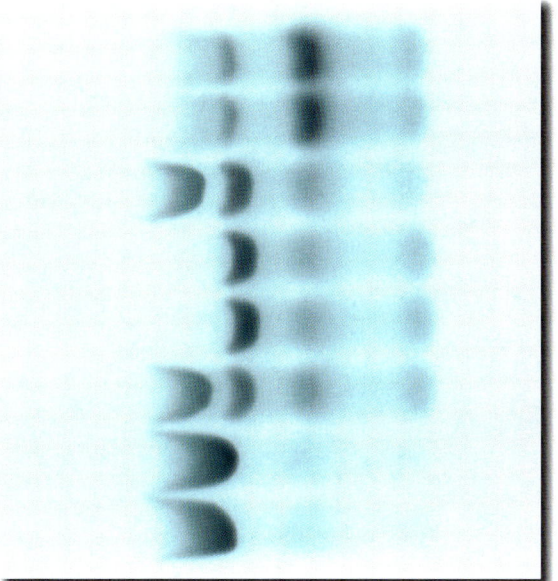

Case 36 Discussion

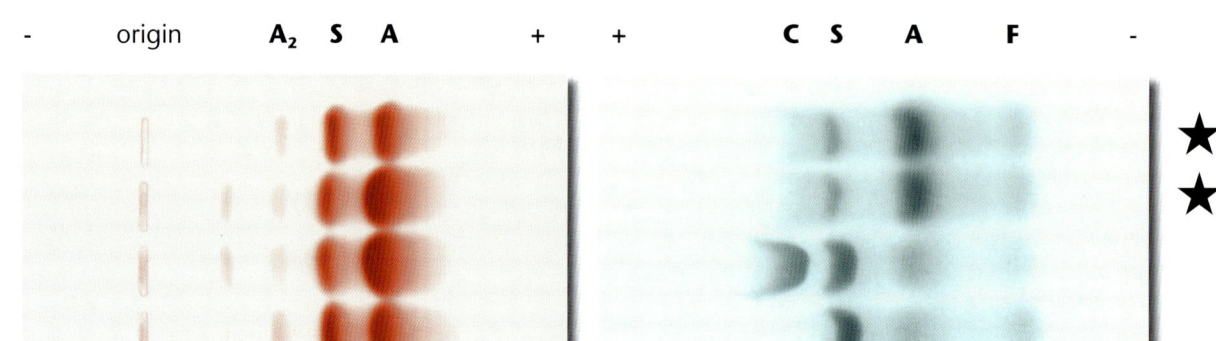

Interpretation

On alkaline electrophoresis, there is a major band in the Hb S region that appears to account for about 25% of the total hemoglobin. There is also a band in the A position. On acid electrophoresis, the abnormal hemoglobin variant migrates slightly anodic to Hb S.

Diagnosis

Hb Hasharon trait.

Performance

Participants in the 1989 survey were not expected to identify Hb Hasharon, but rather to recognize that this is not Hb S and that the specimen contained an unstable hemoglobin. In a subsequent dry lab challenge (1998 – HG-04), 84.5% of participants correctly identified Hb Hasharon.

Discussion

Hb Hasharon is an α chain hemoglobin variant that arises from a mutation in codon 47, resulting in replacement of aspartic acid by histidine (α 47 Asp→His). Hb Hasharon has also been called L-Ferrara, Hb Sinai, and Hb Sealy. Hemoglobin Hasharon is mildly unstable in vitro; the isopropanol test for hemoglobin instability is often positive, although heat stability tests are usually negative. Hb Hasharon is rarely encountered except in Ashenazi Jews (of central European origin) or Italians from the Ferrara district.

Although mildly unstable in vitro, Hb Hasharon is frequently discovered incidentally, as it rarely gives rise to any clinical or hematological manifestations. Rare cases of drug-induced (sulfonamide, dapsone) hemolytic anemia have been associated with Hb Hasharon, and at least one instance of hemolytic disease of the newborn has been described in a neonate with Hb Hasharon. These associations may have been coincidental.

Hb Hasharon has electrophoretic mobilities in alkaline and acid conditions that are very similar to Hb S. Without history or an independent sickling test, this hemoglobin variant may be mistaken for Hb S. An important clue is that Hb Hasharon typically accounts for only 15-20% of the total hemoglobin, which is considerably less than the 35-40% that one would expect to find in uncomplicated Hb S trait.

Italian cases from the Ferrara area have a distinctly higher proportion of Hb Hasharon, in the range of 30-35% of the total hemoglobin. DNA probe studies have shown that these patients have a concurrent α-thalassemia-2 trait, with the Hb Hasharon mutation existing on the single fusion α gene. The cases of Hb Hasharon seen in Ashenazi Jews are not associated with α-thalassemia.

This case exemplifies the problem of spuriously low hemoglobin A_{1c} tests when obtained by resin (ion-exchange) column chromatography in specimens from persons with diabetes mellitus and hemoglobin variants that are electrophoretically slow, such as Hb S, C, D, G, E, and others. The reason that spuriously low values are obtained is that the glycosylated form of Hb Hasharon does not migrate with Hb A_{1c}, and so the total amount of glycosylated hemoglobin is underestimated. This problem is obviated by use of affinity columns for measurement of glycated hemoglobin.

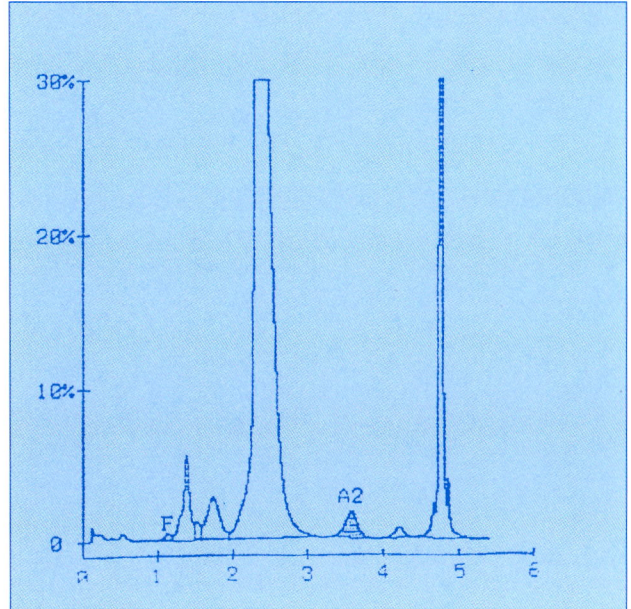

Figure 36.1
An example of Hb Hasharon by HPLC. Hb Hasharon has a retention time of approximately 4.75 minutes, which is usually between the S and C windows.

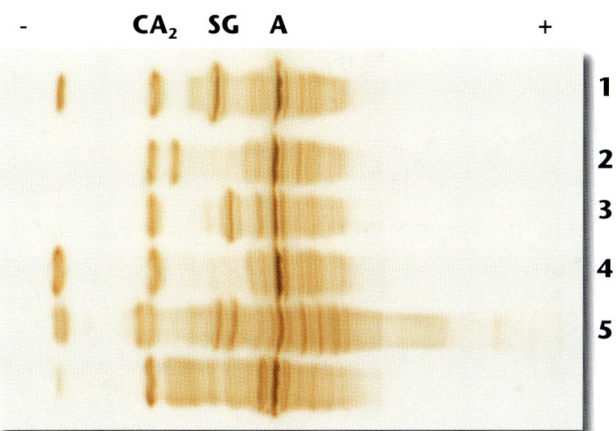

Figure 36.2
An example of Hb Hasharon by isoelectric focusing. (Lane 1) Hb Hasharon migrates slightly cathodal to the Hb S position. Also seen is the delta chain variant of Hb Hasharon cathodal to Hb A_2 ($α^H_2 δ_2$). Lane 2-Hb A_2-Babinga, 3-Hb Lepore trait, 4-Hb A_2', 5-control.

References

Adams JG, Heller P, Abramson RK, Vaithianathan T. Sulfonamide-induced hemolytic anemia and hemoglobin Hasharon. *Arch Int Med.* 1977;137: 1449-1451.

Alberti R, Mariuzzi GM, Marinucci M, et al. Haemoglobin Hasharon in a north Italian community. *J Med Genet.* 1975;12;294-296.

Charache S, Mondzac AM, Gessner V. Hemoglobin Hasharon (α_2^{47} his (CD5) β_2): a hemoglobin found in low concentration. *J Clin Invest.* 1969;48:834-847.

del Senno L, Bernardi F, Marchetti G, et al. Organization of α globin genes and mRNA translation in subjects carrying haemoglobin Hasharon (α^{47} Asp replaced by His) from the Ferrara region (northern Italy). *Eur J Biochem.* 1980;111(1):125-130.

Ganer A, Knobel B, Fryd CH, Rachmilevitz EA. Dapsone induces methemoglobinemia and hemolysis in the presence of familial hemoglobinopathy Hasharon and familial methemoglobin reductase deficiency. *Isr J Med Sci.* 1981;17:61-73.

Halbrecht I, Isaacs WA, Lehman H, et al. Hemoglobin Hasharon (α^{47} aspartic acid histidine). *Isr J Med Sci.* 1967;3:827-831.

Levine RL, Lincoln DR, Duchholz WM, et al. Hemoglobin Hasharon in a premature infant with hemolytic anemia. *Pediatr Res.* 1975;9:7-11.

Case 37

HISTORY
The patient was a 33-year-old woman of English and German origin who had been minimally anemic since early childhood. Her father, paternal aunt, two of her siblings, and two of her children (1 male, 1 female) are also said to be anemic. The physical examination revealed moderate scleral icterus and an enlarged spleen palpable to 3 cm below the left costal margin.

BLOOD COUNT DATA
RBC .... 3.9×10^{12}/L
Hb .... 11.5 g/dL
MCV .... 102 fL
WBC .... 7.8×10^{9}/L
Plt .... 289×10^{9}/L

PERIPHERAL BLOOD SMEAR
Moderate polychromasia, slight hypochromia.

OTHER LABORATORY TESTS
A test for unstable hemoglobin was positive. A Heinz body test was negative. Total serum bilirubin was elevated at 3.6 mg/dL (indirect 3.3 mg/dL). Reticulocytes 200×10^{9}/L (normal: $30-87 \times 10^{9}$/L)

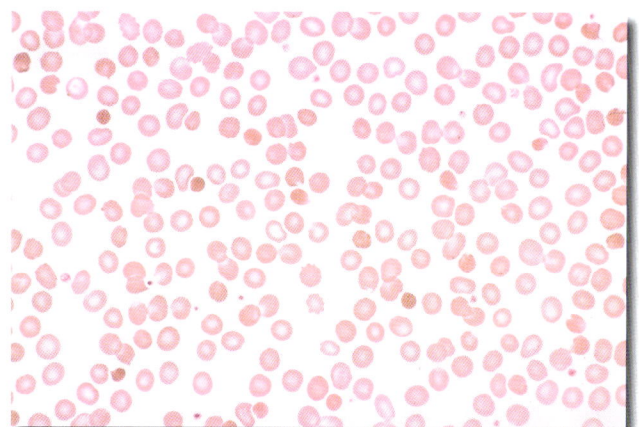

Alkaline Electrophoresis (pH 8.6)

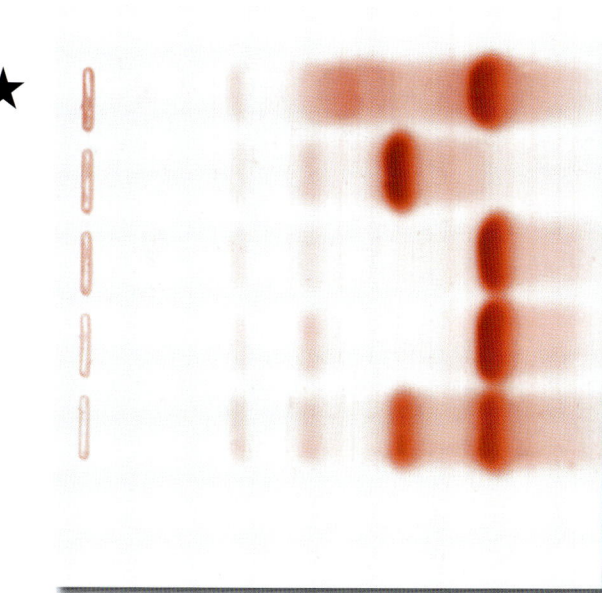

- origin A_2 S   A   +

Acid Electrophoresis (pH 6.2)

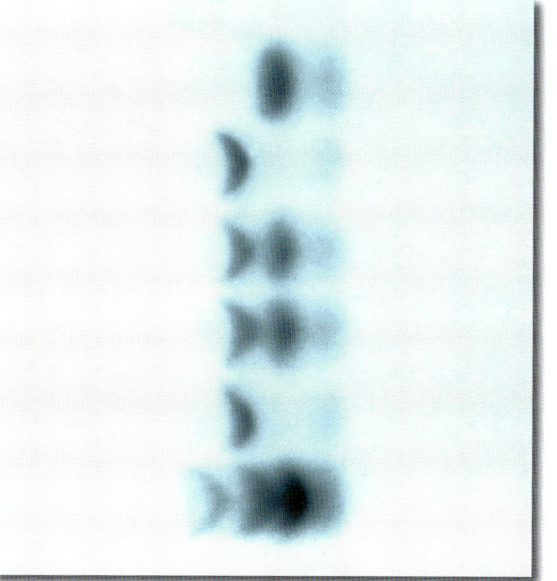

+   C   S   A   F   -

Case Studies

Case 37 Discussion

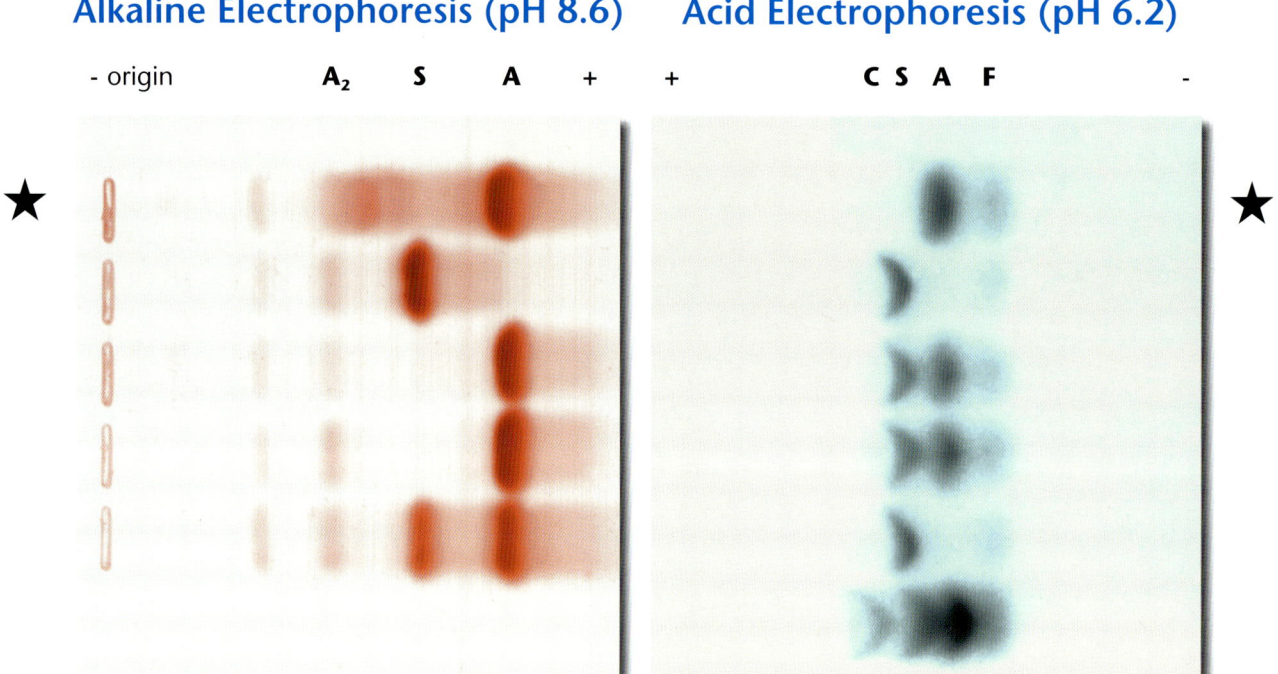

Interpretation

The alkaline electrophoresis demonstrates a broad band or smudge extending from the S region to the C region. Acid electrophoresis demonstrates a normal pattern.

Diagnosis

Hb Köln trait.

Performance

Hb Köln has been used three times in the survey. Most laboratories using both alkaline and acid electrophoresis identified the presence of a slow hemoglobin variant. In the interpretive portion, 55–83% of laboratories correctly identified this as an unstable hemoglobin disorder.

Discussion

Hb Köln results from a valine to methionine substitution at the 98th amino acid position of the β globin chain (β98 Val→Met). Interestingly, the amino acid substitution in Hb Köln does not alter the charge on the hemoglobin molecule, yet this hemoglobin separates from Hb A on alkaline electrophoresis. This results from the fact that the amino acid substitution occurs at a site important for both β chain contact and heme contact. Therefore, besides overall instability of the globin chain tetramer, Hb Köln easily loses heme groups from the abnormal β chains, particularly during electrophoresis, and thus loses negative charges. Interestingly, if excess heme is added to the hemolysate, Hb Köln will migrate with Hb A. The pathophysiology of Hb Köln, as well as other unstable hemoglobins, relates to amino acid substitutions in contact sites that maintain the quaternary structure of hemoglobin. Destabilization of hemoglobin structure results in denaturation and precipitation, with the production of Heinz bodies. Heinz bodies impair red cell deformability and thus shorten the red cell life span. The degree of hemolysis associated with the various unstable hemoglobins ranges from mild to severe. Interestingly, in addition to being unstable, Hb Köln has increased oxygen affinity, and cases associated with erythrocytosis have been reported. All described unstable hemoglobins have been seen in the heterozygous state; homozygous inheritance is presumably incompatible with life. Hb Köln is encountered predominantly in individuals of German or Dutch extraction but has also been found in other ethnic groups. It has been observed as a de novo mutation.

The clinical findings in this case are typical of Hb Köln. As in this case, there is an autosomal dominant mode of familial transmission. Within a given family, the clinical manifestations are quite uniform. The hemolysis is generally mild and well compensated, with minimal or no anemia. However, patients will have evidence of a chronic hemolytic disorder, with scleral icterus, splenomegaly, and reticulocytosis. In addition, hemolysis may be exacerbated in association with infections or with exposure to certain drugs. The blood smear demonstrates macrocytic, hypochromic red cells. (It should be noted that red cell morphology is highly variable across the various unstable hemoglobins, i.e., there is no "typical" red cell morphology associated with unstable hemoglobins in general.) (See Figure 37.1.) Heinz bodies are typically not seen until after splenectomy in these patients. Figure 37.2 compares various disorders associated with Heinz bodies and Heinz-body-like inclusions. Patients with Hb Köln generally require no specific therapy (including splenectomy, which is likely of little value), and this disorder is compatible with a normal life span.

Key to making the appropriate diagnosis in this case is the positive test for hemoglobin instability. Unstable hemoglobins should be suspected when a chronic hemolytic anemia is associated with a heterozygous hemoglobin abnormality, assuming that no other causes of hemolysis are evident. Although more than 100 unstable hemoglobin variants have been described, most are exceedingly rare. Those most commonly encountered are hemoglobins E*, H, Köln, and Hasharon. The electrophoretic findings serve to exclude each of these except Hb Köln: Hb H (β tetramers seen in three-deletion α–thalassemia) is a fast moving hemoglobin on alkaline electrophoresis (more anodal than Hb A); Hb E migrates in the same position as C and A_2; and Hb Hasharon migrates in the S position on both alkaline

* Hemoglobin E is unstable in vitro, but this is not significant in vivo.

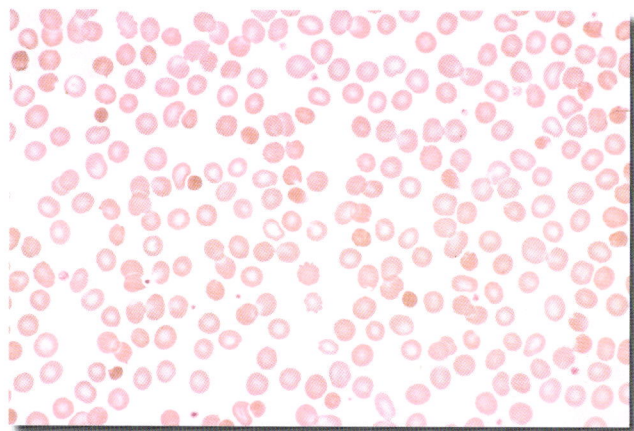
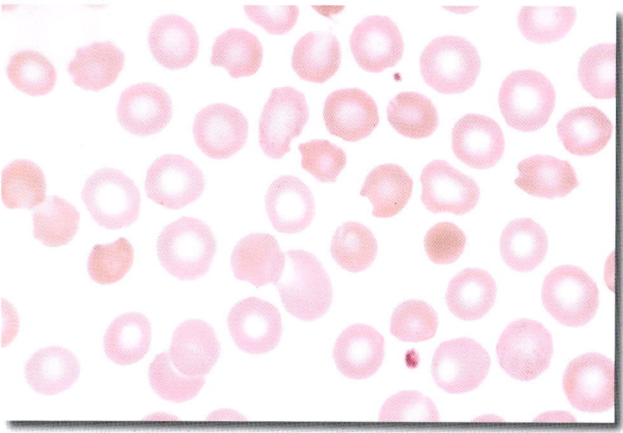

Figure 37.1 (Wright-Giemsa, 160x and 400x)
Low- and high-power views of the peripheral blood smear from a patient with Hb Köln trait. This case shows the presence of bite cells and microspherocytes.

Figure 37.2
Disorders Associated with Precipitated Hemoglobin

Heinz bodies and H bodies, although both derived from hemoglobin, are distinctly different red cell inclusions. Heinz bodies represent precipitated hemoglobin molecules due to either severe oxidant drug reaction in normal individuals or in G-6PD deficiency or unstable hemoglobins.

The size and number of Heinz bodies vary with the ability of the body to handle the oxidative stress. If the red cell enzyme system can barely keep up, the Heinz bodies will be large and few in number. If the oxidative stress completely overwhelms an already weakened HMP shunt, as in G-6PD deficiency or in normal individuals if the amount of drug is excessive, the Heinz bodies will be small and numerous. Even the small variants of Heinz bodies are larger and lack the periodicity seen in hemoglobin H disease.

Unstable hemoglobin disease (also known as congenital Heinz body hemolytic anemia) is an uncommon hereditary hemolytic disorder that is autosomal dominant. Hb Köln is the most common of the 130 variants. Various amino acid substitutions or deletions lead to structural instability that predisposes the hemoglobin molecule to auto-oxidation. Depending on the structural abnormality, the anemia may be mild or dangerously severe. Although the inclusions formed are identical in composition to the Heinz bodies induced by oxidant drugs, they are larger and more irregular in shape. They are also more numerous in reticulocytes, unlike G-6PD deficiency in which reticulocytes are usually free of Heinz bodies.

Heinz bodies attach to the inner surface of the red cell membrane, deforming the skeletal matrix. The rigid structures are excised as the cell navigates through the spleen producing bite deformities and teardrop cells. Heinz bodies are most frequently observed in splenectomized individuals.

In the thalassemia majors, the entire hemoglobin molecule does not precipitate. Instead, excess alpha or beta chains accumulate in the red cell cytoplasm. In hemoglobin H disease, a triple alpha gene deletion results in excess beta globin chains.

Beta-thalassemia major, also known as homozygous β-thalassemia or Cooley's anemia, is a rare congenital severe hemolytic anemia that can result in debilitation and premature death. Homozygous β+-thal accounts for about 90% of cases, while homozygous β⁰-thal is responsible for most of the rest. The complete or near complete lack of beta chain production results in excess alpha hemoglobin chains. About 10% of the hemoglobin in marrow reticulocytes is made up of free α chains. The α hemoglobin chains lose the heme portion, undergo denaturation and oxidation, and precipitate. The number and distribution determine the severity of anemia. The aggregates of insoluble surplus α chains deposit within the nucleus, interfering with cell division, and bind to the inner aspect of the red cell cytoskeleton. The inclusions damage the red cell membrane and limit egress from the marrow. The cells that do make it into the circulation are trapped by the spleen and further pitted and culled from the blood stream. Like Heinz bodies, the alpha chain inclusion bodies are visible by means of supravital stains but not Wright-Giemsa.

Alpha-thalassemia associated with deletion of three of the four α globin genes results in hemoglobin H disease. These inclusions represent excess beta chains which arrange themselves into unstable tetramers (β₄), designated hemoglobin H. They are smaller than Heinz bodies and have an even distribution, likened to the dimples on a golf ball. Although similar in some respects, neither H bodies nor alpha chain inclusions are true Heinz bodies.

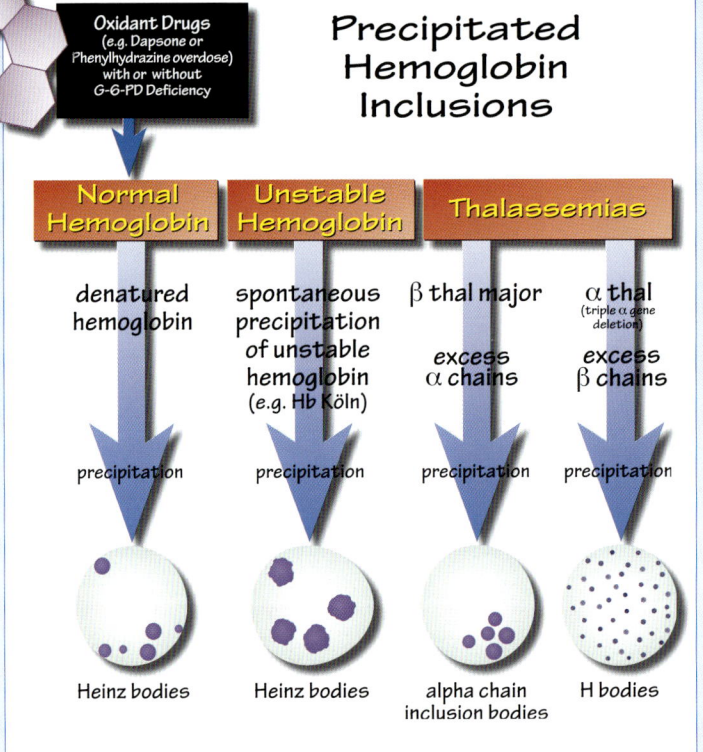

Adapted from Glassy EF, ed. Color Atlas of Hematology. *Northfield, IL: College of American Pathologists; 1998:133.*

and acid electrophoresis. Hb Köln typically produces a broad band or smudge in the general region of Hb S and comprises approximately 25% of the total hemoglobin. This characteristic electrophoretic pattern, in association with evidence of in vitro and in vivo instability, allows a confident diagnosis in most cases. Examples of Hb Köln on HPLC and isoelectric focusing are shown in Figures 37.3 and 37.4.

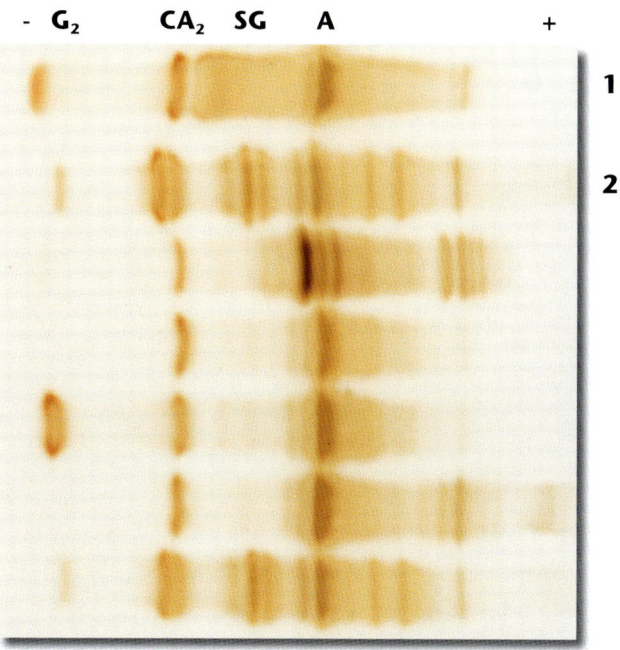

Figure 37.4
An example of Hb Köln by isoelectric focusing (lane 1). A distinct band is not present. However, there is a broad smear between the A and A_2 positions. A band seen cathodal to the A_2 position represents denatured hemoglobin. Lane 2-control.

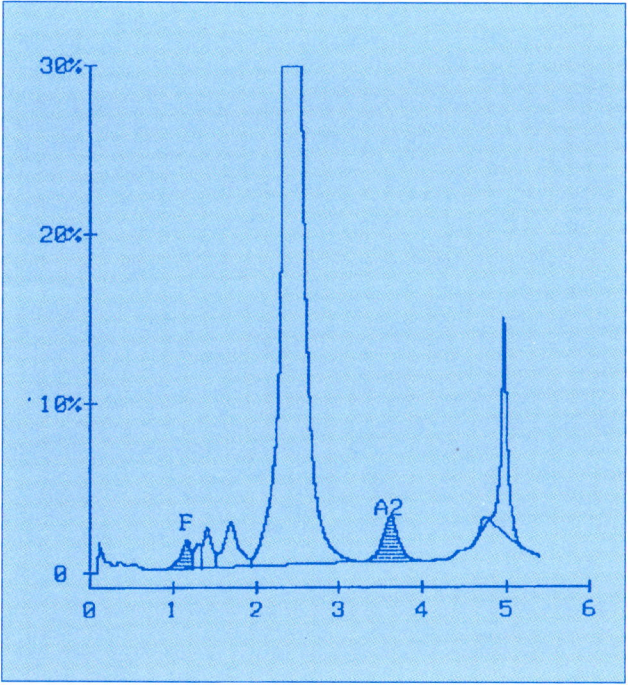

Figure 37.3
An example of Hb Köln by HPLC. In this example, Hb Köln is eluting in the C window at approximately 4.95 minutes; it can also elute between the S and C windows at a slightly slower retention time.

References

Carrell RW, Lehmann H, Hutchison HE. Haemoglobin Köln (beta-98 valine→methionine): an unstable protein causing inclusion-body anaemia. *Nature.* 1966;210:915-916.

Egan EL, Fairbanks VF. Postsplenectomy erythrocytosis in hemoglobin Köln disease. *N Engl J Med.* 1973;288:929-931.

Fairbanks VF, Opfell RW, Burgert EO, Jr. Three families with unstable hemoglobinopathies (Köln, Olmsted and Santa Ana) causing hemolytic anemia with inclusion bodies and pigmenturia. *Am J Med.* 1969;46:344-359.

Ohba Y. Unstable hemoglobins. *Hemoglobin.* 1990;14: 353-388.

Pribilla W, Klesse P, Betke K, Lehmann H, Beale D. [Hemoglobin Koln disease: familial hypochromic hemolytic anemia with hemoglobin anomaly]. *Klin Wochenschr.* 1965;43:1049-1053.

Case 38

HISTORY

The patient is a 23-year-old woman of German/Swiss/English ancestry, who is asymptomatic. At age 16, following a minor surgical procedure, she was prescribed phenazopyridine (Pyridium), in conventional dosage, as a urinary tract analgesic; within 48 hours, she was jaundiced. Hematological examination revealed Hb = 7 g/dL, Hct = 21%, RBC = 2.06×10^{12}/L, reticulocytes = 95×10^9/L (4.6%). Blood smear revealed moderate polychromasia and keratocytes ("bite cells") and occasional pale blue erythrocyte inclusions, approximately 2 microns in diameter. Her serum bilirubin concentration was 4.2 mg/dL indirect, 5 mg/dL total. Upon withdrawal of the phenazopyridine, the hemolysis subsided; blood counts returned to normal and have remained normal except for a slight persistent reticulocytosis.

A few decades earlier, the patient's mother had become jaundiced during pregnancy, after taking sulfonamides for treatment of a urinary tract infection. She had splenomegaly and anemia requiring transfusion. She underwent splenectomy as treatment of the hemolytic anemia. She has subsequently been well, and her hemoglobin concentration, erythrocyte count, and hematocrit are normal. Her physical examination is normal. She has a slight persistent reticulocytosis, and her blood film, following Wright stain, reveals target cells, acanthocytes, Howell-Jolly bodies, polychromasia, and pale blue erythrocyte inclusions. A hemoglobin variant was found in blood obtained from her mother, maternal uncle, and maternal first cousin. None are anemic, and only the mother has had a splenectomy.

BLOOD COUNT DATA

RBC .... 4.35×10^{12}/L
Hb .... 14.5 g/dL
MCV .... 101 fL
WBC .... 8.4×10^9/L
Plt .... 343×10^9/L

PERIPHERAL BLOOD SMEAR

Slight polychromasia, occasional pale blue erythrocyte inclusions, approximately 2 microns in diameter.

OTHER LABORATORY TESTS

A stain for Heinz bodies confirmed that the erythrocyte inclusions stain with crystal violet. Measurement of erythrocyte glucose-6-phosphate dehydrogenase activity indicated normal values. The solubility test for sickling hemoglobin was negative.
Reticulocytes = 97×10^9/L (2%) (normal: $30\text{-}87 \times 10^9$/L)

Alkaline Electrophoresis (pH 8.6)

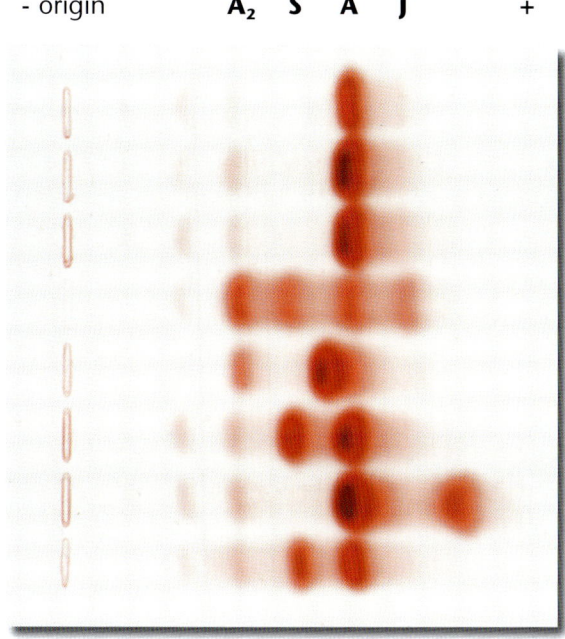

Acid Electrophoresis (pH 6.2)

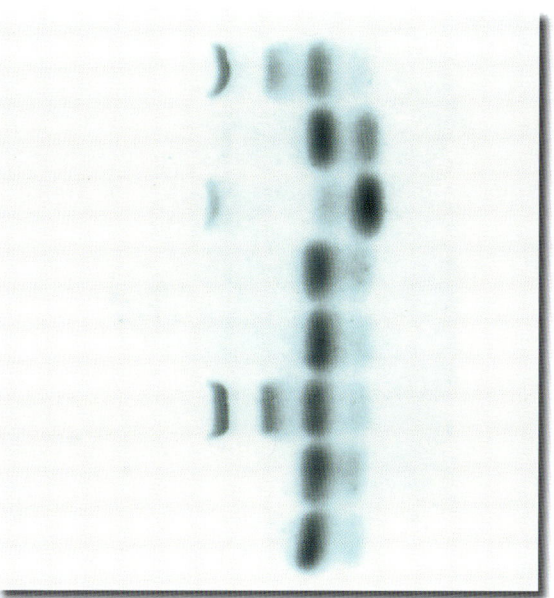

Case 38 Discussion

Alkaline Electrophoresis (pH 8.6) Acid Electrophoresis (pH 6.2)

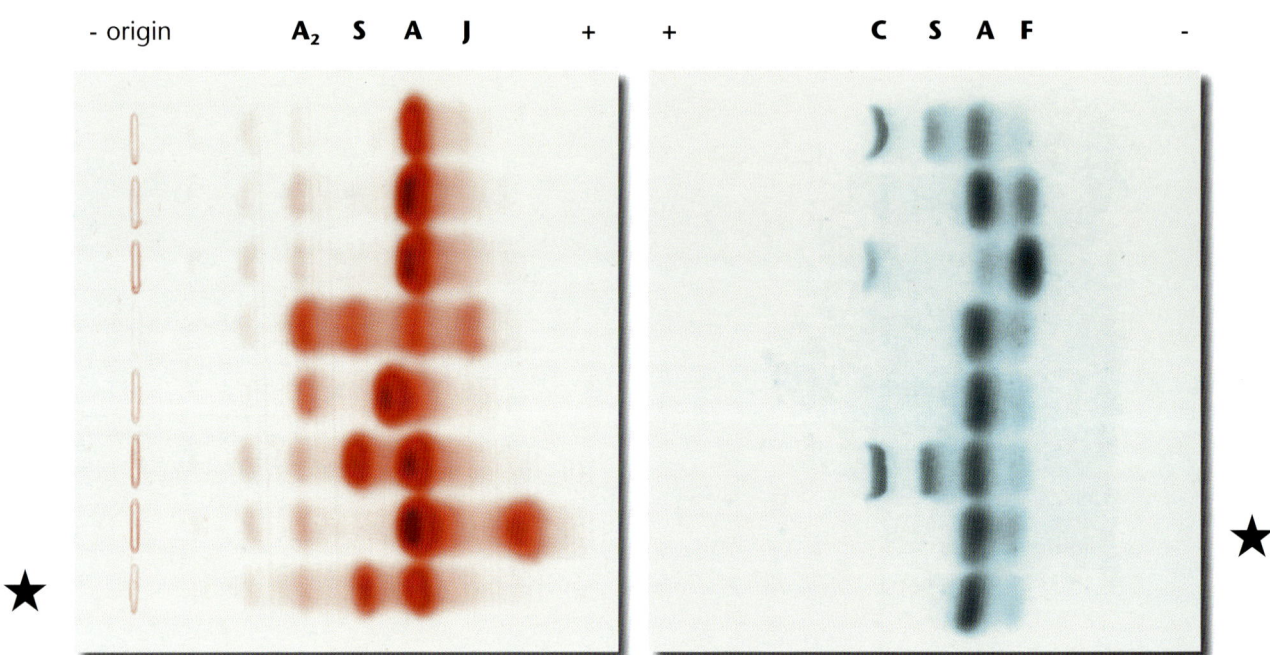

Interpretation

On alkaline electrophoresis, there are two bands seen, one in the A position and one in the S position. On acid electrophoresis, however, there is only a band in the A position. The quantitative measurement for Hb A_2 was slightly elevated at 3.7%. Further testing, including globin chain electrophoresis, isoelectric focusing, HPLC, and DNA sequencing, identified the variant as Hb Zürich.

Diagnosis

Hb Zürich trait.

Performance

Exact identification of the variant was not required; 69.3% of laboratories correctly reported the presence of an unstable hemoglobin.

Discussion

Hb Zürich is a rare unstable hemoglobin variant that results from a histidine to arginine substitution at the 63rd position of the β globin chain (β63 His→Arg). This position in the β chain is a critical heme contact, as it is the site of the normal "distal histidine," which participates in configurational changes that occur with oxygenation and deoxygenation. Normally, the imidazole side chain of the histidine at this position swings away from the heme group to permit the entry of oxygen and back toward the heme group when oxygen leaves the heme pocket. The replacement of histidine by arginine results in a shift in the amino acids in this helical region and also in an increase in oxygen affinity. The introduction of a more hydrophilic amino acid at this site contributes to the destabilization of binding of heme to globin, and thereby instability of the hemoglobin molecule. The substitution at this site of tyrosine for histidine (in methemoglobin M-Saskatoon), is associated with methemoglobinemia, and it would not be surprising if some degree of methemoglobinemia existed in persons with Hb Zürich. Indeed, the patient in the current case had a slightly elevated methemoglobin concentration. Hb Zürich is seen primarily in those of Swiss ancestry but has also been reported from Japan.

As in congenital deficiency of glucose 6-phosphate dehydrogenase, hemolysis in Hb Zürich is induced or exacerbated by exposure to oxidant drugs. These include sulfonamides, sulfones, phenacetin-like analgesics, and most of the local anesthetics. Typically, patients with Hb Zürich have recurrent bouts of acute hemolysis precipitated by treatment with drugs or by acute respiratory infections. Otherwise, they are well and asymptomatic. During a hemolytic episode, numerous Heinz bodies are demonstrable in most of the red cells. Oddly, the Heinz bodies associated with Hb Zurich are seen with routine Giemsa stains, whereas in other Heinz body hemolytic anemias, they are invisible unless supravital stains are applied. Other unstable hemoglobin variants that respond similarly to oxidant stress include hemoglobins H, Hasharon, Mequon, Shepherd's Bush, Bushwick, Peterborough, Torino, Buenos Aires, and possibly others. However, it is prudent to advise patients and their physicians that any of the unstable hemoglobin disorders might have an exacerbation of hemolysis following exposure to these substances.

Hb Zurich migrates in the S position on alkaline electrophoresis and in the A position on acid electrophoresis. It typically represents 22-35% of total hemoglobin (all patients described have been heterozygous). Definitive identification of this variant is not possible with routine methods. However, a key study is the demonstration of in vitro instability. As in the current case, unstable hemoglobins (particularly Hb Tacoma) are sometimes associated with elevations of Hb A_2 and do not imply concurrent β-thalassemia trait.

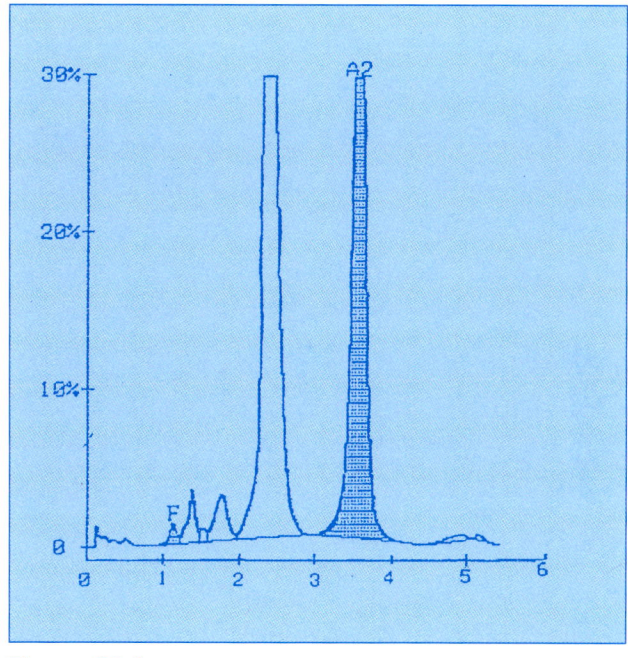

Figure 38.1
An example of Hb Zürich trait by HPLC. Hb Zürich elutes in the A_2 position, with a retention time of approximately 3.55 minutes.

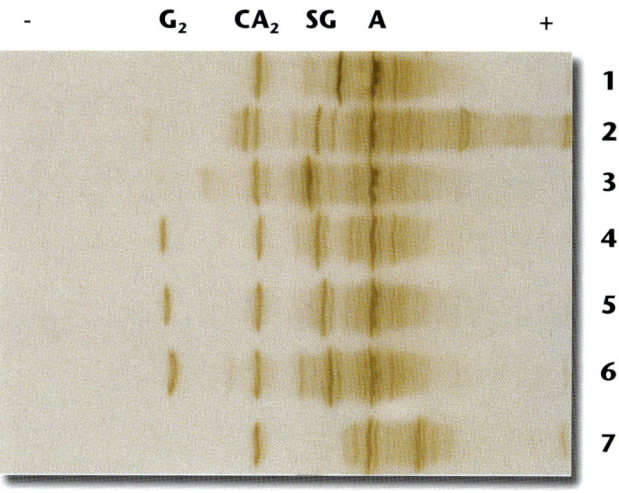

Figure 38.2
An example of Hb Zürich by isoelectric focusing (lane 3). Hb Zürich migrates slightly cathodal to the Hb S position. Lane 1- Hb G-San Jose, 2-control, 4-Hb Hasharon, 5-Hb Q-Iran, 6-Hb G-Philadelphia, 7-Hb N-Baltimore.

Case Studies

References

Aguinaga NDP, Wright CPJ, Roa PD, et al. Molecular characterization of hemoglobin Zürich (β63 His→Arg) identifies a CAT→CGT change at the DNA sequence. *Eighteenth Annual Meeting of the National Sickle Cell Disease Program.* 1993;110A.

Bachmann F, Marti HR. Hemoglobin Zürich, II: physiochemical properties of the abnormal hemoglobin. *Blood.* 1962;20:272-286.

Dickerman JD, Holtzman NA, Zinkham WH. Hemoglobin Zürich. *Am J Med.* 1973;55:638-642.

Frick PG, Hitzig WH, Betke K. Hemoglobin Zürich, I: a new hemoglobin anomaly associated with acute hemolytic episodes with inclusion bodies after sulfonamide therapy. *Blood.* 1962;20:261-271.

Frick PG, Hitzig WH, Stauffer U. Das Hämoglobin -Zürich-Syndrome. *Schweiz Med Wchnschr.* 1961;91:1203-1205.

Giacometti GM, Brunori M, Antonini E, Di Iorio EE, Winterhalter KH. The reaction of hemoglobin Zürich with oxygen and carbon monoxide. *J Biol Chem.* 1980;255(13):6160-6165.

Hitzig WH, Frick PG, Betke K, Huisman THJ. Hemoglobin Zürich: eine neue Hämoglobinanomalie mit sulfonamidinduzierter Innenkörperan-5mie. *Helv PJd Act.* 1960;15:399-513.

Muller CJ, Kingma S. Haemoglobin Zürich: $\alpha_2\beta_2$ 63Arg. *Biochim Biophys Acta.* 1961;40:595-596.

Rieder RF, Zinkharn WH, Holtzman NA. Hemoglobin Zürich: clinical, chemical and kinetic studies. *Am J Med.* 1965;39:4-20.

Tucker PW, Phillips SEV, Perutz MF, Houtchens R, Caughey WS. Structure of hemoglobins Zürich, β63 [βHis E7 63 His→Arg] and Sydney, β67 [E11] Val→Ala and role of the distal residues in ligand binding. *Proc Natl Acad Sci USA.* 1978;75:1076-1080.

Winterhalter KH, Anderson NM, Amiconi G, Antonini E, Brunori M. Functional properties of hemoglobin Zürich. *Eur J Biochem.* 1969;11:435-440.

Zinkham WH, Houtchens RA, Caughey WS. Relation between variations in the phenotypic expression of an unstable hemoglobin disorder (hemoglobin Zürich) and carboxyhemoglobin levels. *Am J Med.* 1983;74(1):23-29.

Zinkham WH, Liljestrand JD, Dixon SM, Hutchison JL. Observations on the rate and mechanisms of hemolysis in individuals with Hb Zürich, β63 (E7) His→Arg, II: thermal denaturation of hemoglobin as a cause of anemia during fever. *Johns Hopkins Med J.* 1979;144: 109-116.

Zinkham WH, Rieder RIF, Holtzman NA. Hemoglobin Zürich: chemical and kinetic studies. *J Clin Invest.* 1963;42:996.

Case 39

HISTORY

The patient is a 43-year-old male of Swiss ancestry who was seen for evaluation of polycythemia. He was asymptomatic. He stated that he had always had quite a rosy-pink complexion and that some of his brothers, sisters and cousins were being treated by phlebotomy for polycythemia

The physical examination was unremarkable except for facial plethora. The spleen was not palpable.

BLOOD COUNT DATA

RBC .... 6.8 x 10^{12}/L
Hgb .... 19.8 g/dL
MCV .... 89 fL
WBC .... 7.8 x 10^9/L
Plt .... 256 x 10^9/L

PERIPHERAL BLOOD SMEAR

Unremarkable except for slight crowding of erythrocytes.

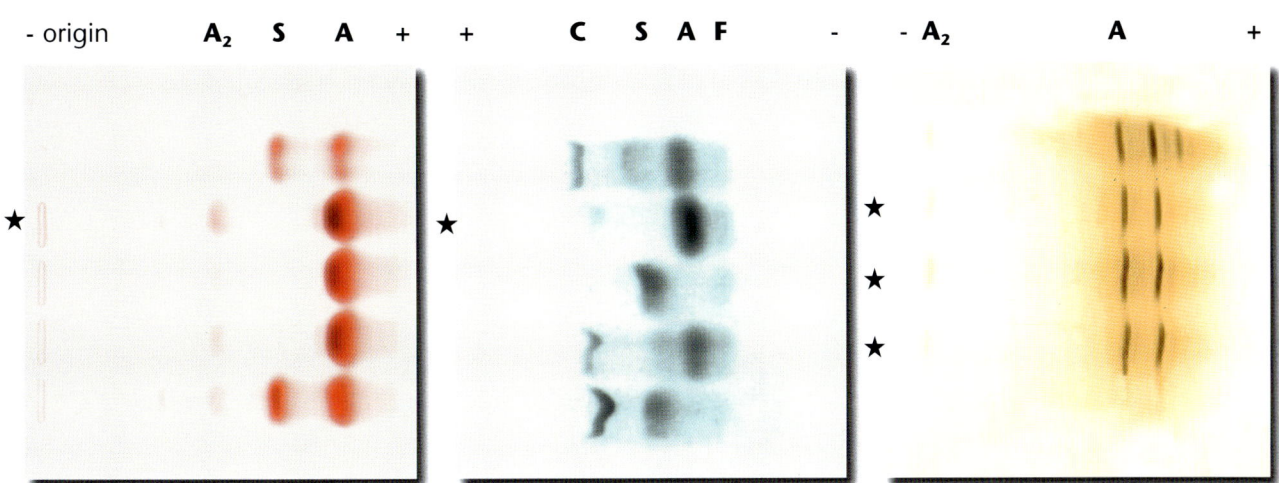

Alkaline Electrophoresis (pH 8.6)   Acid Electrophoresis (pH 6.2)   Isoelectric Focusing

Case 39 Discussion

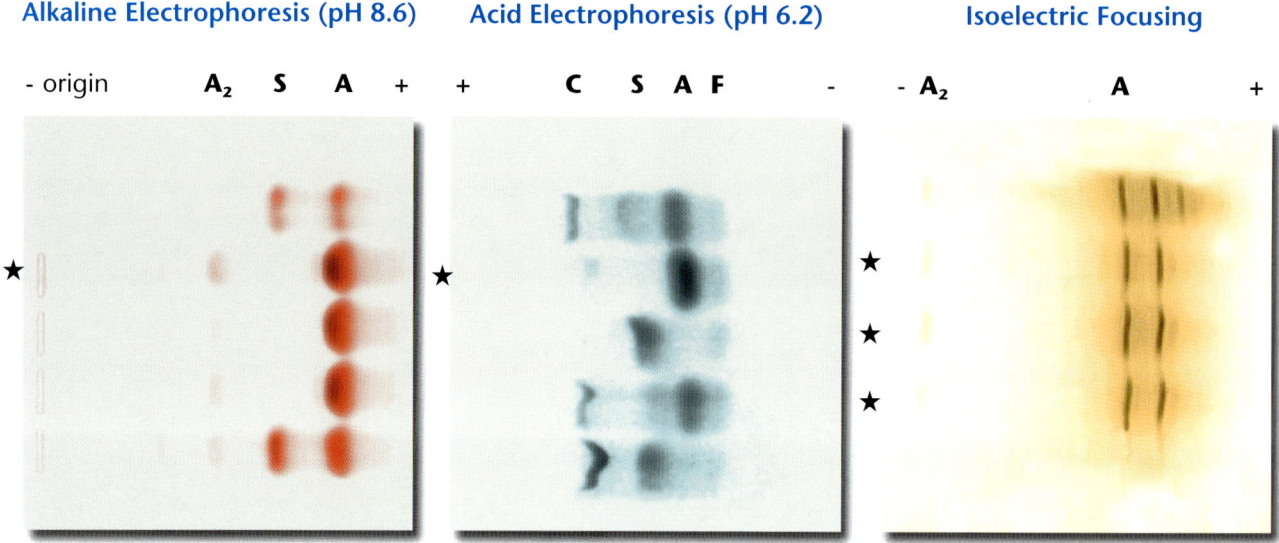

Interpretation

On alkaline and acid electrophoresis, there are no abnormal bands seen. However, on isoelectric focusing, there is a second band seen which is slightly anodal to Hb A. Other ancillary procedures, such as globin chain electrophoresis and HPLC, identify this variant as Hb Malmö.

Diagnosis

Hb Malmö trait.

Performance

Hb Malmö has been included in the survey twice. Exact identification was not required. However, 53% and 56.9% of laboratories correctly reported the presence of a high oxygen affinity hemoglobin variant.

Discussion

Hb Malmö is one of over 100 high oxygen affinity hemoglobin variants that have been described. It is characterized by the substitution of a glutamine for a histidine at the 97th amino acid of the β chain (β97 His→Gln). The mutation in Hb Malmö is at a critical site in the FG segment of the β globin chain, at which movement normally occurs during oxygenation and deoxygenation. The FG segment, also called the *FG corner*, acts like a switch in the communication between α and β globin chains, so that the uptake and release of oxygen can be properly coordinated. The substitution of glutamine for histidine at this critical site tends to lock the affected αβ dimer into the oxy-configuration; it is unable to release oxygen efficiently. Another segment of the β chain that is critical to normal function of the hemoglobin molecule is the short C-terminal nonhelical region of the β globin chain. Mutations in or near this site are also typically associated with impaired oxygen release (high oxygen affinity). These substitutions appear to inhibit deoxygenation by impairing 2,3 DPG binding at positions β 143 and β 146. The importance of these regions to regulation of oxygen affinity is exemplified by the effects of changes in the amino acid sequences in the HC segment or the FG corner of the β globin chain, as shown in Tables 39.1 and 39.2. Amino acid substitutions in the analogous regions of the α globin chain are also associated with polycythemia.

When hemoglobin has an abnormally high affinity for oxygen, the oxygen saturation remains high even at very low levels of oxygen tension. Measurement of the oxygen affinity of whole blood that contains Hb Malmö shows a markedly leftward-shifted curve (p50 of about 13 torr compared to normal values of 26-30 torr) with a hyperbolic rather than sigmoidal shape. A hemoglobin that cannot unload oxygen is essentially nonfunctional, and at normal levels of venous hemoglobin concentration or hematocrit, persons with Hb Malmö are functionally anemic. As a result, there is a compensatory increase in erythropoietin production, which produces erythrocytosis. All described patients with Hb Malmö have been heterozygous, as the homozygous state is likely to be incompatible with life (although one reported patient with Hb Malmö/β°-thalassemia had a hematocrit of 90%!). Thus, the pattern of inheritance is autosomal dominant, as is evident in the current case.

Hb Malmö was first described from southern Sweden. Hb Malmö has been described in two families in Sweden, one in Sicily, and two very large families in the United States. Neither of the American families is known to have Swedish or Sicilian ancestry.

The laboratory data shown in the case summary are typical for patients with Hb Malmö. There is likely to be an increase in blood viscosity in patients with any of the hemoglobinopathies that are associated with erythrocytosis. Most patients are asymptomatic, have no impairment in physical capacity, and have normal longevity. However, some patients have fatigue, headaches, or light-headedness, which are alleviated by phlebotomy. In addition, the frequency of strokes and myocardial infarctions seems to be higher than in the general population, particularly in those patients who also smoke (thereby making the erythrocytosis more pronounced and the viscosity of blood higher). It is prudent to advise all persons with high oxygen affinity hemoglobins to refrain from smoking and avoid other forms of chronic carbon monoxide exposure; those who are symptomatic may benefit from periodic phlebotomy. Whether all persons with these hemoglobinopathies who have erythrocytosis should undergo phlebotomy regularly is a question that is as yet unresolved.

Hemoglobin Malmö is not seen on alkaline electrophoresis with commonly used media. However, it is readily demonstrated by other techniques, including HPLC (Figure 39.1) and isoelectric focusing. In the heterozygous state, Hb Malmö accounts for approximately 48% of the total hemoglobin. While Hb Malmö will not be detected by routine methods, the presence of familial erythrocytosis inherited in an autosomal fashion is nearly diagnostic for a high oxygen affinity hemoglobin.

Table 39.1 β Chain Variants in FG "Corner" and G Helix

Position	Helical #	Substitution	Name	Effect
94	FG1	Asp→His	Barcelona	polycythemia
		Asp→Asn	Bunbury	normal
95	FG2	Lys→Asn	Detroit	normal
		Lys→Glu	N-Baltimore	normal
97	FG4	His→Gln	Malmö	polycythemia
		His→Leu	Wood	polycythemia
98	FG5	Val→Met	Köln	hemolysis (high O_2 affinity)
		Val→Gly	Nottingham	hemolysis
		Val→Ala	Djelfa	(?)
99	G1	Asp→Asn	Kempsey	polycythemia
		Asp→His	Yakima	polycythemia
		Asp→Ala	Radcliffe	polycythemia
		Asp→Tyr	Ypsilanti	polycythemia
		Asp→Gly	Hotel Dieu	polycythemia
		Asp→Val	Chemilly	polycythemia
100	G2	Pro→Leu	Brigham	polycythemia
101	G3	Glu→Gly	Alberta	polycythemia
		Glu→Gln	Rush	hemolysis
		Glu→Asp	Potomac	polycythemia
		Glu→Lys	British Columbia	polycythemia
102	G4	Asn→Lys	Richmond	normal
		Asn→Thr	Kansas	cyanosis
		Asn→Ser	Beth Israel	cyanosis
		Asn→Tyr	Saint Mandé	cyanosis
103	G5	Phe→Leu	Heathrow	polycythemia

Table 39.2 β Chain Variants Near the C-Terminus

Position	Helical #	Substitution	Name	Effect
143	H21	His→Arg	Abbruzzo	polycythemia
		His→Gln	Little Rock	polycythemia
		His→Pro	Syracuse	polycythemia
		His→Asp	Rancho Mirage	(?)
		His→Tyr	Old Dominion	normal CBC, slight increased O_2 affinity
144	HC1	Lys→Asn	Andrew-Minneapolis	polycythemia
		Lys→Glu	Mito	polycythemia
145	HC2	Tyr→His	Bethesda	polycythemia
		Tyr→Cys	Rainier	polycythemia
		Tyr→Asn*	Osler	polycythemia
		Tyr→Stop	McKees Rocks	polycythemia
146	HC3	His→Asp	Hiroshima	polycythemia
		His→Pro	York	polycythemia
		His→Arg	Cochin-Port Royal	(?)
		His→Leu	Cowtown	polycythemia
		His→Gln	Kodaira	polycythemia

* Originally reported as Asp

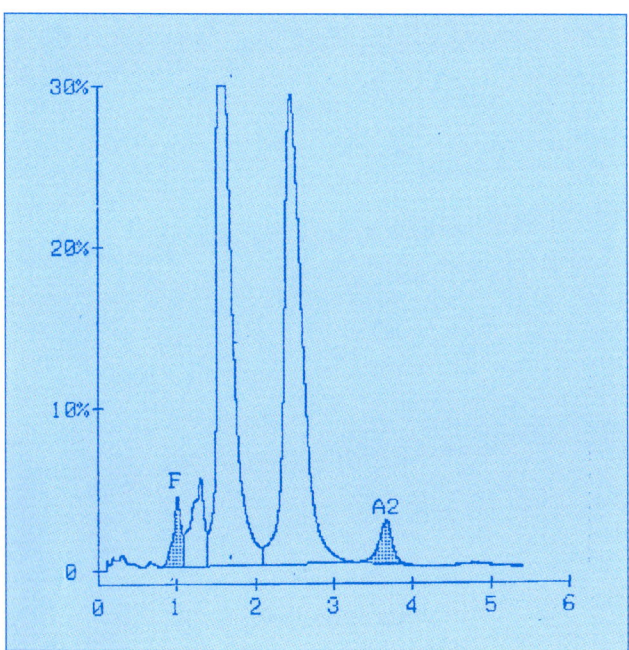

Figure 39.1
An example of Hb Malmö trait by HPLC. Hb Malmö elutes ahead of Hb A at approximately 1.60-1.70 minutes. This is usually in the P3 window.

References

Boyer SH, Charache S, Fairbanks VF, Maldonado JE, Noyes A, Gayle EE. Hemoglobin Malmö-97 (FG4) histidine→glutamine: a cause of polycythemia. *J Clin Invest.* 1972;51:666-676.

Fairbanks VF, Maldonado JE, Charache S, et al. Familial erythrocytosis due to electrophoretically undetectable hemoglobin with impaired oxygen dissociation (hemoglobin Malmö, $\alpha_2\beta_2$ 97 glu). *Mayo Clin Proc.* 1971;46:721-727.

Girino M, Riccardi A, Mosca A, Paleari R, Bonomo P. Double heterozygosity for hemoglobin Malmö [β97 (FG4) His→Glu] and β-thalassemia traits. *Haematologica.* 1989;74:187-190.

Landin B, Berglund S, Wallman K. Two different mutations in codon 97 of the beta-globin gene cause Hb Malmö in Sweden. *Am J Hematol.* 1996;51:32-36.

Lorkin PA, Lehmann H, Fairbanks VF, Berglund G, Leonhardt T. Two new pathologic hemoglobins: Olmsted [beta 141 (H9) Len→Arg] and Malmö [beta 97 (FG4) His→Glu]. *Biochem J.* 1970;119:68.

McCormack NK, Zak SJ, Geller GR, et al. A new kindred with hemoglobin Malmö (beta 97 His→Gln) (letter). *J Pediatr.* 1976;88:1061-1063.

Zak SJ, Geller GR, Krivit W, et al. A hypothesis for the increased oxygen affinity in haemoglobin Malmö. *Br J Haematol.* 1976;33:101-107.

Case 40

HISTORY
The patient is a 35-year-old white male who presented to his local medical doctor because of easy fatigability. He was otherwise asymptomatic. He was not a smoker. The physical examination showed that other than facial rubor, no abnormalities were noted. Specifically, there was no hepatomegaly nor splenomegaly, and he had no tremor or ataxia.

BLOOD COUNT DATA
RBC ....7.1 x 10^{12}/L
Hgb ....22.0 g/dL
MCV ....92.0 fl
WBC ....6.0 x 10^9/L
Plt ....250.0 x 10^9/L

PERIPHERAL BLOOD SMEAR
Mild crowding of erythrocytes.

OTHER LABORATORY TESTS
Arterial blood gas study revealed pO_2 110 mm Hg, 98% O_2 saturation, and 0.2% carboxyhemoglobin.

Alkaline Electrophoresis (pH 8.6)

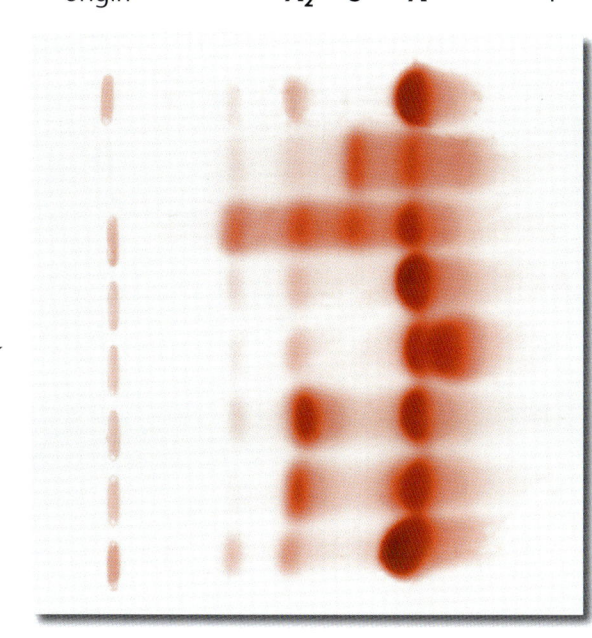

Acid Electrophoresis (pH 6.2)

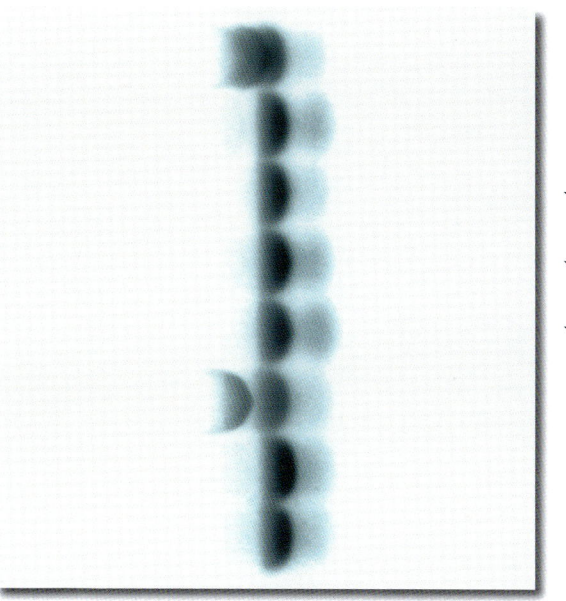

Case Studies

Case 40 Discussion

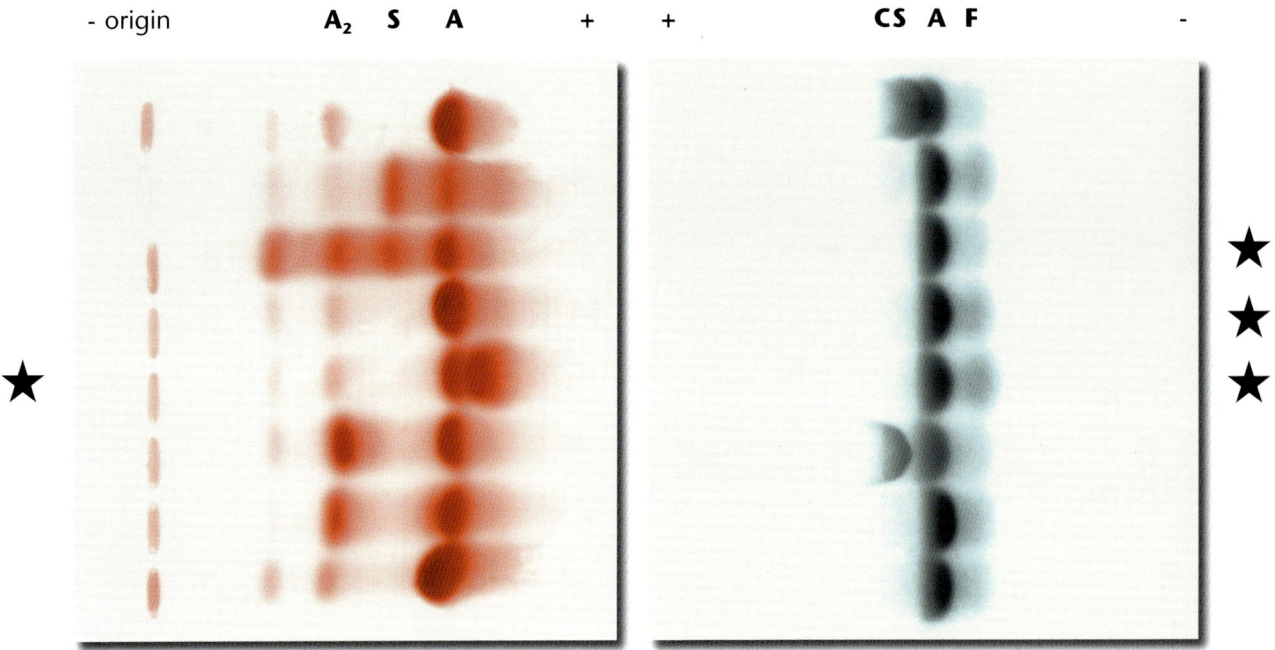

Interpretation

On alkaline electrophoresis, there are two bands seen, one is in the A position and a fast band anodal to Hb A. On acid electrophoresis, there is only a band in the A position. Other methods identified the hemoglobin variant as Hb Andrew-Minneapolis.

Diagnosis

Hb Andrew-Minneapolis trait.

Performance

Laboratories were not expected to identify the hemoglobin variant; 79.3% of laboratories correctly identified the presence of a high oxygen affinity hemoglobin variant.

Discussion

Hb Andrew-Minneapolis is another example of a high oxygen affinity hemoglobin. This variant results from a lysine to asparagine substitution at the 144th position of the beta chain (β144 Lys→Asn). Hb Andrew-Minneapolis is one of several Hb variants with amino acid alterations in or near the short C-terminal nonhelical region of the β globin chain that result in high oxygen affinity (see Case 39). Cases of Hb Andrew-Minneapolis have been reported in a family from Minnesota of German descent as well as in patients from Japan, Bulgaria, and Germany.

The clinical history and laboratory data that were provided are typical for high oxygen affinity Hb disorders as a group (see Case 39) as well as for persons with Hb Andrew-Minneapolis. Patients with Hb Andrew-Minneapolis typically have hematocrits in the range of 52-57%.

The electrophoretic findings in this case are typical of Hb Andrew-Minneapolis. Typically, the abnormal band comprises approximately 45% of total hemoglobin. While additional studies are required to definitively identify this variant, the fact that it represented a high oxygen affinity hemoglobin was strongly suggested by the clinical history. Examples of Hb Andrew-Minneapolis trait on HPLC and isoelectric focusing are shown in Figures 40.1 and 40.2.

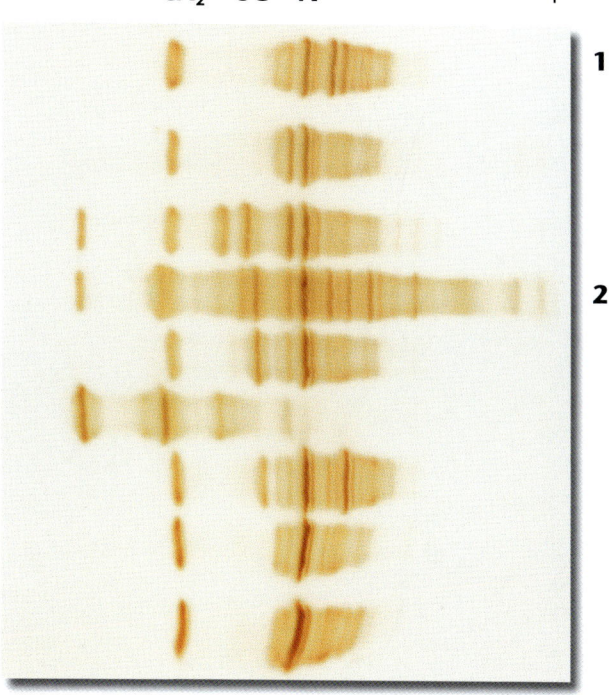

Figure 40.2
An example of Hb Andrew-Minneapolis trait by isoelectric focusing (lane 1). Hb Andrew-Minneapolis appears as a band anodal to Hb A. Lane 2 is the control.

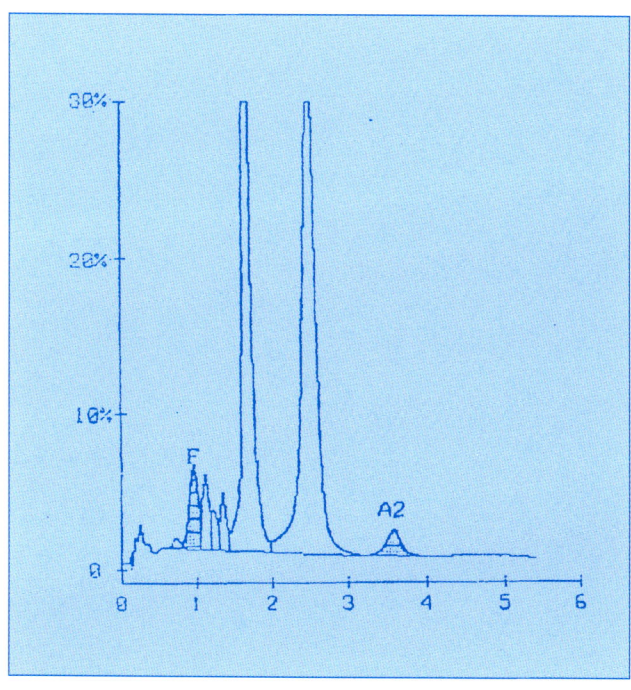

Figure 40.1
An example of Hb Andrew-Minneapolis trait by HPLC. Hb Andrew-Minneapolis elutes ahead of Hb A at approximately 1.65-1.70 minutes. This is usually in the P3 position.

References

Ahmed A, Jahan M, Braunitzer G, et al. Hb Andrew-Minneapolis [β144(HCl)Lys→Asn] in a German family. *Hemoglobin.* 1989;13:189-192.

Gomi T, Ikeda T, Harano T. Hemoglobin Andrew-Minneapolis [β144(HCl)Lys→Asn] in a Japanese family. *Intern Med.* 1992;31:659-661.

Hebbel RP, Kroenberg RS, Eaton JW. Hypoxic ventilatory response in subjects with normal and high oxygen affinity hemoglobins. *J Clin Invest.* 1977;60: 1211-1215.

Tasheva ES, Zareva ZZ, Toupuzova ST, Molchanova TP. Hb Andrew-Minneapolis [β144(HCl)Lys→Asn] in a Bulgarian family. *Hemoglobin.* 1990;14:227-228.

Zak SJ, Brimhall B, Jones RT, Kaplan ME. Hemoglobin Andrew-Minneapolis $\alpha_2^A\beta_2$144Lys→Asn: a new high oxygen-affinity mutant human hemoglobin. *Blood.* 1974;44:543-549.

Case 41

HISTORY
The patient is an asymptomatic 38-year-old Caucasian male, except that his skin exhibited a persistent generalized erythema. No abnormalities were noted on physical examination. He is not a smoker. Two of his five siblings were also known to have polycythemia.

BLOOD COUNT DATA
RBC..................7.2 x 10^{12}/L
Hb....................19.5 g/dL
MCV..................89.0 fL
WBC..................7.8 x 10^9/L
Plt.....................320 x 10^9/L

PERIPHERAL BLOOD SMEAR
Slight "crowding" of erythrocytes. Otherwise, unremarkable.

Alkaline Electrophoresis (pH 8.6)

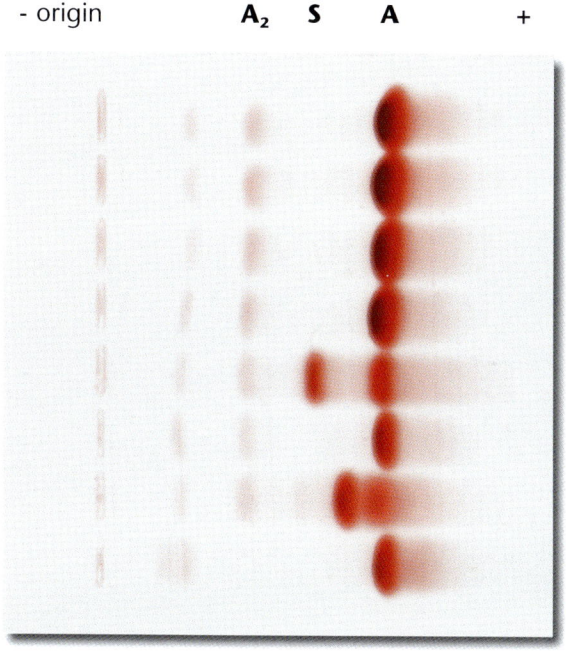

Acid Electrophoresis (pH 6.2)

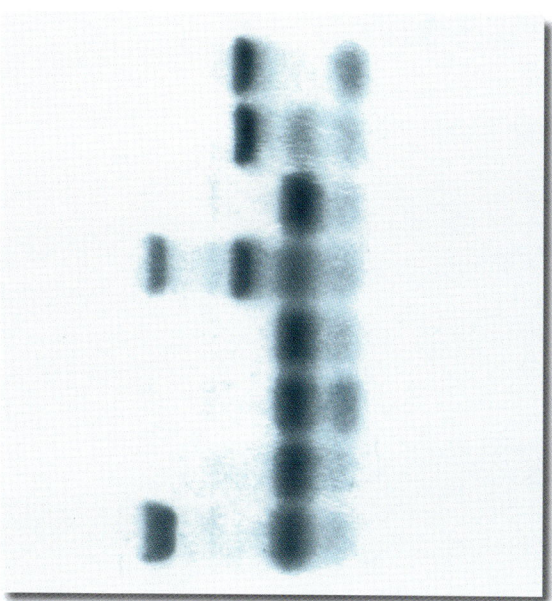

Case 41 Discussion

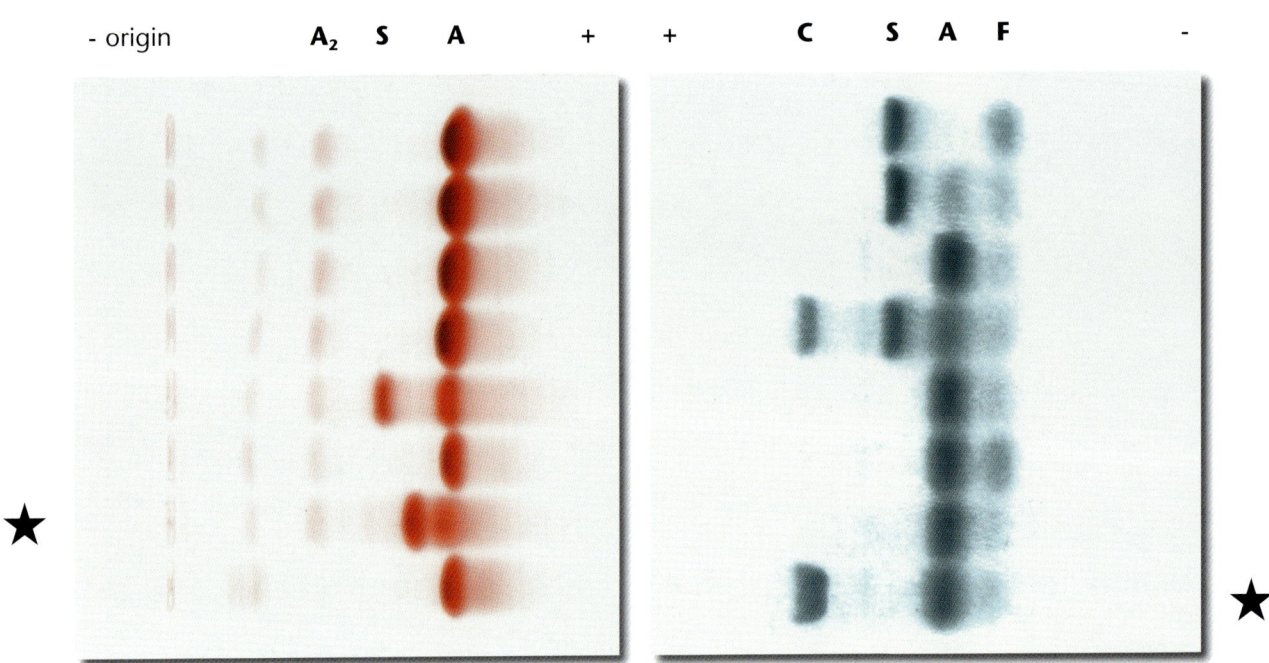

Alkaline Electrophoresis (pH 8.6)   Acid Electrophoresis (pH 6.2)

Interpretation

On alkaline electrophoresis, there are two major bands seen, one in the A position and one between the A and S positions. The band in the A position appears broad. On acid electrophoresis, there is a band in the A position and one in the C position. Other methods identified the variant as Hb British Columbia.

Diagnosis

Hb British Columbia trait.

Performance

Exact identification of the variant was not required; 83% of laboratories were correct in identifying the presence of a high oxygen affinity Hb variant.

Discussion

Hb British Columbia is a rare high oxygen affinity β chain variant resulting from a glutamic acid to lysine substitution at the 101st amino acid [β101 (G3) Glu→Lys]. The p50 of whole blood in this case was 14 mm Hg, with a dissociation curve that appeared nearly hyperbolic. Heterozygotes for Hb British Columbia have mild erythrocytosis.

Although hemoglobin British Columbia has the same type of amino acid substitution as Hb C, it does not behave as one might predict on alkaline electrophoresis, since it migrates between the Hb S and Hb A position. The aberrant Hb band seems to predominate, e.g., in a ratio to Hb A of about 60:40. The separated $β^A$ and $β^{BrCo}$ globin chains, however, are in the ratio of approximately 1:1. On isoelectric focusing, three bands may be seen; but with prolonged focusing, the middle band gradually diminishes. The cause of these peculiarities is the formation of a relatively stable, asymmetrical hybrid $α_2β^Aβ^{BrCo}$ that migrates on alkaline electrophoresis in the position demonstrated in this case. There are several other hemoglobin variants that exist as asymmetrical hybrids in dilute hemoglobin solutions. These include hemoglobins Richmond, Yakima, Kempsey, Rush, Alberta, and Ypsilanti (five of these are also high oxygen affinity hemoglobins; Richmond and Rush are not). It is of interest to note that all six of these hemoglobin variants are due to amino acid substitutions in the region β99-102, all in the G helix. Each of these hemoglobin variants, when present with Hb A, displays three bands on electrophoresis, of which the middle band is the hybrid.

Within intact erythrocytes, all—or nearly all—hemoglobin variants probably form asymmetrical hybrids with the Hb A dimer. In conditions such as Hb S trait the hybrid may comprise approximately half the hemoglobin content of the erythrocyte, hemoglobins A and S each being approximately 25% of the total. The formation of hybrids has important consequences. For example, the $α_2β^Aβ^S$ hybrid in Hb S trait does not co-polymerize with $α_2β^S_2$ to cause sickling, whereas the $α_2β^Sβ^C$ hybrid may. The fact that we usually do not see hybrids on electrophoresis merely reflects the artificial conditions of electrophoresis, i.e., dilution and high oxygen tension, which result in dissociation of tetramers and reassociation of fast-migrating dimers with fast-migrating dimers, slow-moving dimers with slow-moving dimers. In Hb British Columbia trait, the tetrameric hybrids seem to dissociate very slowly to yield $αβ^A$ and $αβ^{BrCo}$.

References

Jones RT, Brimhall B, Gray G. Hemoglobin British Columbia [$α_2β_2^{101}$(G3)Glu→Lys]: a new variant with high oxygen affinity. *Hemoglobin.* 1976-77;1:171-182.

Stinson RA. Asymmetric hybrids formed with hemoglobin British Columbia [$α_2β_2^{101}$(G3)Glu→Lys]. *Hemoglobin.* 1984;8:483-496.

Case 42

HISTORY
The patient is a 31-year-old woman of Irish origin evaluated for erythrocytosis. She commented that she was concerned that some of her family members had had strokes or heart attacks at relatively early ages. She was asymptomatic. She was aware that her complexion had always been "rosy." She denied use of tobacco. The physical examination revealed no abnormalities. There was no splenomegaly.

BLOOD COUNT DATA
RBC .... $5.82 \times 10^{12}/L$
Hb .... 17.9 g/dL
MCV .... 92.8 fL
WBC .... $7.8 \times 10^9/L$
Plt .... $278 \times 10^9/L$

PERIPHERAL BLOOD SMEAR
Normal.

OTHER LABORATORY TESTS
Test for unstable Hb was negative. Arterial O_2 saturation was 98%, pO_2 100 mm Hg. Carboxyhemoglobin was <1%.

Alkaline Electrophoresis (pH 8.6)

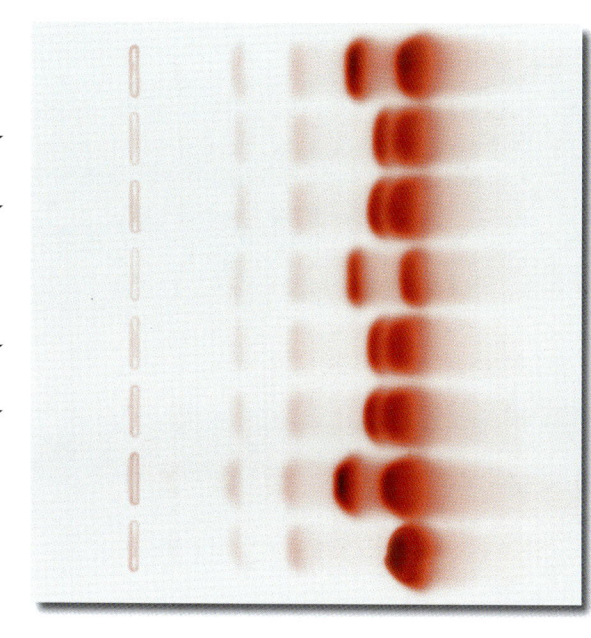

Acid Electrophoresis (pH 6.2)

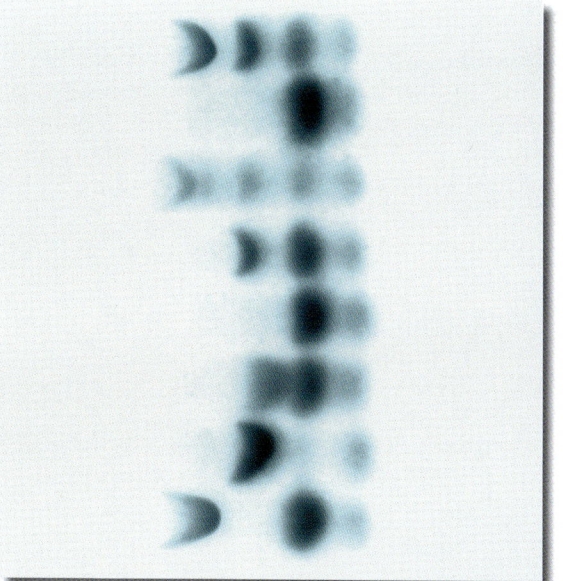

Case 42 Discussion

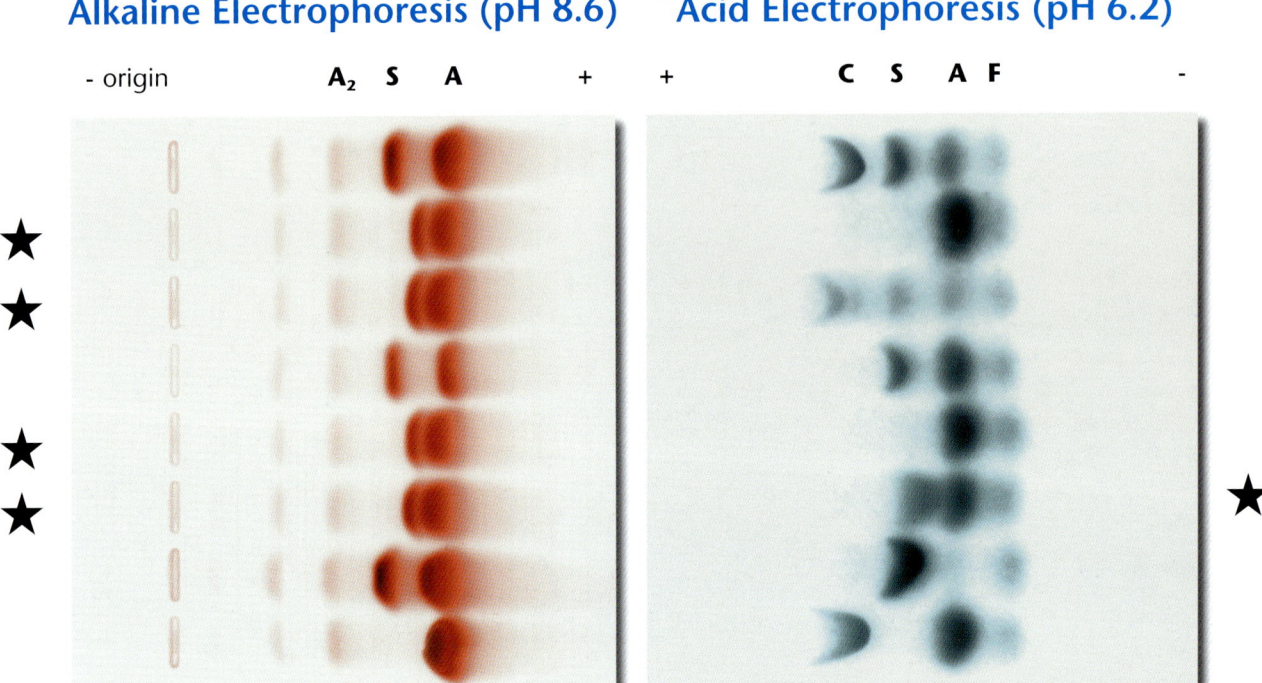

Interpretation

On alkaline electrophoresis, there are two apparent bands seen, one in the A position and one between the A and S positions, approximately in the Hb F position. However, in comparison to other normal specimens seen on this gel, the band in the A position appears much broader. Acid electrophoresis shows a band in the A position and a band between the A and S positions. A band in the F position is not seen, and a quantitative measurement for Hb F showed a normal Hb F level. Other testing identified the hemoglobin variant as Hb Kempsey.

Diagnosis

Hb Kempsey trait.

Performance

Laboratories were not expected to definitely identify the variant; 83% laboratories were correct in identifying the presence of a high oxygen affinity hemoglobin variant.

Discussion

Hb Kempsey results from an aspartic acid to asparagine substitution at the 99th position of the β chain (β99 Asp→Asn). Hb Kempsey is a high oxygen affinity hemoglobin (see Cases 39, 40, and 41). Interestingly, the substitution for Hb Kempsey is near that for Hb Malmö (β97 His→Gln) and Hb Köln (β99 Val→Met), two other variants that are included in this atlas. Hemoglobin Kempsey has been described in many families of Irish ancestry. Patients heterozygous for Hb Kempsey have erythrocytosis, with hematocrits in the range of 52-63%.

As with Hb British Columbia, Hb Yakima, and Hb Ypsilanti, which are also high O_2 Hb variants, electrophoresis of a specimen that contains Hb Kempsey may be observed to exhibit three hemoglobin bands, of which the most anodic is Hb A, the most cathodic is Hb Kempsey, and the intermediate band is presumed to be the asymmetric hybrid $\alpha_2/\beta^A/\beta^{Kempsey}$. The hybrid molecule is seen because it is unusually stable and does not dissociate as readily into α/β dimers as do Hb A and most hemoglobin variants (see Case 40). In this case, two separate bands are not seen; rather the Hb A band appears very broad on alkaline electrophoresis. Examples of Hb Kempsey on HPLC and isoelectric focusing are shown in Figures 42.1 and 42.2.

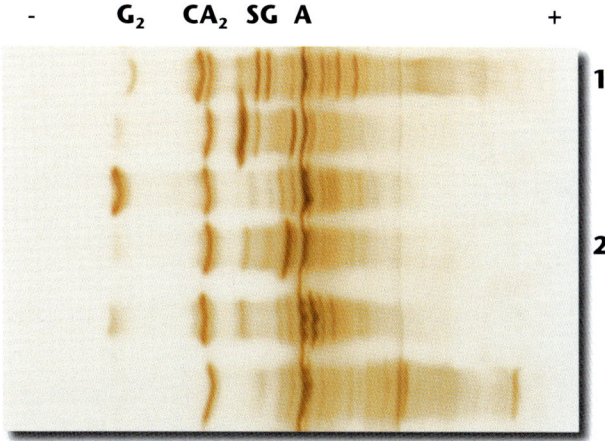

Figure 42.2
An example of Hb Kempsey trait by isoelectric focusing (lane 2). Hb Kempsey appears as a band slightly cathodal to the F position. Lane 1-control.

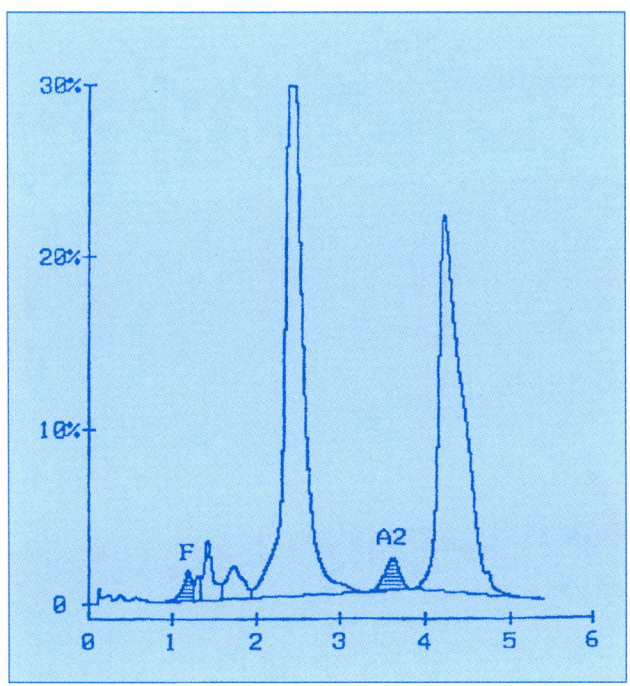

Figure 42.1
An example of Hb Kempsey trait by HPLC. Hb Kempsey elutes in the D window at approximately 4.2 minutes.

References

Bunn HF, Wohl RC, Bradley TB, et al. Functional properties of Hemoglobin Kempsey. *J Biol Chem.* 1974;249:7402-7409.

Reed CS, Hampson R, Gordon S, et al. Erythrocytosis secondary to increased oxygen affinity of a mutant hemoglobin, Hemoglobin Kempsey. *Blood.* 1968;31:623-632.

Case 43

HISTORY
The patient is a 29-year-old African-American woman who sustained multiple fractures and internal injuries in a motor vehicle accident. She underwent exploratory laparotomy with removal of an enlarged, ruptured spleen. She received several units of blood before and during the surgery. No previous clinical history was available.

BLOOD COUNT DATA
RBC .... $2.71 \times 10^{12}/L$
Hb .... 7.5 g/dL
MCV .... 80.7 fL
WBC .... $5.2 \times 10^9/L$
Plt .... $200 \times 10^9/L$

PERIPHERAL BLOOD SMEAR
Moderate erythrocyte anisocytosis and occasional target cells.

Alkaline Electrophoresis (pH 8.6)

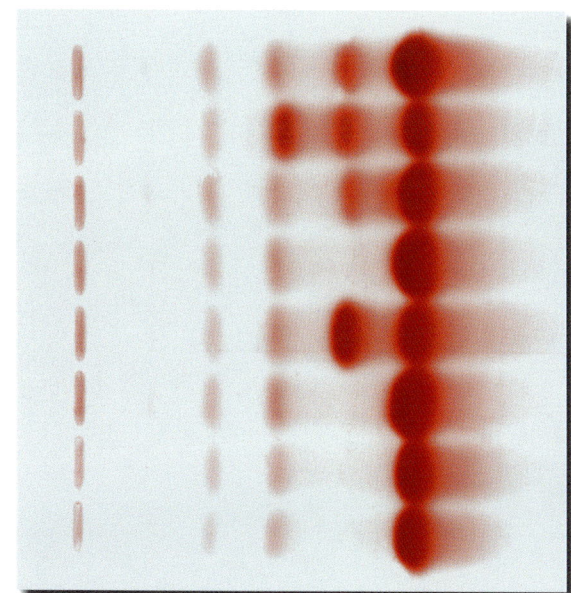

Acid Electrophoresis (pH 6.2)

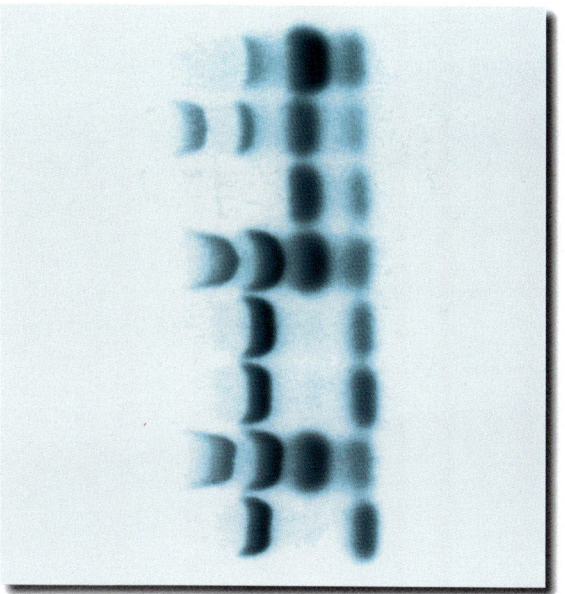

Case 43 Discussion

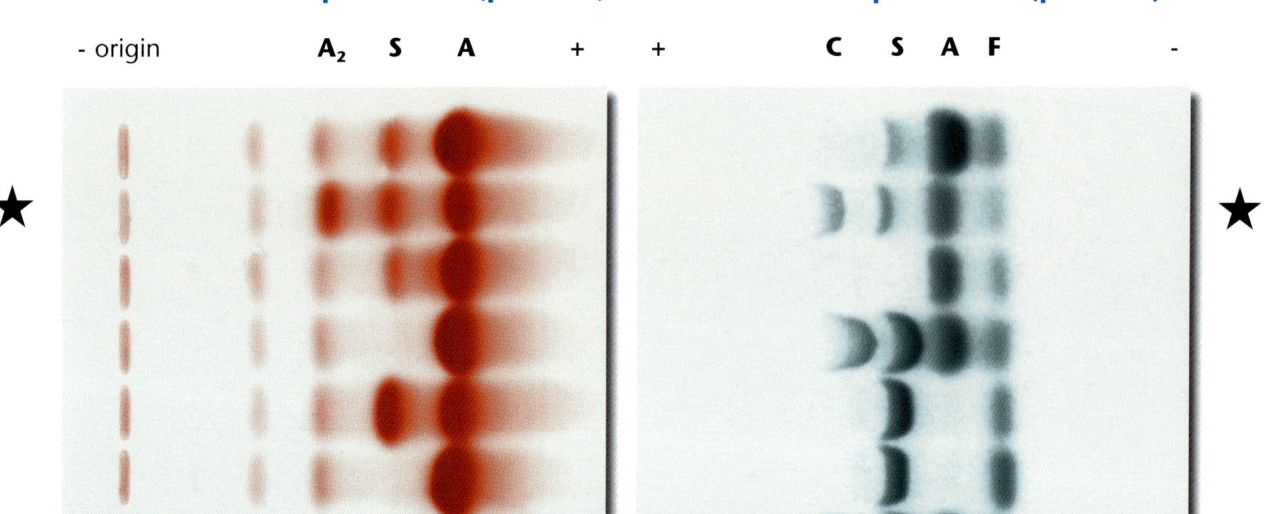

Interpretation

On alkaline electrophoresis, there are three major bands in the A, S, and C positions. Similarly, on acid electrophoresis, there are bands in the A, S, and C positions.

Diagnosis

Hb S/C disease, after transfusion.

Performance

This type of specimen has been used twice in the survey, with 94.3% and 89.7% of laboratories giving the correct response of Hb S/C/A recently transfused.

Discussion

When, as in this case, one finds Hb A, Hb S, and Hb C all present in a single specimen, there are only two possibilities: 1) the patient has been transfused and Hb A, Hb S, or Hb C was received in the transfusion; or 2) two or more specimens were inadvertently mixed (a rare occurrence, but not impossible). A similar pattern may be seen on alkaline electrophoresis only in specimens from patients who have both Hb S trait and Hb G-Philadelphia trait (see Case 19, page 93). However, in such cases, acid electrophoresis demonstrates no abnormal hemoglobin in the Hb C position. The relative proportions of Hb A, "S," and "C" in Hb S/G-Philadelphia is often 2:3:1, respectively. The band in the C position on alkaline electrophoresis is the S/G hybrid. These proportions are quite different from those seen in Case 19.

Case 44

HISTORY
The patient is a 23-year-old Caucasian male who has been of ashen-blue complexion all of his life. There was no family history of cyanosis. Although formerly a smoker, he had stopped smoking three months prior to this examination. He had no other known exposure to carbon monoxide. He was taking no medications. There was also concern about polycythemia, as his venous hemoglobin concentration was usually about 18 g/dL. Despite the cyanosis, he was asymptomatic. The physical examination revealed no abnormalities.

BLOOD COUNT DATA
Hb..................................18.4 g/dL
MCV...............................89.0 fL
WBC..............................6.4 x 10^9/L
Plt..................................241 x 10^9/L

PERIPHERAL BLOOD SMEAR
No abnormalities.

OTHER LABORATORY TESTS
Reticulocytes 5%.
Blood gas studies (using a Co-oximeter): O_2 saturation of hemoglobin 60%, Co-Hb 22%, Met-Hb 0.7%.

TREATMENT
The patient was treated with 100% oxygen by face mask for four hours. At the end of this time, the blood gas studies were repeated; the same results were obtained. He was still asymptomatic and still blue.

Alkaline Electrophoresis (pH 8.6)

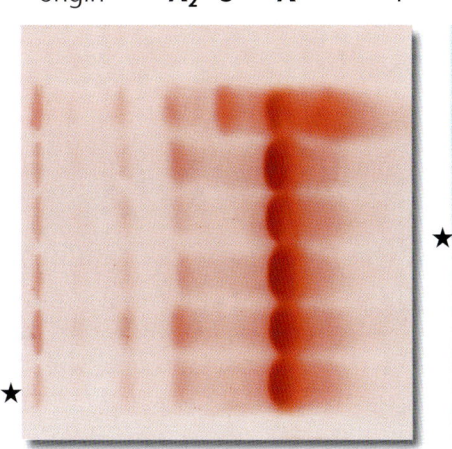

Acid Electrophoresis (pH 6.2)

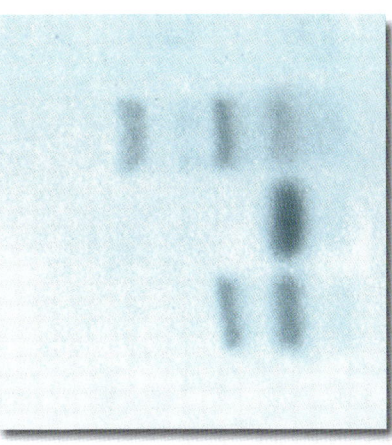

Isoelectric Focusing

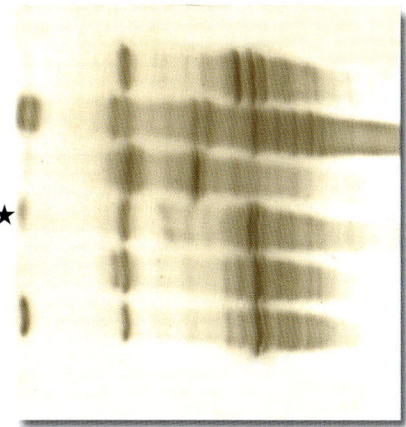

Case 44 Discussion

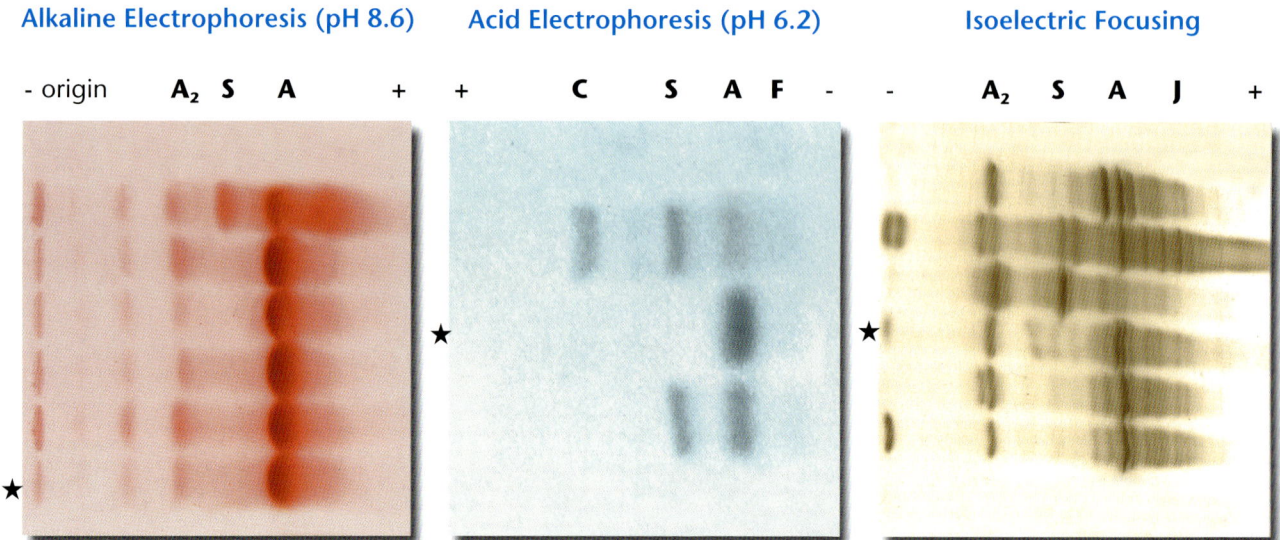

Interpretation

Both alkaline and acid electrophoresis do not show an abnormal band. However, on isoelectric focusing, there is an abnormal band slightly cathodic to Hb A. Other techniques were necessary to identify this variant, including DNA sequencing of the β globin gene.

Diagnosis

Hb M-Saskatoon trait.

Performance

Identification of this specimen was problematic for many laboratories since M hemoglobins are rarely encountered. Laboratories which performed only alkaline and acid electrophoresis did not see any abnormal bands. Those laboratories that performed isoelectric focusing or HPLC did see an abnormal band peak. Approximately 12% of laboratories identified this as a case of congenital methemoglobinemia.

Discussion

Methemoglobinemia is most often due to ingestion of drugs, such as dapsone, phenazopyridine, or sulfonamides, or administration of a local anesthetic, such as benzocaine. Methemoglobinemia may also result from ingestion of nitrite in food (as a preservative in sausage) or from ingestion of well water that has high nitrate content. Much less commonly, methemoglobinemia is due to congenital deficiency of the erythrocyte enzyme methemoglobin reductase (also known as DNH diaphorase or cytochrome B_5 reductase), which is responsible for regenerating hemoglobin from the methemoglobin under normal physiologic conditions. Least common by far as a cause of methemoglobinemia is congenital methemoglobinemia due to Hb M variants.

Case 44 is a case of congenital methemoglobinemia due to Hb M-Saskatoon, as confirmed by DNA sequencing of the β globin gene. Hb M Saskatoon results from a substitution of tyrosine for histidine at the 63rd amino acid of the β chain. Hb M-Saskatoon is one of seven M hemoglobins. These include α, β, and γ chain variants (Table 44.1). All of the M hemoglobins have mutations near the heme pocket that stabilize methemoglobin (hemoglobin containing ferric rather than ferrous iron in the heme group), a form of hemoglobin that is incapable of binding oxygen. All patients with M hemoglobins have been heterozygous, as homozygous inheritance is likely incompatible with life. Hb M-Saskatoon has been the most frequently reported of the M hemoglobins. Many cases of this variant are believed to have been due to new mutations.

The M-hemoglobin variants of the α and β chains, with one exception, result from substitutions of tyrosine for histidine at either the proximal or distal histidine. The exception is the very rare variant Hb M-Milwaukee-1 (Table 44.1). The proximal histidines (α87 and β92, both at the helical position F8) are tightly bound to the iron atom at the center of the heme moiety. The distal histidines (α58 and β63, both at the helical position E7), are not bound to iron or to heme, but move outward as oxygen enters the heme pocket, and inward as oxygen is released; they participate in the coordinated movement of the globin chains with oxygenation and deoxygenation. Substitution of either distal or proximal histidine by tyrosine prevents the normal uptake and release of oxygen, results in oxidation of iron to the ferric form, and destabilizes the hemoglobin by introducing a hydrophilic group into the normally hydrophobic heme pocket. Thus, these variants typically exhibit impaired oxygen transport, methemoglobinemia, and hemoglobin instability.

Table 44.1 The M Hemoglobins

Names*	Positions	Synonyms
α-chain variants		
M-Boston	α58Tyr	M-Osaka M-Gothenberg M-Norin M-Kiskunhalas
M-Iwate	α87Tyr	M-Kankakee M-Oldenburg M-Sendai M-Leipzig II (?)
β-chain variants		
M-Saskatoon	β63Tyr	M-Chicago M-Erlangen Hörlein-Weber M-Arhus I M-Radom Novi Sad M-Emory M-Hida M-Kurume M-Hamburg M-Leipzig 1
M-Milwaukee-1	β67Glu	
M-Milwaukee-2	β92Tyr	M-Hyde Park M-Akita
γ-chain variants		
F-M-Osaka	Gγ63Tyr	
F-M-Fort Ripley	Gγ92Tyr	

*Generic names assigned on basis of priority of description.

The clinical consequence of an M hemoglobin is cyanosis. The onset of cyanosis is at birth in the α chain variants and at approximately 9 months of age in the β chain variants. Aside from cyanosis, patients are well and require no treatment. Gamma chain variants manifest cyanosis at birth, which resolves in the first year of life. The hematologic features of the M hemoglobins are somewhat variable. Both Hb M-Saskatoon and Hb M-Milwaukee-2 are unstable to isopropanol and may be associated with mild hemolysis. Hb M-Saskatoon is associated with reticulocytosis, both in Case 44 and in many published cases, but usually not with anemia. As with other unstable hemoglobin disorders, sulfonamide ingestion may precipitate more severe hemolysis. With few exceptions, the published cases of Hb M-Saskatoon have had hemoglobin concentration and hematocrit values ranging from normal to slightly elevated, as in Case 44. It may seem paradoxical that in most cases of congenital methemoglobinemia, there is no

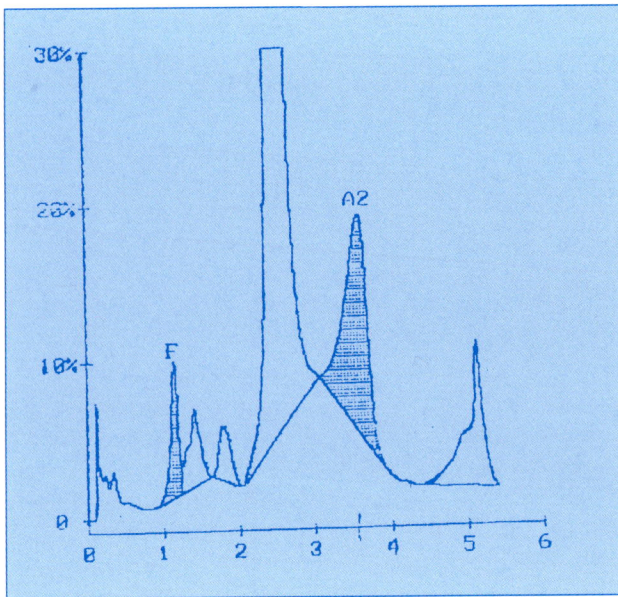

Figure 44.1
An example of Hb M-Saskatoon trait by HPLC. This hemoglobin variant produces a very unusual HPLC pattern. In addition to a large peak which is generally in the A_2 position, there is also a separate peak which elutes in the C window. Several examples of Hb M-Saskatoon have given this same type of HPLC chromatogram.

erythrocytosis, since oxygen transport is impaired. The presence of methemoglobin A may reduce the oxygen affinity of the normal hemoglobin, causing it to deliver oxygen more efficiently, as has been observed in patients with low oxygen affinity hemoglobin variants. There have been few studies of oxygen affinity in cases of Hb M. In Case 44, the whole blood oxygen affinity was measured by conventional means using spectrophotometry to estimate oxygen saturation of hemoglobin. A markedly left-shifted, hyperbolic curve was observed with a p50 of 15 torr. It is not clear, however, to what extent these results may also have been compromised by the peculiar absorbance spectrum of Hb M-Saskatoon. Other studies have shown that approximately half of the Hb M-Saskatoon molecules are in the reduced or ferroheme state and thus may transport oxygen.

Like all the M hemoglobins, Hb M-Saskatoon is quite rare. Unfortunately, M hemoglobins migrate with Hb A, precluding diagnosis with routine electrophoresis. However, in individuals with lifelong cyanosis, an M hemoglobin should be suspected as a possible cause, and appropriate studies initiated. Diagnostic methods that may be used to help establish a diagnosis of an M hemoglobin are illustrated in Figures 44.1 and 44.2. Figure 44.1 shows the results that were observed in Case 44 with weak cation exchange chromatography.

The Hb M elutes in a broad band later than Hb A. Figure 44.2 compares isoelectric focusing results, as have been observed for Hb M-Saskatoon (Case 44) and other Hb M variants that have been studied. Hb M-Saskatoon separates well from Hb A, about 0.7 nm cathodic to Hb A.

Another technique that may be used to demonstrate an M hemoglobin is to convert all Hb A to Met Hb A by addition of potassium ferricyanide to the hemolysate prior to electrophoresis. Met Hb A may thus be separated as a band cathodic to Hb M-Saskatoon or Hb M-Milwaukee-2.

The strange values given in Case 44 for arterial oxygen saturation, CO-hemoglobin, and methemoglobin require explanation. Such values seem to be typical for Hb M-Saskatoon, as well as for other M hemoglobins. They result from the peculiar absorbance spectra exhibited by the M hemoglobins (Figure 44.3). None of these variants has a peak at 630-635 nm, which is usually associated with methemoglobinemia (either drug-induced or due to methemoglobin reductase deficiency). Therefore, conventional spectrophotometric measurements of methemoglobin are in the normal range, as in this case. Furthermore, these same peculiar absorbance properties of the M hemoglobins prevent accurate measurement of oxygen saturation and CO-Hb. The most characteristic absorbance anomaly of the M hemoglobins is a high absorbance peak at 600 nm, a wavelength at which normal hemoglobin and its methemoglobin derivative have low absorbance. The CO-Oximeter, which is widely used in blood gas laboratories, measures absorbance at 594.5 nm to estimate concentrations of CO-Hb, methemoglobin, and percent oxygen saturation. This is quite close to the anomalous 600 nm peak of the M hemoglobins, and it is for this reason that spectrophotometric measurement by CO-Oximeter, or similar instruments, is unreliable in the presence of an M hemoglobin.

Measurement of hemoglobin pigments, or any pigments, by spectrophotometry requires that the number of wavelength absorbencies analyzed, and their

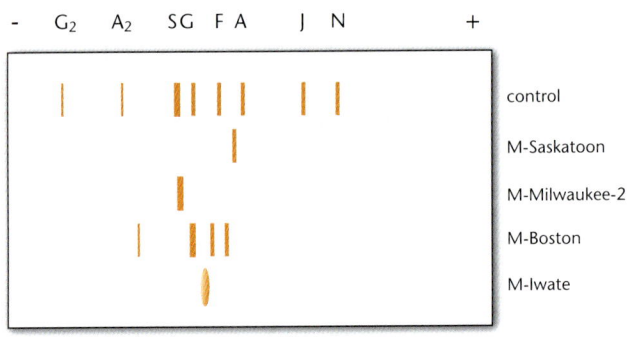

Figure 44.2
Isoelectric focusing comparison of the M hemoglobins.

coefficients, must be equal to the number of pigments in a solution. Thus, if only Hb A is present, all other pigments being in negligible amount, one can quantify it with absorbance measurement at only one wavelength. If both oxyhemoglobin and deoxyhemoglobin are present—but no other pigment—absorbance measurements at two wavelengths suffice to determine percent oxygen saturation. If oxyhemoglobin, deoxyhemoglobin, and carboxyhemoglobin are present, then absorbance measurements at three wavelengths are required to quantify all three pigments, but only if no other pigment is present in significant quantity. The rule therefore is that for every additional pigment, one needs an additional absorbance measurement at an additional wavelength, and the corresponding absorptivity coefficients at that additional wavelength for each pigment present. Current models of the CO-Oximeter assume that no more than four pigments will be present in a blood specimen. The basic equations for the assays of four pigments are as follows, where a, b, c, d, e, f, g, h, i, j, k, l, m, n, o, p are empirically determined coefficients for each of these four pigments at the four stated wavelengths:

Principle of CO-Oximeter

$$OxyHb = a(A_{535}) + b(A_{582.5}) + c(A_{594.5}) + d(A_{626.5})$$

$$Deoxy\ Hb = e(A_{535}) + f(A_{582.5}) + g(A_{594.5}) + h(A_{626.5})$$

$$CO\ Hb = i(A_{535}) + j(A_{582.5}) + k(A_{594.5}) + l(A_{626.5})$$

$$Met\ Hb = m(A_{535}) + n(A_{582.5}) + o(A_{594.5}) + p(A_{626.5})$$

$$O_2\ Sat = \frac{100 \times Oxy\ Hb}{Oxy\ Hb + Deoxy\ Hb + CO\text{-}Hb + Met\ Hb}$$

The software for the CO-Oximeter is programmed with these coefficients and automatically calculates the results.

Clearly, therefore, the reason that the CO-Oximeter blood gas studies were wrong in Case 44 is that the instrument could not correct for the presence of the M hemoglobin with its peculiar absorbance characteristics. Unfortunately, this is not only a problem for M hemoglobins. Extreme hyperlipidemia also causes spurious results, as does extreme hyperbilirubinemia. For example, cases have been observed in which 30% methemoglobin was reported spuriously as a result of marked hyperlipidemia, and 30% methemoglobin has been reported spuriously as a result of sulfhemoglobinemia. This is not a problem just of the CO-Oximeter, but of all similar instruments.

Inspection of the absorbance scan of oxyhemoglobin in a whole blood hemolysate in cases of M hemoglobins reveals, at most, a slight elevation of the descending limb of the absorbance curve in the range 587-620 nm. This is quite subtle and may not be recognized. A reliable screening test for the M hemoglobins would obviously be desirable. In 1961, Dr. Klaus Betke proposed a screening test that depends principally on the anomalous Hb M absorbance peak at 600 nm, and compares it with the absorbance of methemoglobin derived from Hb A by treatment with ferricyanide. He wrote, "From the practical standpoint, it is sufficient to compare the absorbances at 630 nm and 500 nm with that at 600 nm. At pH 7.0, the quotient A630/A600 should (normally) be not less than 1.25, and the quotient A500/A600 should be not less than 2.8. Thus, one may recognize all the presently known types of Hb M with one exception; Met-Hb M Milwaukee-1 is so similar to methemoglobin A that one must examine the spectrum very precisely." The Mayo Clinic experience with this method is provided in Table 44.2. It is evident that Betke's absorbance ratio method works quite well. The normal ratios have a very narrow range that is quite different from the ratios observed for specimens that contain M hemoglobins. However, the ratios cannot distinguish Hb M variants from toxic sulfhemoglobinemia.

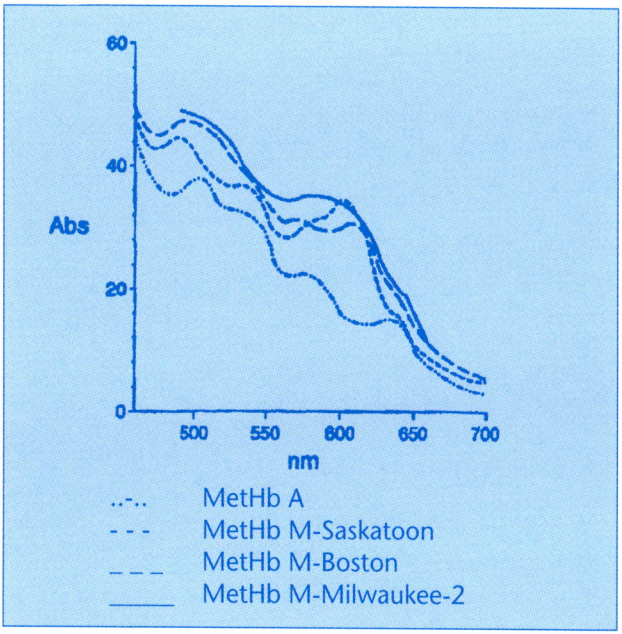

Figure 44.3
Absorbance spectra for three M hemoglobins compared with methemoglobin A.

Table 44.2

Absorbance Ratios for M Hemoglobins, Methemoglobin, and Sulfhemoglobin

	n	A500/A600			A630/A600			%Met	%Sulf
		mean	median	SD	mean	median	SD	mean	mean
Normal Persons	47	1.37	1.37	0.02	2.92	2.91	0.11	<1.0	<1.0
Methemoglobinemia	10	1.32	1.32	0.04	2.80	2.78	0.13	7.1	<1.0
Sulfhemoglobinemia	6	1.14	1.26	0.27	2.52	2.40	0.18	0.5	15.5
M-Boston	4	1.08	1.07	0.10	2.45	2.40	0.12	0.7	10.1
M-Saskatoon	5	0.86	0.80	0.13	1.90	1.72	0.37	3.6	3.0
M-Milwaukee-2 (M-Hyde Park, M-Akita)	4	1.00	0.98	0.10	2.28	2.31	0.09	2.9	6.7
M-Iwate	3	1.01	1.06	--	2.26	2.50	--	1.2	7.7

The numbers in the table are ratios, except where indicated otherwise. The absorbance values for calculation of absorbance ratios were obtained using clear hemolysate that was treated with potassium ferricyanide to convert all normal hemoglobin to methemoglobin. The M hemoglobins are quite rare, and data are available from only a small number of cases. However, in these cases, observed over many years, the results shown were quite consistent, with little difference in ratios from case to case. The cases shown as methemoglobinemia were either due to toxic drug effects (or nitrite ingestion) or due to congenital methemoglobin reductase deficiency. Those shown as sulfhemoglobinemia were the result of exposure to drugs, such as dapsone, flutamide, or phenazopyridine. Note that for persons with M hemoglobins, traditional tests for methemoglobin (next-to-last column) may yield normal results, and results of assay for sulfhemoglobin (last column) are typically high. If there is a lack of clinical information concerning duration of cyanosis, congenital methemoglobinemia that is due to an M hemoglobin may either not be recognized or may be mistaken for toxic sulfhemoglobinemia. Hb M-Milwaukee-1, so rare that we have not encountered a case, has properties like those of methemoglobin A and thus would be readily mistaken for toxic drug exposure (or nitrite ingestion) or congenital methemoglobin reductase deficiency.

References

Betke K, Hämoglobin M. Typen und ihre differenzierung (Übersicht). In: Lehmann H, Betke K, eds. *Haemoglobin-Colloquium.* Wien 31.8.1961, Georg Thieme Verlag, Stuttgart; 1962:39-47.

Betke K, Kleihauer E, Gehring-Milller R, Braunitzer G, Jacobi J, Schmidt I. HbM Hamburg, eine β-Ketten-Anomalie: $\alpha_2\beta_2^{63Tyr}$(=HbM Saskatoon). *Klin Wschr.* 1966;44:961-966.

Bychova V, Wajcman H, Labie D, Travers F. Hemoglobin M Saskatoon: further data on biophysics and oxygen equilibrium. *Biochim Biophys Acta.* 1971;243:117-125.

Efremov GD, Huisman THJ, Stanulovic M, Zurovec M, et al. Haemoglobin M-Saskatoon and haemoglobin M-Hyde Park in two Yugoslavian families. *Scand J Haemat.* 1974;13:48-60.

Gerald PS, Efron ML. Chemical studies of several varieties of Hb M. *Proc Natl Acad Sci.* 1961;47:1758-1767.

Hobolth N. Haemoglobin M Arhus 1: clinical family study. *Acta Paed Scand.* 1965;54:357-362.

Josephson AM, Weinstein HG, Yakulis BJ, Singer L, Heller P. A new variant of hemoglobin M disease: hemoglobin M Chicago. *J Lab Clin Med.* 1962;59:918-925.

Kohne E, Grosse HP, Versmold H, Kley HP, Kleihauer E. Hb M Erlangen: $\alpha_2\beta_2$ 63 (E7) Tyr. Eine neue mutation mit hämolyse und diaphorasemangel. *Z Kinderheilk.* 1975;120:69-78.

Murawski K, Szymanowski Z, Kozlowska J. A new variant of abnormal methaemoglobin: Hb M Radom. *Biochim Biophys Acta.* 1963;69:442-444.

Nagai M, Mawatari K, Nagai Y, et al. Studies of the oxidation states of hemoglobin M Boston and hemoglobin M Saskatoon in blood by EPR spectroscopy. *Biochem Biophys Res Comm.* 1996;210:483-490.

Pik C, Raine DN. The chemical identification of two cases of Hb M (Hb M Boston and Hb M Saskatoon) occurring in England. *Clin Chim Acta.* 1964;10:90-92.

Shibata S, Miyaji T, Iuchi I, Ueda S. A comparative study of hemoglobin M Iwate and hemoglobin M Kurume by means of electrophoresis, chromatography and analysis of peptide chains. *Acta Haematol Jpn.* 1961;24:486-494.

Stavem P, Stromme J, Lorkin PA, Lehmann H. Haemoglobin M Saskatoon with slight constant haemolysis markedly increased by sulphonamides. *Scand J Haematol.* 1972;9:566-571.

Suryantoro P, Takeshima Y, Haryanto A, Matsuo M. C to T transition at the first nucleotide of codon 63 of the β-globin gene corresponding to hemoglobin M-Saskatoon in an Indonesian boy. *Jpn J Hum Genet.* 1995;40:195-201.

Vella F, Kamuzora H, Lehmann H, Duncan B, Harold W. A second family with hemoglobin M Saskatoon in Saskatchewan. *Clin Biochem.* 1974;7:186-191.

Case 45

HISTORY
An asymptomatic 30-year-old Caucasian male was found to have an elevated fasting blood glucose. Further investigation confirmed diabetes mellitus. Although the elevation in blood glucose was mild and became well-controlled with insulin, he had persistent elevation of Hb A_{1c}, ranging from 40-50%. Because this was inconsistent with the apparent mildness of his diabetes, an abnormal hemoglobin was suspected, and further studies were undertaken. He was hematologically normal, and no abnormalities had been found on the physical examination. The patient's father has Wilson's disease, and he also has an elevated Hb A_{1c} of 45%, although his blood glucose concentration is normal.

BLOOD COUNT DATA
RBC .... 4.16×10^{12}/L
Hb .... 13.0 g/dL
MCV .... 89.0 fL
WBC .... 6.0×10^9/L
Plt .... 270×10^9/L

PERIPHERAL BLOOD SMEAR
No abnormalities.

OTHER LABORATORY TESTS
The solubility test for sickling hemoglobin is negative.

Alkaline Electrophoresis (pH 8.6)

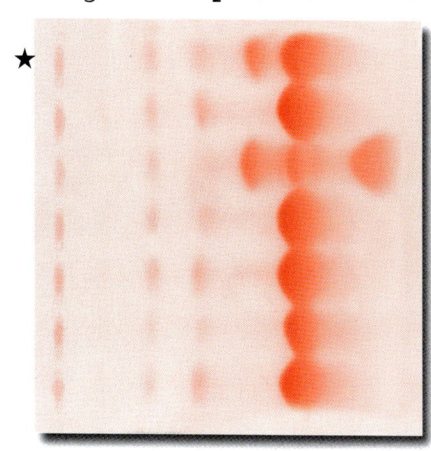

Acid Electrophoresis (pH 6.2)

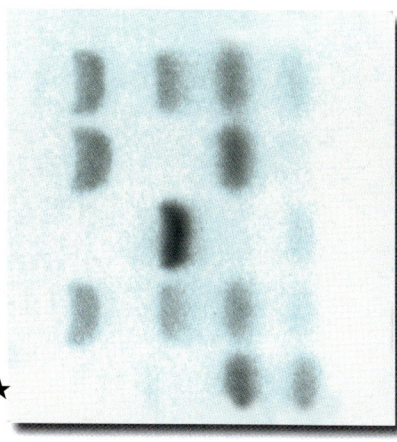

Isoelectric Focusing

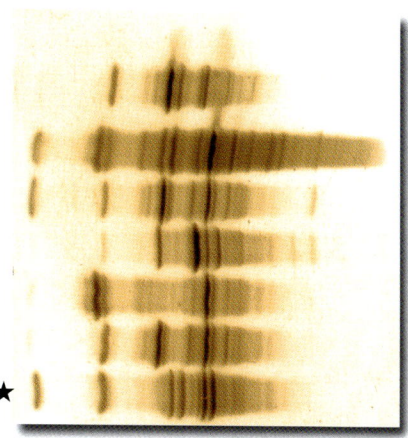

Case Studies

Case 45 Discussion

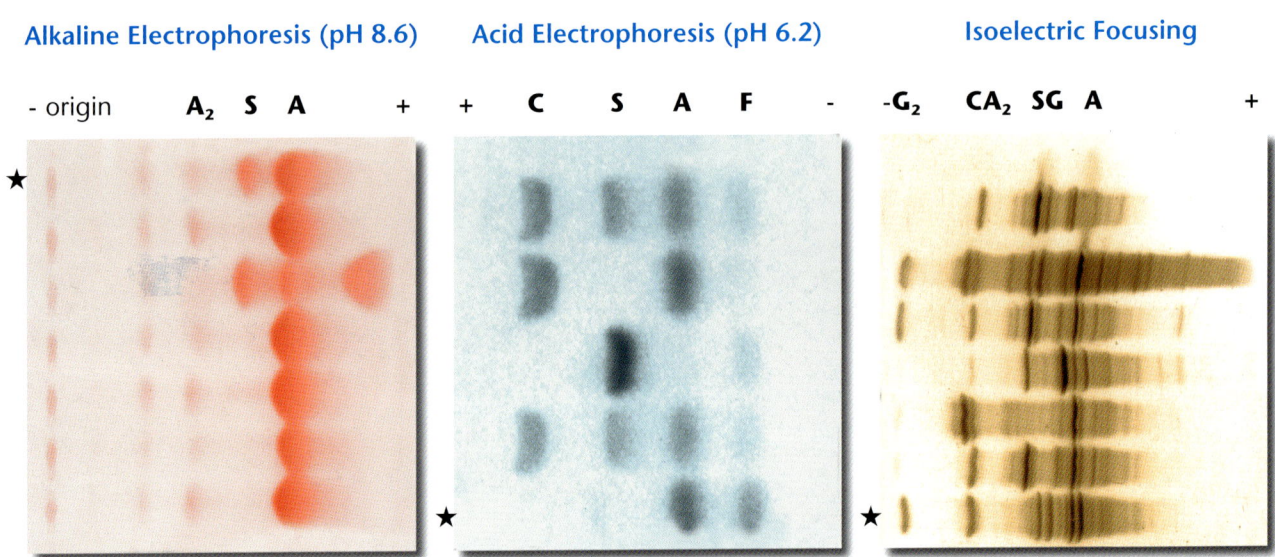

Interpretation

On alkaline electrophoresis, there are two bands seen, one in the A position and one in the S position which accounts for approximately 20% of the total hemoglobin. On acid electrophoresis, there is a band in the A position and a band in the F position. Those laboratories that used isoelectric focusing observed several bands, including two in the approximate S position and one slightly anodal to Hb A. Additional studies were necessary to identify the presence of both an α chain variant (Hb Russ) and β chain variant (Hb Raleigh).

Diagnosis

Hb Russ/Hb Raleigh.

Performance

Exact identification was not expected, although 48.1% of laboratories recognized that a hemoglobin variant was present which was affecting the Hb A_{1c} measurement; 4% of laboratories actually wrote in and correctly identified Hb Raleigh.

Discussion

Hb Raleigh results from a valine to acetyl alanine mutation at the first amino acid of the β globin chain (β1 Val→ac-Ala). It is the classic example of a Hb variant that compromises measurement of Hb A_{1c}. Although Hb Raleigh is reported to have reduced oxygen affinity, it is not associated with any hematologic abnormality. Hb Raleigh has been reported in persons of northern European origin.

The only significance of Hb Raleigh is that it leads to spuriously high Hb A_{1c} values when measured by ion exchange chromatography. In contrast with some other Hb variants that compromise Hb A_{1c} measurement, such as Hb J or Hb I, Hb Raleigh is not seen on alkaline electrophoresis. In the heterozygous state, Hb Raleigh accounts for approximately 45% of the total hemoglobin. It elutes in the Hb A_{1c} position on weak cation exchange chromatography or from a BioRex 70 column (as originally employed in the measurement of Hb A_{1c}) (Figure 45.1). It also separates as a distinct band slightly anodic to Hb A on isoelectric focusing (IEF) (Figure 45.2). On acid electrophoresis, Hb Raleigh co-migrates with Hb F, as should have been observed by laboratories that performed this procedure. Twenty-seven hemoglobin variants are known to compromise the measurement of Hb A_{1c} by ion exchange resin method; these are listed in Table 45.1.

The second abnormal hemoglobin present in this sample was Hb Russ. This is an α chain variant resulting from a glycine to arginine substitution at the 51st amino acid position of the α chain [α51 (CE9) Gly→Arg]. Hb Russ is not associated with any clinical or hematologic abnormalities. Like Hb Raleigh, Hb Russ has been reported in persons of Northern European origin. In addition, it has been reported from China. Case 45 and his father both had Hb Raleigh and Hb Russ in their specimens. Since Hb Raleigh is a β chain variant, and Hb Russ is an α chain variant, the transmission of both variants from father to son is not particularly unlikely: it has a probability of 25% for any sibling within this family. The likelihood is infinitesimal, however, that both of these rare variants occur together in persons of apparently unrelated families. The originally reported case of Hb Raleigh also had Hb Russ, as in Case 45 and his father. Careful inquiry established that the patient in Case 45 is not known to be related to previously reported cases of either Hb Raleigh or Hb Russ. We know of no genetic mechanism to explain this astonishing coincidence.

Hb Russ constitutes 10-13% of hemoglobin in the heterozygous state. It migrates with Hb S on alkaline

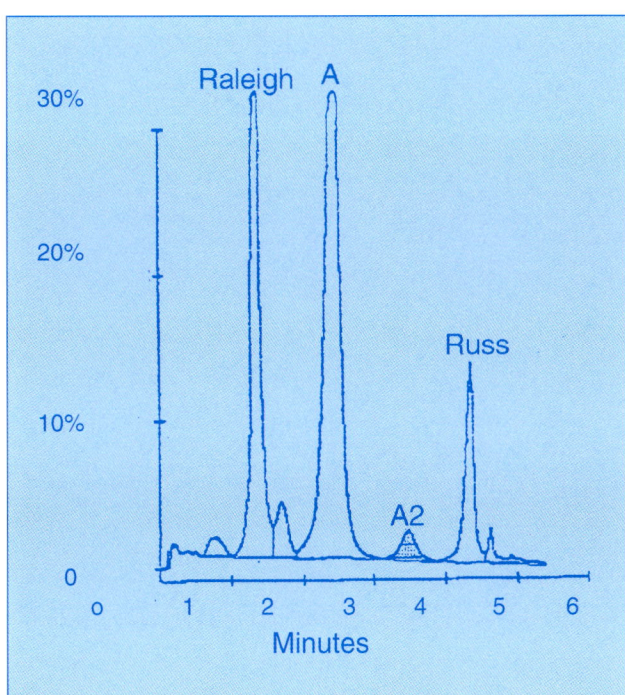

Figure 45.1
Weak cation exchange HPLC for this case.

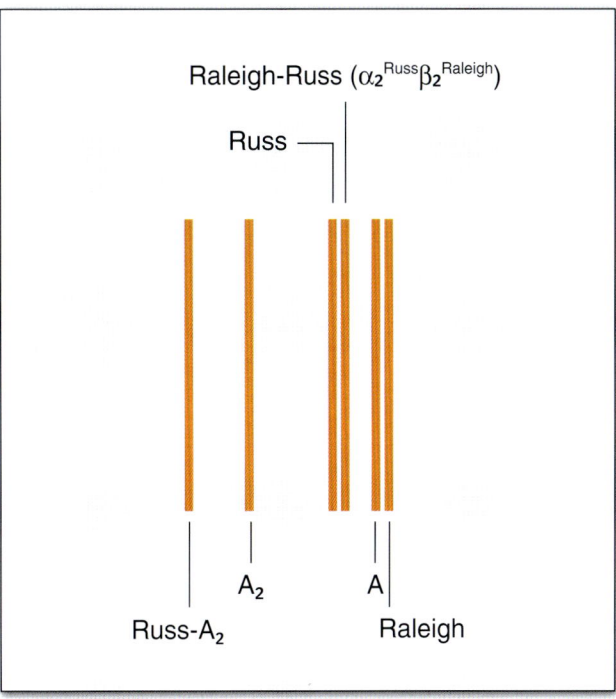

Figure 45.2
Diagram of isoelectric focusing for this case.

Table 45.1 Twenty-seven Hemoglobin Variants That Interfere With Measurement of Glycated Hemoglobin by Ion-Exchange Chromatography

Variant	Reference
F* J K Bart's H N I	References to these variants may be found in textbooks.
Hope Raleigh South Florida Deer Lodge Okayama Marseille/Long Island Andrew-Minneapolis Osler Sherwood Forest Fukuyama Tatras Lisbon Malmo Tacoma Fannin-Lubbock Olomouc Hifiyama Le Lamentin Graz Hokusetsu	Source listed in Elder et al.

electrophoresis and with Hb A on acid electrophoresis. Its significance in the current case relates to the confusion it may cause in interpretation. First, it is important to realize at initial interpretation that Hb Russ is not responsible for the spurious Hb A_{1c} value. Further confusing interpretation in this case is the complex pattern observed on isoelectric focusing due to the co-existence of α and β chain variants. The multiple bands seen are a result of the various possible combinations of normal and abnormal α and β chains. On isoelectric focusing, one observes six bands. These were, in order from anode, Raleigh, A, Russ-Raleigh ($\alpha_2^{Russ} \beta_2^{Raleigh}$), Russ, A_2, Russ-A_2 ($\alpha_2^{Russ} \delta_2$). In mm relative to Hb A, these were, respectively, +1.1, 0, -3.0, -4.5, -14.5, -24.5 (Figure 45.2).

The measurement of glycated Hb by affinity method, using 2-amino boronate resin, circumvents the problem of spurious results for Hb A_{1c}. For Case 45, Hb A_{1c} by ion exchange chromatography was 40%, compared with 7.8% glycated Hb by affinity chromatography.

Diabetic patients may be found to have 0.0% Hb A_{1c} (or "Hb A_{1c} not measurable") by ion exchange method, but high glycated Hb by 2-amino boronate affinity method, because they have no Hb A. If there is no Hb A, there cannot be any Hb A_{1c}. This would be true of those who are homozygous for Hb S, C, E, or D, or β-thalassemia, or are compound heterozygotes for any two of these conditions. Each of these common Hb variants has a glycated form, such as Hb S_{1c}, Hb C_{1c}, Hb E_{1c}, and Hb D_{1c}, that will not be measured as Hb A_{1c} by ion exchange method but is measured as glycated Hb by affinity method. This is not usually a problem for specimens from heterozygotes when ion exchange methods are used that measure Hb A_{1c} as a percent of total Hb A. We are aware of only one Hb variant that may seriously compromise measurement of glycated Hb by the affinity method. The rare Hb Setif [A94(G1) Asp→Tyr], that occurs predominantly in north African and Middle Eastern populations (but also in Spain and Malta), spuriously elevates glycated Hb by the 2-amino boronate affinity method, but not by ion exchange chromatography.

There are many newer assays for Hb A_{1c} that utilize a monoclonal antibody that recognizes the first five amino acids of the terminal end of the beta globin chain (as well as the glucose molecule attached). Interestingly, patients with Hb Raleigh will show a spuriously low value for Hb A_{1c} by these methods. Due to the amino acid substitution at the first position, the monoclonal antibody will not combine with β chains that have the Hb Raleigh mutation.

References

Elder GE, Lappin TRJ, Horne AB, Fairbanks VF, et al. Hemoglobin Old Dominion/Burton-upon-Trent, β143 (H21) his→tyr, codon 143 CAC→TAC – a variant with altered oxygen affinity that compromises measurement of glycated hemoglobin in diabetes mellitus: structure, function and DNA sequence. *Mayo Clin Proc.* 1998;73:321-328.

Landin B, Jeppsson J-O. Rare β chain variants found in Swedish patients during Hb A_{1C} analysis. *Hemoglobin.* 1993;17:303-318.

Moo-Penn WF, Bechtel KC, Schmidt RM, et al. Hemoglobin Raleigh (β1 val replaced by acetylalanine): structure and functional characterization. *Biochemistry.* 1977;16:4872 4879.

Section III: Dry Lab Challenges

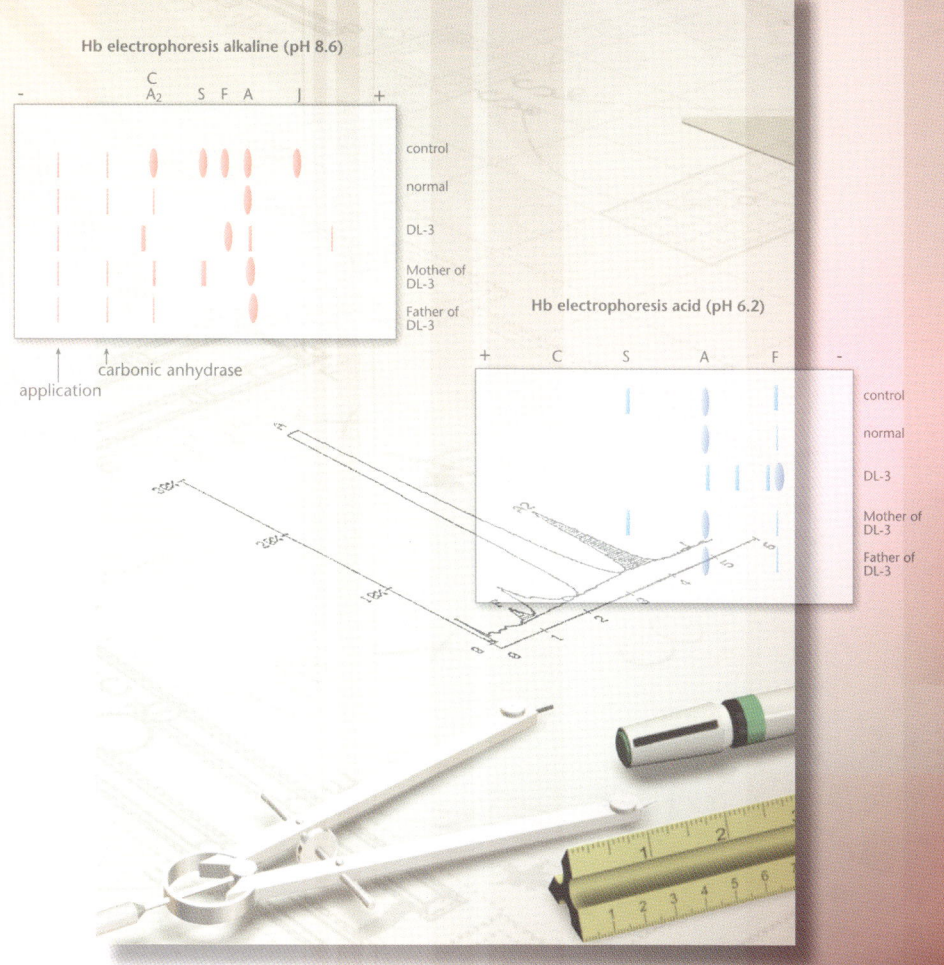

DL-1

HISTORY
The patient is a 33-year-old woman of Laotian ancestry who was examined for anemia and jaundice. She has mild splenomegaly.

BLOOD COUNT DATA
RBC .... 4.5 x 10^{12}/L
Hb .... 8.5 g/dL
MCV .... 57.8 fL
WBC .... 6.3 x 10^9/L
Plt .... 268 x 10^9/L

OTHER LABORATORY TESTS
The isopropanol hemoglobin stability test was positive.

PERIPHERAL BLOOD SMEAR
Hypochromia, target cells, coarse basophilic stippling.

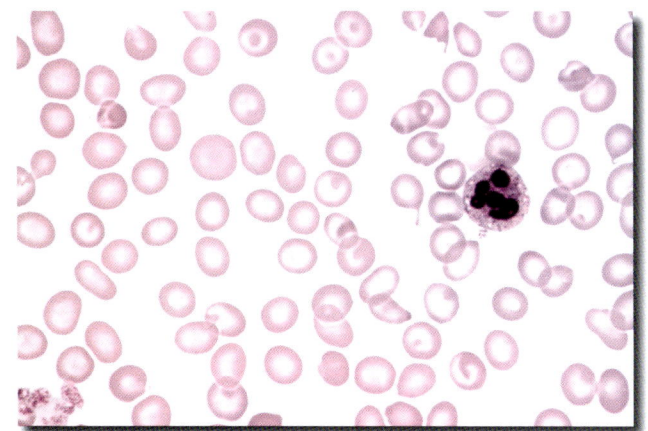

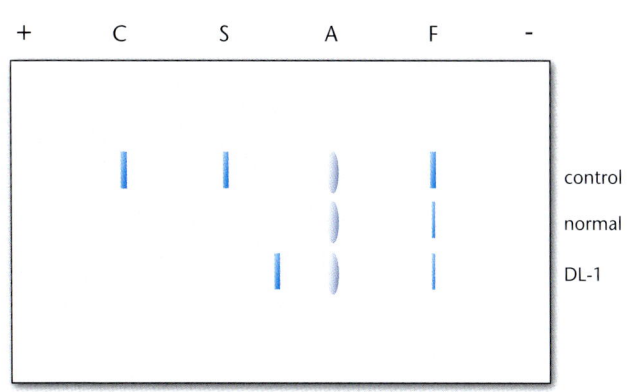

Hb electrophoresis alkaline (pH 8.6)

Hb electrophoresis acid (pH 6.2)

Dry Lab Challenges

Case DL-1 Discussion

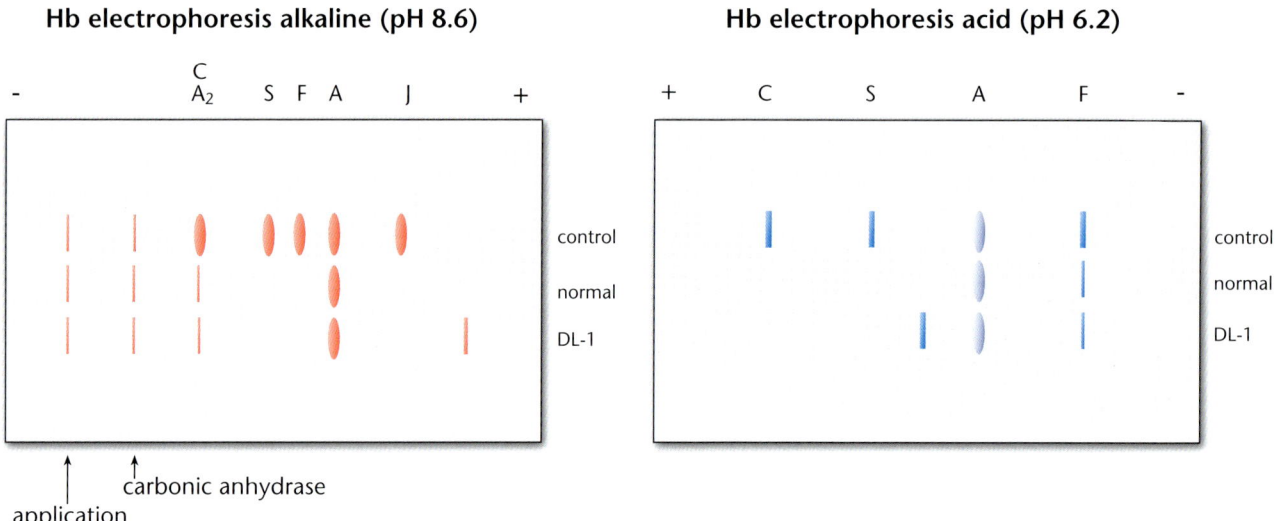

Interpretation

The alkaline electrophoresis demonstrates a single, abnormal, fast moving band that is located approximately twice as far from Hb A as the Hb J control. This fast band accounts for approximately 5-10% of the total hemoglobin. Acid electrophoresis demonstrates an abnormal band between the A and S positions.

Diagnosis

Hb H disease.

Performance

Hb H disease has been used once as a dry lab challenge. More than 90% of laboratories correctly identified this as an example of Hb H disease and recognized that it causes chronic hemolytic anemia.

Discussion

Aside from the hydrops fetalis form of α-thalassemia, which causes death in utero or shortly thereafter, Hb H disease is the most severe form of α-thalassemia (see *A Closer Look At...Alpha-Thalassemia,* page 18). It results when only one of four α globin genes is functional. The disease has two major genotypes in Southeast Asia, where the disease is predominantly seen. The first, seen in about half of Southeast Asian patients with Hb H disease, is double heterozygosity for α-thalassemia-1 (--) and α-thalassemia-2 (-α), resulting in deletion of three of four α genes (--/-α). The other 50% of cases demonstrate co-inheritance of α-thalassemia-1 and Hb Constant Spring (--/$α^{cs}α$) (see case DL-12, page 261). Hb H disease is virtually unheard of in the black population because of the rarity of the α-thalassemia-1 mutation in this population.

Inactivation of three α genes results in an excess of β chains, which tetramerize to form Hb H. Hb H is soluble and thus does not precipitate in the erythroblasts to cause the intramedullary cell death that is a prominent feature of severe β-thalassemias. However, Hb H is unstable and will eventually precipitate in the erythrocytes, shortening red cell survival. Therefore, the anemia of hemoglobin H disease is predominantly hemolytic. Note also that Hb H is ineffective in delivering oxygen, and thus the oxygen carrying capacity in these patients is worse than would be anticipated from the hemoglobin level.

Patients with Hb H disease have a chronic moderate hemolytic anemia, with hemoglobin levels ranging from 7-11 g/dL. The disease is compatible with a normal life span, although patients may suffer from complications of chronic hemolysis such as gallstones, splenomegaly, jaundice, leg ulcers, and susceptibility to infection. The peripheral blood smear demonstrates moderate anisopoikilocytosis with hypochromia, polychromasia and many target cells (Figure DL-1.1). Incubation of red cells with brilliant cresyl blue demonstrates numerous pale blue Hb H inclusions in all red cells. Heinz bodies are usually only demonstrable after splenectomy.

Examination of the alkaline electrophoresis schematic provided with this challenge reveals a very fast moving abnormal hemoglobin band located anodal to the Hb J band present in the control. The abnormal

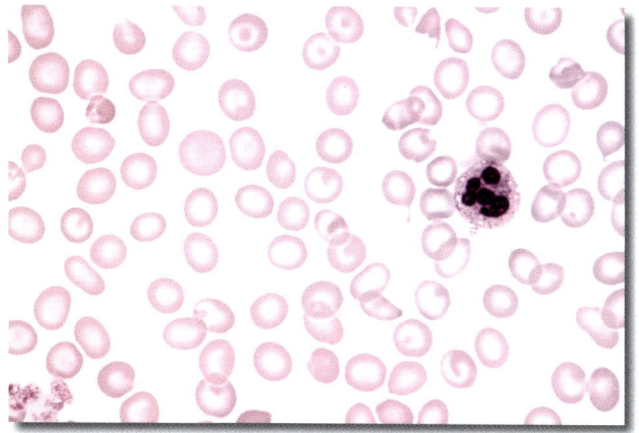

Figure DL-1.1 (Wright-Giemsa, 200x)
The peripheral blood smear from a patient with Hb H disease. There is mild to moderate anisopoikilocytosis with increased target cells.

band is approximately as far from Hb J as Hb J is from Hb A. This is the approximate position of hemoglobins H and I, which are the fastest moving abnormal hemoglobins seen on alkaline electrophoresis. These cannot be distinguished solely based on their alkaline electrophoretic mobilities. On acid electrophoresis, Hb I migrates with Hb A, whereas Hb H migrates between Hb A and Hb S. (In some systems, Hb H migrates near the C position.) However, acid electrophoresis was not required in this case to distinguish between these two possibilities for the following reasons. First, hemoglobin I produces no hematologic manifestations, whereas the patient in this example had a lifelong anemia of moderate severity. Second, the hemoglobin stability test was positive, consistent with Hb H. While Hb I -Toulouse is, in fact, an unstable hemoglobin which produces a mild chronic hemolytic anemia, this is an exceedingly rare variant. Third, the percentage of the hemoglobin variant (5-10%) is that typically seen with Hb H. Hb I, being an α chain variant, usually accounts for 25% of the total hemoglobin. Isoelectric focusing will also help to distinguish these variants, as Hb H disease characteristically produces multiple bands (usually two), whereas Hb I produces a single band on isoelectric focusing. Examples of Hb H disease by HPLC (Figure DL-1.2) and isoelectric focusing (Figure DL-1.3) are given.

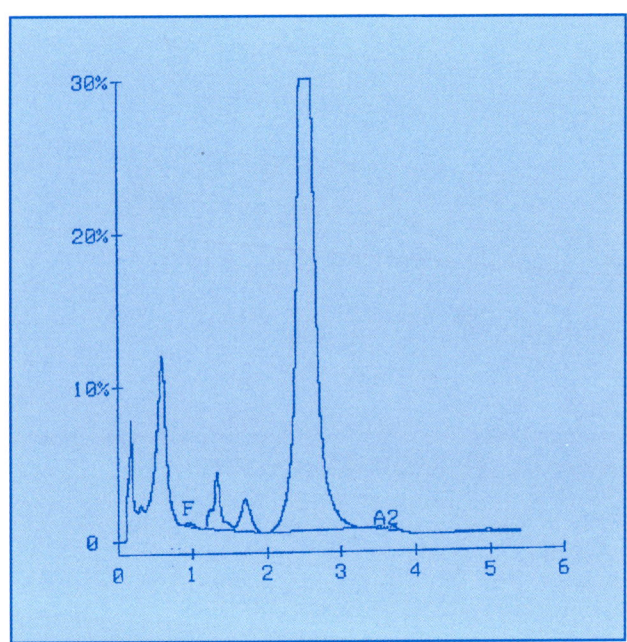

Figure DL-1.2
An example of Hb H disease by HPLC. Hb H elutes very fast from the column, usually at approximately 0.5 minutes. It is not possible to quantitate Hb H by HPLC, as this retention time is before the machine begins to quantitate the hemoglobin fractions.

References

Bunn HF, Forget BG. *Hemoglobin: Molecular, Genetic, and Clinical Aspects.* Philadelphia, PA: WB Saunders Co;1986:329, 331.

Fairbanks VF. *Hemoglobinopathies and Thalassemias. Laboratory Methods and Case Studies.* New York, NY: Brian C. Decker; 1980;231-233,188-191.

Luken JN. The thalassemias and related disorders; quantitative disorders of hemoglobin synthesis. In: Lee GR, Foerster J, Lukens J, et al, eds. *Wintrobe's Clinical Hematology.* 10th ed. Baltimore, MD: Williams and Wilkins; 1999:1405-1448.

Orkin SH, Nathan DG. The thalassemias. In: Nathan DG, Orkin SH, eds. *Hematology of Infancy and Childhood.* 5th ed. Philadelphia, PA: WB Saunders Co; 1998:811-886.

Weatherall DL, Clegg JB. *The Thalassemia Syndromes.* 4th ed. Oxford, England: Blackwell Science, Ltd; 2001:493-507.

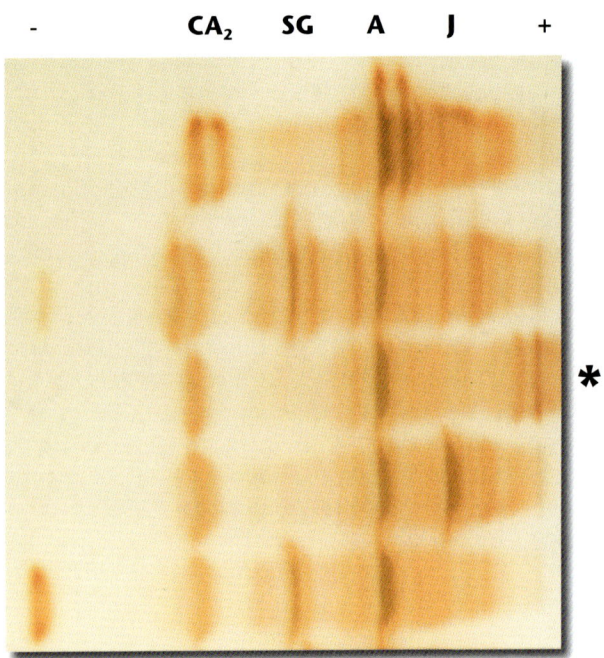

Figure DL-1.3
A case of Hb H disease by isoelectric focusing (*). On IEF, Hb H often appears as a doublet.

DL-2

SPECIMEN HG-02
The specimen is from a one-month-old African-American male. An abnormality was seen on a newborn screening sample.

BLOOD COUNT DATA
Not available.

Hb electrophoresis alkaline (pH 8.6)

Hb electrophoresis acid (pH 6.2)

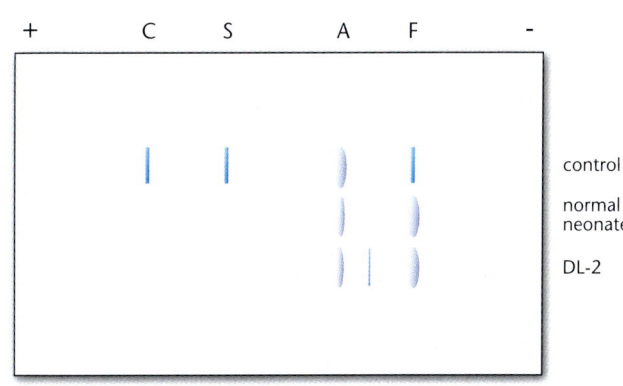

Case DL-2 Discussion

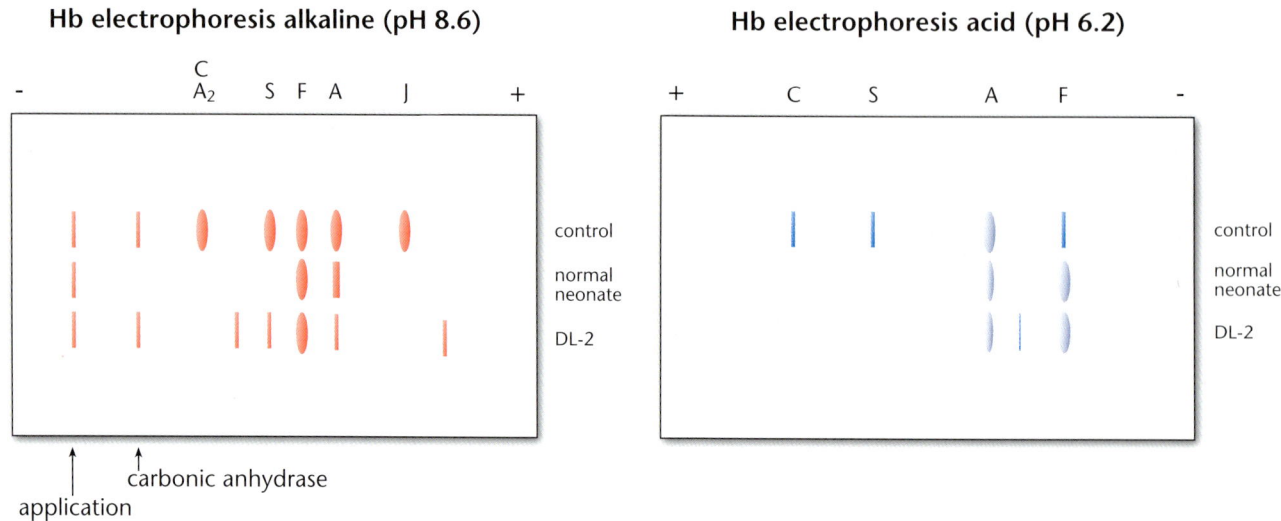

Interpretation

On alkaline electrophoresis, in addition to Hb F and a small amount of Hb A, there is a small band in the S position. There is also a band behind Hb S, consistent with the gamma hybrid of an alpha chain variant ($\alpha^V_2\gamma_2$), as well as a fast band consistent with Hb Bart's.

Diagnosis

1) Hb G-Philadelphia.
2) Hb Bart's indicating concurrent α-thalassemia-2 trait.

Performance

76.3% of laboratories correctly identified the presence of G α trait. Although 48.0% of laboratories recognized the presence of Hb Bart's, only 28.7% of laboratories indicated the presence of α-thalassemia trait.

Discussion

Hb G-Philadelphia trait has already been discussed in Case 13 (page 65). This dry lab exercise, however illustrates two important points. When Hb G-Philadelphia is seen in combination with a β chain variant, the result is an array of multiple bands. Similarly, Hb G-Philadelphia in a neonate will combine with the normal gamma chains to produce multiple bands as well. Thus, the four bands see in this case are Hb A ($\alpha_2\beta_2$), Hb F ($\alpha_2\gamma_2$), Hb G-Philadelphia ($\alpha^G_2\beta_2$), and the F/G hybrid ($\alpha^G_2\gamma_2$). These multiple bands are also seen on HPLC (Figure DL-2.1) and isoelectric focusing (Figure DL-2.2). As discussed in Case 13, Hb G-Philadelphia is usually inherited with α-thalassemia-2 trait. The presence of Hb Bart's in this case is a nice illustration of that fact. Hb Bart's is seen as a fast band which migrates not quite as far as Hb H on alkaline electrophoresis and isoelectric focusing. Hb Bart's can also be seen as a faint band between A and F on acid electrophoresis.

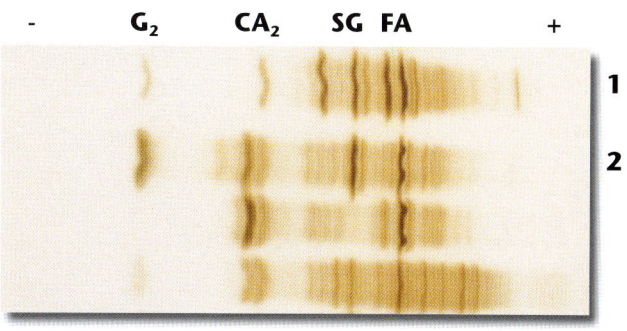

Figure DL-2.2
The same infant as presented in Figure DL-2.1 by isoelectric focusing (lane 1). There are four major bands seen representing Hb A, Hb F, Hb G-Philadelphia$_2$ ($\alpha^G_2\beta^A_2$), and the F/G hybrid ($\alpha^G_2\gamma_2$). Hb A$_2$ as well as the G$_2$ variant is also seen. There is also a very small fast band present consistent with Hb Bart's. This indicates a concurrent α-thalassemia trait. Also seen on this gel is an example of Hb C in combination with Hb G-Philadelphia (lane 2).

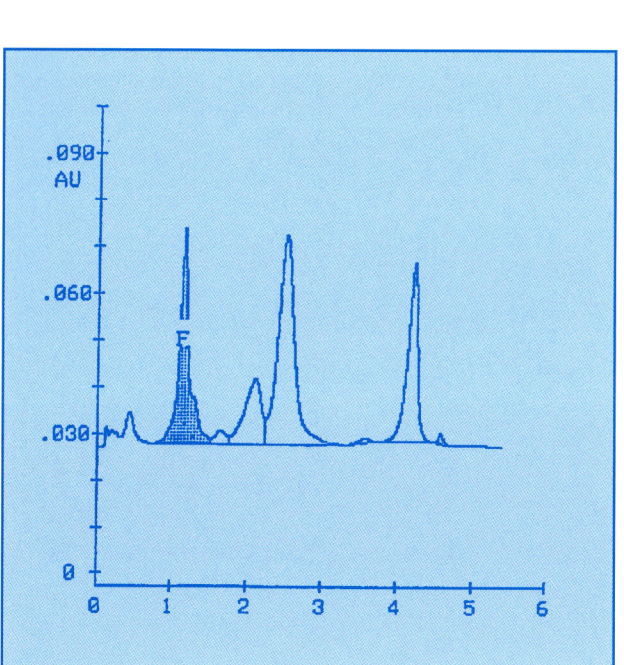

Figure DL-2.1
An example of Hb G-Philadelphia in a month-old child. In addition to Hb A and Hb F, the Hb G-Philadelphia peak elutes in the D window at approximately 4.2 minutes. There is also a small peak slightly ahead of Hb A at approximately 2.1 minutes, which represents the F/G hybrid ($\alpha^G_2\gamma_2$).

References

Milner PF, Huisman TJH. Studies on the proportion and synthesis of haemoglobin G-Philadelphia in red cells of heterozygotes, a homozygote, and a heterozygote for both haemoglobin G and α-thalassemia. *Br J Haematol.* 1976;34:207-220.

Sciaratta GV, Sansome G, Ivaldi G, Felice AE, Huisman TJH. Alternate organization of Hb G-Philadelphia globin genes among US black and Italian caucasian heterozygotes. *Hemoglobin.* 1984;8(6):537-547.

DL-3

SPECIMEN HG-04
The specimen is from a one-week-old infant. The specimen was sent due to abnormalities found on newborn screening.

BLOOD COUNT DATA
Not available.

PERIPHERAL BLOOD SMEAR
The peripheral blood smear shows no abnormalities

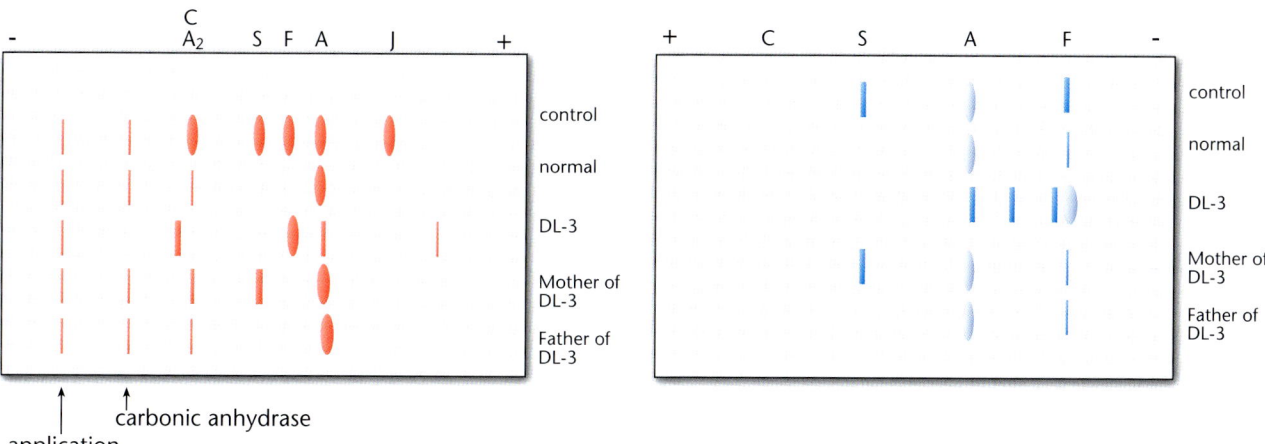

Hb electrophoresis alkaline (pH 8.6)

Hb electrophoresis acid (pH 6.2)

Case DL-3 Discussion

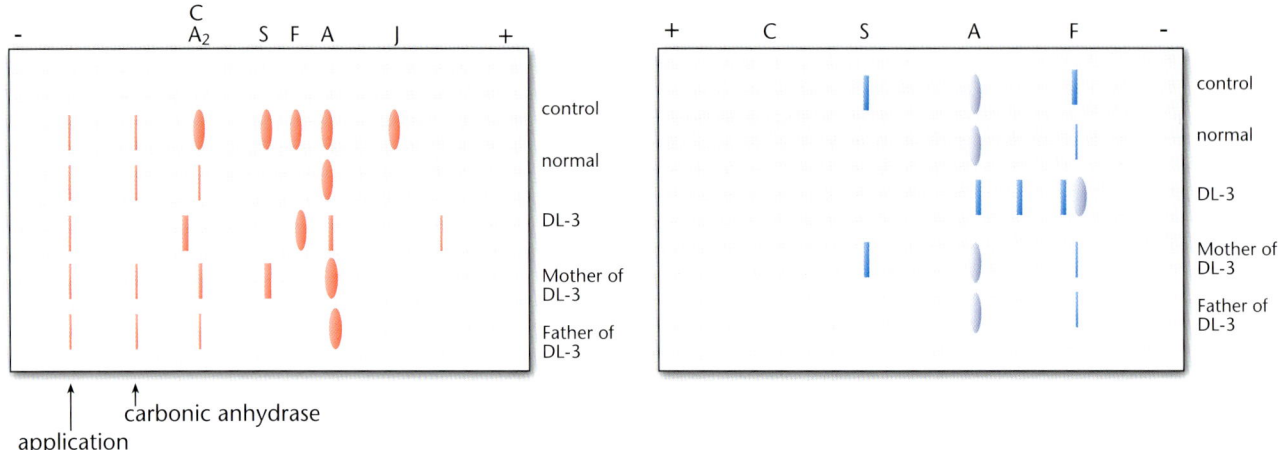

Interpretation

In addition to Hb A and Hb F, there is a band which migrates slightly slower than the A_2 position. On alkaline electrophoresis, there is also a very small fast band present.

Diagnosis

1) Gamma chain variant, most likely Hb F-Texas I.
2) Hb Bart's consistent with alpha-thalassemia trait.

Performance

90% of laboratories recognized the presence of hemoglobins A and F, with 56.4% of laboratories also recognizing the presence of Hb Bart's. Only 17.5% of laboratories recognized the other band as being a gamma chain variant; 38.9% of laboratories considered this an alpha chain variant, and 23.8% of laboratories identified this as an embryonic hemoglobin variant.

Discussion

This represents a case of a gamma chain variant, most consistent with Hb F-Texas I. This variant results from a glutamic acid to lysine substitution at the 5th position of the $^A\gamma$ chain ($^A\gamma$5 Glu→Lys). Thus, because it has the same amino acid substitution as Hb C, it shows a similar electrophoretic position on cellulose acetate electrophoresis. Hb F-Texas I has no clinical or hematologic effects. It is probably one of the more common gamma chain variants, as it has been seen many times in newborn screening programs. It is typically found in African-American babies. An example of Hb F-Texas I by HPLC is shown in Figure DL-3.1 and by isoelectric focusing in Figure DL-3.2.

With the advent of newborn screening programs, many laboratories may encounter gamma chain variants. The presence of a hemoglobin variant in the newborn period usually indicates either a gamma or alpha chain variant. A helpful feature with gamma chain variants is that the percentage of the variant is greater than the percentage of Hb A present. If an alpha chain variant is present, the main abnormal band/peak seen is due to the abnormal alpha chain in combination with the normal gamma chains ($\alpha^V_2\gamma_2$). One should also be able to find a small peak which corresponds to the abnormal alpha chains combining with the normal beta chains ($\alpha^V_2\beta_2$), particularly by such techniques as IEF or HPLC. The previous dry lab challenge of Hb G-Philadelphia in a neonate illustrated these various combinations. Exact identification of most gamma chain variants is not necessary, as they are asymptomatic and will disappear as Hb F production decreases and Hb A production increases. Thus, a repeat specimen at six months to one year of age is adequate to check for disappearance of the abnormal band/peak. If the abnormal bands persist, further workup can be performed at that time.

Although the vast majority of gamma chain variants have no clinical or hematologic effects, a few have been associated with clinical manifestations. Hb F-Poole is unstable and has been associated with neonatal hemolytic anemia. Two fetal M-Hemoglobins have been reported. Similar to the other M-Hemoglobins, they involve substitutions of either the proximal (Hb F-M-Fort Rippley $^G\gamma$92 His→Tyr) or distal (Hb F-M-Osaka $^G\gamma$63 His→Tyr) histidine by tyrosine. Thus, Hb M-Fort Rippley and Hb F-M Osaka are analogous to Hb M-Hyde Park and Hb M-Saskatoon, respectively. Both of these fetal M-Hemoglobins are associated with neonatal cyanosis, which resolves as the child gets older.

Table DL-3.1 and Figure DL-3.3 attempt to summarize the information present in the literature concerning many gamma chain variants. This information is at best incomplete, as many of these variants have been incompletely characterized. The figure is based on alkaline electrophoresis, but similar findings are expected by isoelectric focusing. Also shown for comparisons are several alpha chain variants in the newborn period.

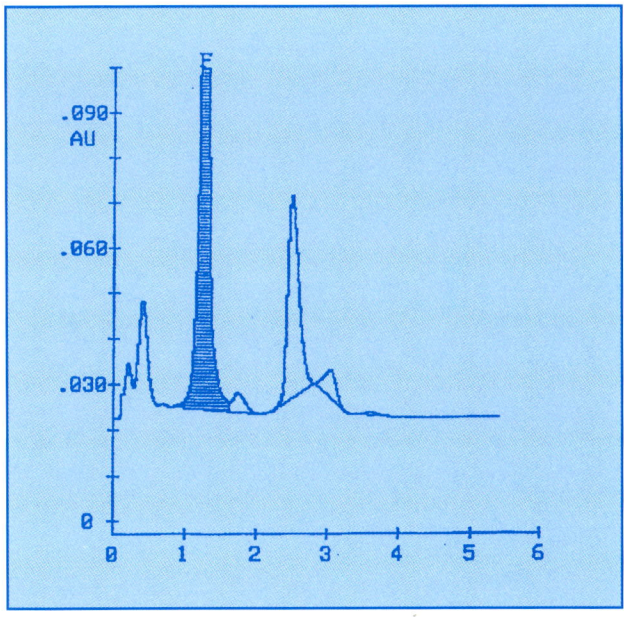

Figure DL-3.1

An example of Hb F-Texas by HPLC. Hb F-Texas elutes as a peak at approximately 3.0 minutes. Due to overlap with the Hb A peak, it is difficult to quantitate this variant by HPLC.

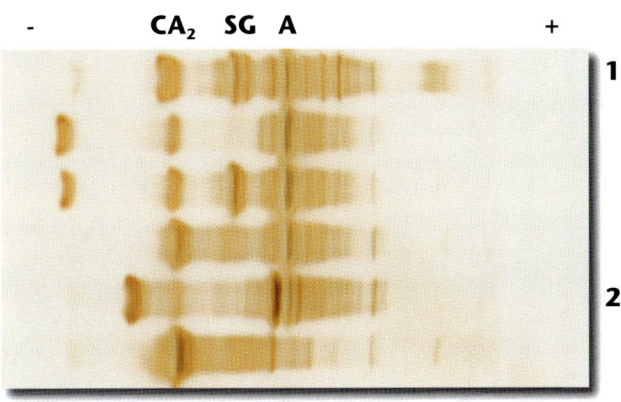

Figure DL-3.2

An example of Hb F-Texas by isoelectric focusing. Hb F-Texas appears as a band cathodal to the A_2 band (lane 2). Lane 1- control specimen.

Dry Lab Challenges

Table DL-3.1 Gamma Chain Variants

Name	Substitution			Charge†	Position*	Ancestry
F-Malaysia	$^G\gamma$	1	gly→cys	N	Like K-Woolwich	Chinese
F-Texas-I	$^A\gamma$	5	glu→lys	+2	Slower than C	African-American
F-Texas-II	γ	6	glu→lys	+2	Slower than C	British
F-Meinohama	$^A\gamma$	5	glu→gly	+1	Between S and F	Japanese
F-Kotobuki	$^A\gamma$	6	glu→gly	+1	Slightly slower than S	Japanese
F-Pordenone	$^A\gamma$	6	glu→gly	+1	Slightly slower than S	Italian
F-Auckland	$^G\gamma$	7	asp→asn	+1	S position	British
F-Alexandra	γ	12	thr→lys	+1	Just in front of C	Greek, Swiss
F-Calluna	$^A\gamma$	12	thr→arg	+1	Between S and C	Black/Caucasian
F-Melbourne	$^G\gamma$	16	gly→arg	+1	Slightly slower than S	Spanish/Australian
F-Kuala Lumpur	$^A\gamma$	22	asp→gly	+1	Between S and C	East Indian
F-Oakland	$^G\gamma$	26	glu→lys	+2	Slower than C	Chinese/Black
F-Tokyo	$^G\gamma$	34	val→ile	N	No separation from F	Japanese
F-Prendergrass	$^A\gamma$	36	pro→arg	+1	S position	European
F-Bonaire – GA	$^A\gamma$	39	gln→arg	+1	Between S and C	English/Vietnamese
F-Lodz	$^G\gamma$	44	ser→arg	+1	Between S and C	Polish/American
F-Beech Island	$^A\gamma$	53	ala→asp	-1	Slightly faster than A	Black/Caucasian
F-Kingston	$^G\gamma$	55	met→arg	+1	Between S and C	Jamaican/Spanish
F-Emirates	$^G\gamma$	59	lys→glu	-2	I position	Arabic
F-Jamaica	$^A\gamma$	61	lys→glu	-2	Slower than Bart's	African/Indian/Caucasian
F-M-Osaka	$^G\gamma$	63	his→tyr	-1	No separation from F	Japanese
F-Clarke	$^G\gamma$	65	lys→asn	-1	Slightly faster than A	Hispanic
F-Shanghai	$^G\gamma$	66	lys→arg	N	No separation from F	Chinese
F-Iwata	$^A\gamma$	72	gly→arg	+1	Slightly slower than S	Japanese
F-Sardinia	$^A\gamma$	75	ile→thr	N	No separation from F	Mediterranean/Dutch (30%)
F-Kennestone	$^A\gamma$	77	his→arg	+1	Between S and C	Caucasian
F-Dammam	$^A\gamma$	79	asp→asn	+1	Between S and C	Arab
F-Victoria Jubilee	$^A\gamma$	80	asp→tyr	+1	S position	Black
F-Marietta	$^A\gamma$	80	asp→asn	+1	Slightly slower than S	Caucasian
F-M-Fort Rippley	$^G\gamma$	92	his→tyr	-1	No separation from F	Caucasian
F-Columbus – GA	$^G\gamma$	94	asp→asn	+1	Between S and C	Caucasian
F-Dickinson	$^A\gamma$	97	his→arg	+1	S position	British
F-LaGrange	$^G\gamma$	101	glu→lys	+2	Between S and F	Caucasian
F-Malta	$^G\gamma$	117	his→arg	+1	Between S and C	Maltese (1%)
F-Caltech	$^G\gamma$	120	lys→gln	-1	Like K-Woolwich	Caucasian
F-Hull	$^A\gamma$	121	glu→lys	+2	Slower than C	Black/Caucasian
F-Carlton	$^G\gamma$	121	glu→lys	+2	Slower than C	Italian/Australian
F-Port Royal	$^G\gamma$	125	glu→ala	+2	Between S and C	Black
F-Poole	$^G\gamma$	130	trp→gly	N	No separation from F	Black/Caucasian
Doubly Substituted Variants						
F-Forest Park	$^A\gamma$	73	asp→asn	+1	Between S and C	Caucasian
	$^A\gamma$	75	ile→thr	N		
F-Yamaguchi	$^A\gamma$	75	ile→thr	N	Between S and C	Japanese
	$^A\gamma$	80	asp→asn	+1		
F-Siena	$^A\gamma$	75	ile→thr	N	Slower than C	Italian
	$^A\gamma$	121	glu→lys	+2		

† +1 means that the substitution causes a net charge change of +1, e.g., from Glu- to Val° or Thr° to Arg+. N = neutral, i.e., no charge change. +2, -1, and –2 indicate charge changes of +2, -1, and -2, respectively.

*Position on alkaline electrophoresis. Mobilities of many γ chain variants have been incompletely described. Acid electrophoresis mobilities in most of the γ chain variants have not yet been described. Only three have been reported as separating from Hb F: Hbs F-Texas-I, F-Poole, and F-Dickinson migrate between the Hb F and Hb A positions in this medium.

Figure DL-3.3
Gamma chain variants by alkaline electrophoresis.

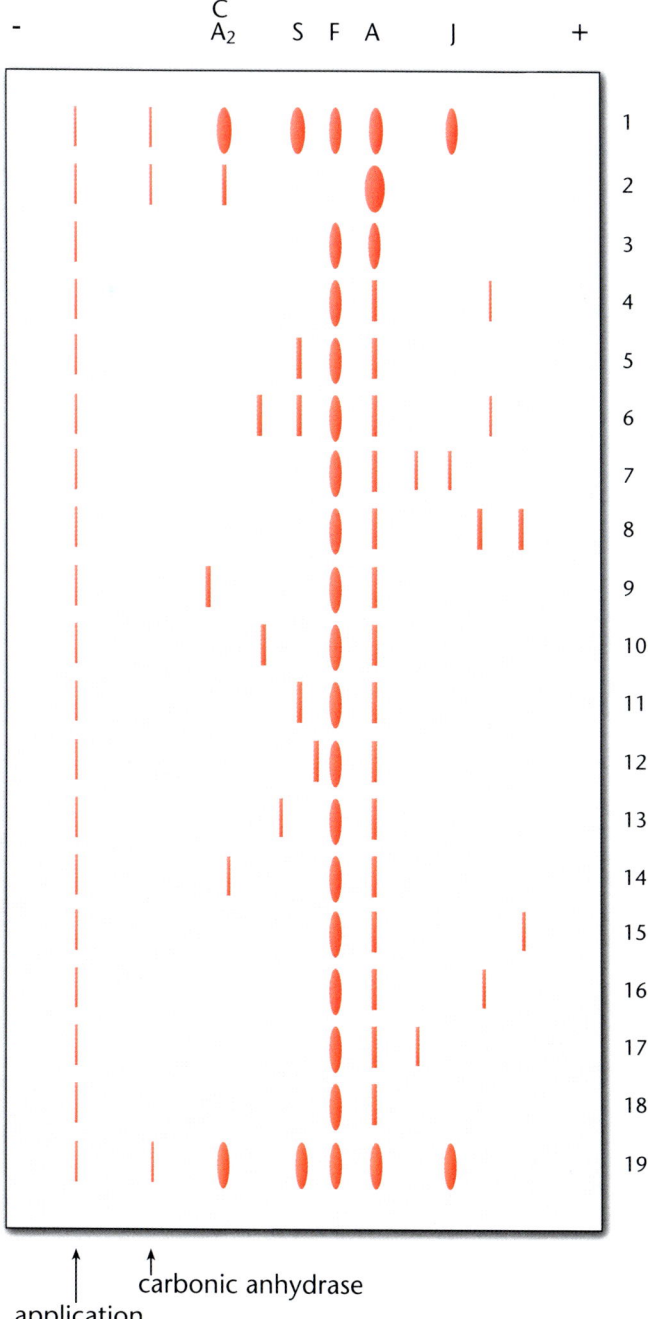

LANE 1	Control mixture of Hemoglobins J, A, F, S, and C
LANE 2	Specimen from a normal adult
LANE 3	Specimen from a neonate, showing nearly equal amounts of hemoglobins A and F
LANE 4	Specimen from a neonate with α-thalassemia trait in which Hb Bart's is present
LANE 5	Specimen from a neonate with Hb S trait
LANE 6	Specimen from a neonate with Hb G-Philadelphia trait, four major bands are present (from anodic to cathodic): Hb A, Hb F, Hb G-Philadelphia, and the F/G hybrid (i.e., $\alpha_2^G\gamma_2$). Hb Bart's is also present, indicating concurrent α-thalassemia trait
LANE 7	Specimen from a neonate with Hb J α trait (such as Hb J-Oxford). The four bands seen are (from anodic to cathodic): Hb J α, the F/J hybrid ($\alpha_2^J\gamma_2$), Hb A, and Hb F
LANE 8	Specimen from a neonate with Hb I trait. The four bands are (from anodic to cathodic): Hb I, the F/I hybrid ($\alpha_2^I\gamma_2$), Hb A, and Hb F
LANE 9:	Gamma chain variants which migrate slower than Hb C: F-Texas I, F-Texas II, F-Oakland, F-Hull, F-Carlton, F-Siena
LANE 10:	Gamma chain variants which migrate between S and C: F-Calluna, F-Kuala Lumpur, F-Lodz, F-Kingston, F-Malta, F-Forest Park
LANE 11	Gamma chain variants which migrate in the S position: F-Prendergrass, F-Victoria Jubilee, F-Dickinson, F-Auckland
LANE 12	Gamma chain variants which migrate between S and F: F-Meinohama, F-LaGrange
LANE 13	Gamma chain variants which migrate slightly slower than S: F-Kotobuki, F-Pordenone, F-Marietta, F-Iwata, F-Melbourne
LANE 14	Gamma chain variants which migrate just in front of C: F-Alexandra
LANE 15	Gamma chain variants which migrate similar to Hb I: F-Emirates
LANE 16	Gamma chain variants which migrate slightly slower than Bart's: Hb F-Jamaica
LANE 17	Gamma chain variants which migrate similar to Hb K-Woolwich: F-Malaysia, F-Caltech
LANE 18	Gamma chain variants which do not separate from Hb F: F-Tokyo, F-M-Osaka, F-Shanghai, F-Sardinia, F-M-Fort Rippley, F-Poole
LANE 19	Control mixture of Hemoglobins J, A, F, S, and C

References

Husiman THJ. Gamma chain abnormal human fetal hemoglobin variants. *Am J Hematol.* 1997;55:159-163.

Huisman THJ, Carver MFH, Efremon GD. *A Syllabus of Human Hemoglobin Variants.* 2nd ed. Augusta, GA: Sickle Cell Anemia Foundation; 1998:281-313.

Jenkins GC, Beace D, Black AJ, et al. Hemoglobin F Texas ($\alpha_2{}^A\gamma_2$ glu→lys): a variant of haemoglobin F. *Br J Haematol.* 1967;13:252-255.

Schneider RG, Jones RT. Hemoglobin F-Texas: gamma chain variant. *Science.* 1965;148:240-241.

DL-4

HISTORY
The specimen is from a 23-year-old woman of Cambodian ancestry who was examined because of fatigue. On physical examination, she was small in stature and build, and had icteric sclera. The spleen was palpable 3 cm below the left costal margin.

BLOOD COUNT DATA
RBC .... 4.2 x 10^{12}/L
Hb .... 7.5 g/dL
MCV .... 59 fL
WBC .... 11.1 x 10^9/L
Plt .... 392 x 10^9/L

OTHER LABORATORY TESTS
Reticulocytes 11.0%.
Isopropanol test for unstable hemoglobin was positive.
Total serum bilirubin 3.6 mg/dL.

PERIPHERAL BLOOD SMEAR
The red blood cells are notable for polychromasia, hypochromia, microcytosis, and moderate target cell formation.

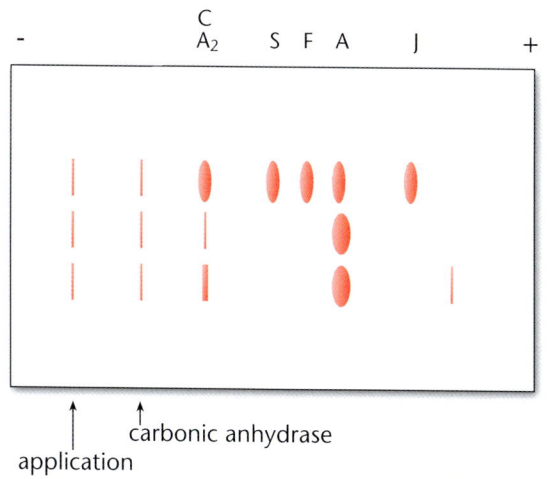

Hb electrophoresis alkaline (pH 8.6)

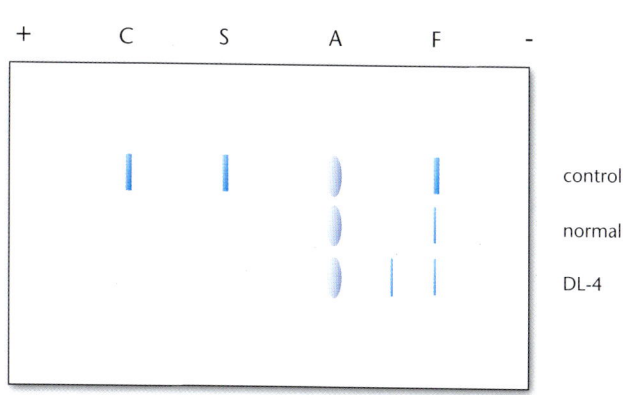

Hb electrophoresis acid (pH 6.2)

Dry Lab Challenges

Case DL-4 Discussion

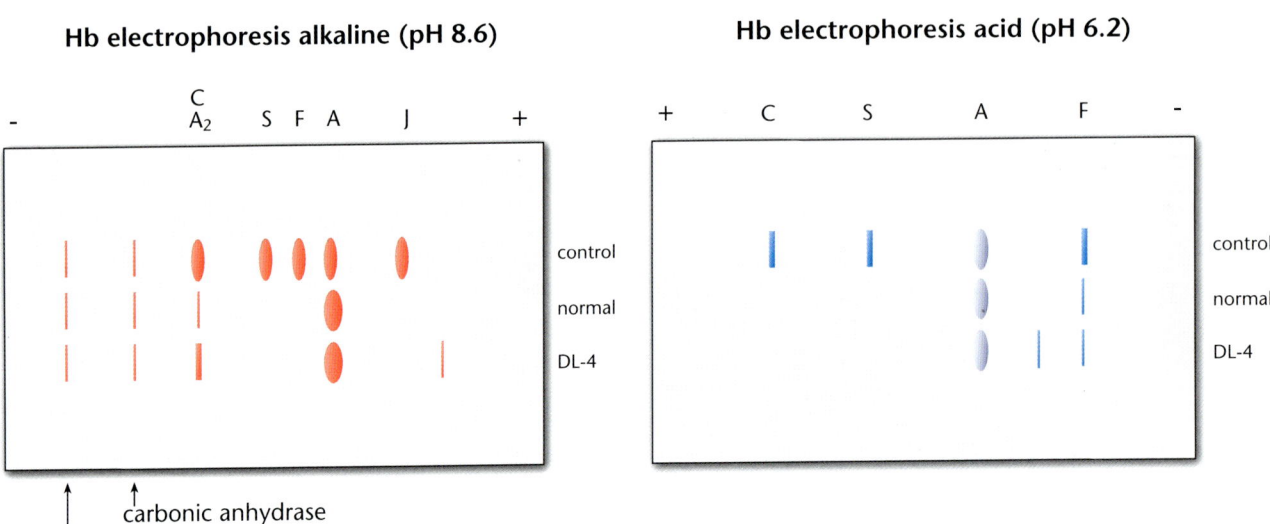

Interpretation

On alkaline electrophoresis, in addition to Hb A, there is a major band in the A_2 position which accounts for 10-15% of the total hemoglobin. There is also a small fast band that migrates slightly ahead of the J position. On acid electrophoresis, there is a small band between the A and F positions.

Performance

81.0% of laboratories correctly identified the presence of Hb E. Only 19.2% of laboratories identified the fast band as Hb Bart's; 67.9% of laboratories identified this band as Hb H. However, 77.2% of laboratories were correct that this case is consistent with Hb H disease with Hb E trait.

Diagnosis

Hb AE-Bart's disease.

Discussion

This dry lab exercise illustrated the combination of Hb E trait with a three alpha chain deletion. Thus, this condition is equivalent to Hb H disease, as this patient's history and CBC data indicate. However, the typical Hb H band is not present. The presence of Hb E trait causes an overall decreased production of normal beta chains. Therefore, the β_4 tetramers are not produced in sufficient quantity to be seen on alkaline electrophoresis (although a small Hb H band is usually seen on isoelectric focusing). Hb Bart's is seen instead. Thus, this condition has also been called "Hb AE-Bart's disease."

A previous study from Thailand involving 25 patients showed that 21 of the 25 patients also had Hb Constant Spring. Thus, there was a combination of α-thalassemia-1 trait on one chromosome 16 and a nondeletional α-thalassemia mutation (Hb Constant Spring) on the other chromosome (--/α^{CS}-). Hb Constant Spring is discussed more fully in a separate dry lab challenge (see case DL-12). The severity of disease is worse when Hb Constant Spring is present. An example of Hb A+E+Bart's+Constant Spring is shown on HPLC (Figure DL-4.2) and on IEF (Figure DL-4.2).

Figure DL-4.2
The same patient as presented in Figure DL-4.1 by isoelectric focusing (lane 1). Hb Constant Spring is identified as a band cathodal to the A_2 position, which in this case is increased due to the presence of Hb E. By isoelectric focusing, one often sees, in addition to the Hb Bart's peak, a slightly faster band representing a small amount of Hb H. This specimen also shows a slight increase in Hb F. Lane 2-control specimen.

References

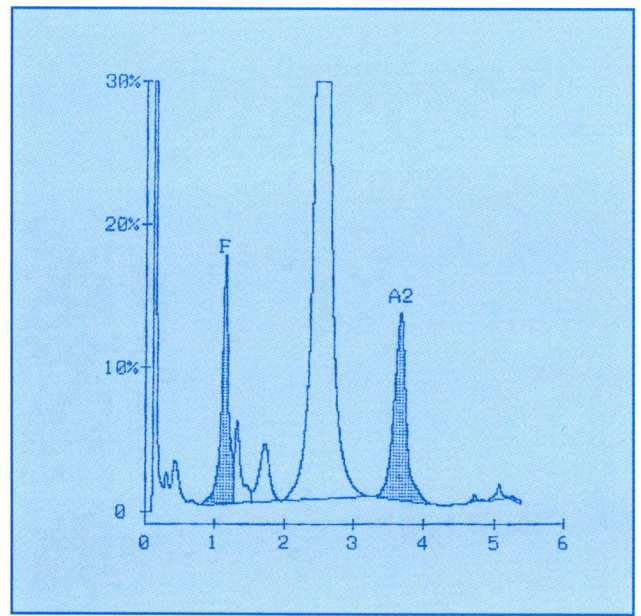

Figure DL-4.1
An example of Hb A+E+Bart's+Constant Spring by HPLC. There is a peak which elutes from the column almost instantaneously (0.1 minutes) which represents Hb Bart's. There is also a prominent Hb A_2 peak representing Hb E, and a very small peak in the C window at approximately 5.1 minutes representing Hb Constant Spring.

Fucharoen S, Winichagoon P, Prayoonwiwat W, et al. Clinical and hematologic manifestations of AE-Bart's disease. *Birth Defects*. 1988;23:327-332.

Thonglairuam V, Winichagoon P, Fucharoen S, et al. The molecular basis of AE-Bart's disease. *Hemoglobin*. 1989;13:117-124.

Wasi P, Sookanek M, Pootrakul S, et al. Haemoglobin E and alpha-thalassemia. *Br Med J*. 1967;4:29-32.

DL-5

HISTORY
Specimens were received from fraternal twins (one month old) in a neonatal screening program. Both specimens are represented along with those of the parents. Both twins appeared healthy at the time of examination, and neither had been transfused. Twin A is case DL-5.

BLOOD COUNT DATA

	Father	Mother
RBC (x 10^{12}/L)	6.60	3.64
Hb (g/dL)	14.1	10.2
MCV (fL)	64.0	84.0
WBC (x 10^9/L)	5.8	6.3
Plt (x 10^9/L)	253	224

OTHER LABORATORY TESTS
None.

PERIPHERAL BLOOD SMEAR
The peripheral blood smear of both twins showed slight microcytosis for age. The father's smear showed microcytosis, target cells, and basophilic stippling. The mother's smear showed rare sickle cells, occasional target cells, and clam-shaped cells.

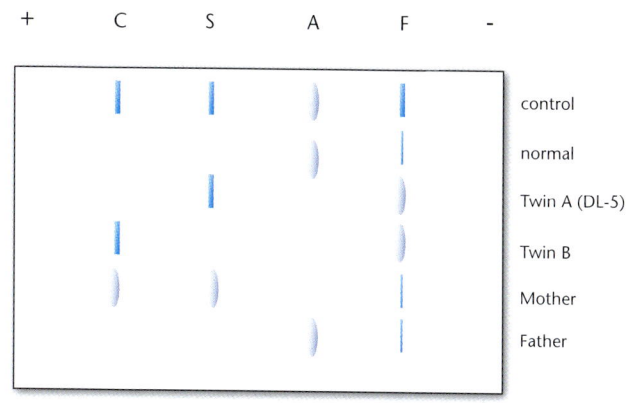

Case DL-5 Discussion

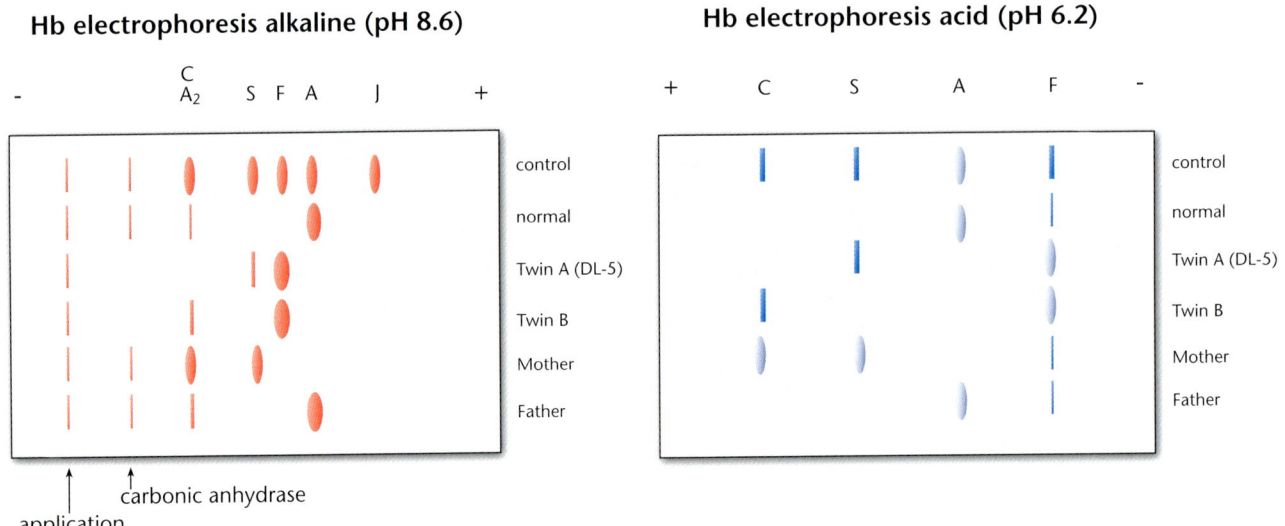

Interpretation

The alkaline electrophoresis of twin A shows no Hb A present. There is a large amount of Hb F and a small band in the S position. There is no Hb A_2 present, which is normal for this age. On acid electrophoresis, there is a band in the S position confirming the presence of Hb S, and a band in the F position.

Diagnosis

Hb S/β^0-thalassemia in a neonate.

Performance

Laboratories were not required to identify the condition in twin A, but 99.5% of laboratories correctly identified the presence of Hb S, and 99.3% the presence of Hb F.

Discussion

This dry lab challenge illustrates the value of performing family studies in unusual or confusing cases. Neither twin A nor twin B has any Hb A. In addition to Hb F, twin A has only Hb S, and twin B Hb C. Examination of the mother's hemoglobin electrophoresis shows results consistent with Hb S/C disease. The father's hemoglobin electrophoresis and his CBC results are consistent with β-thalassemia trait. Thus, each twin has a hemoglobin variant inherited from the mother (either Hb S or Hb C) and β-thalassemia trait from the father. Furthermore, the absence of Hb A in both twins indicates that this must be a $β^0$-thalassemia mutation.

The β-thalassemia mutation seen in this family was analyzed by molecular methods. These revealed a 532 bp deletion of a portion of the β globin gene nucleotide −454 to +78. This deletion includes the promoter region and part of the first exon (Figure DL-5.1).

This mutation is unusual in that most β-thalassemia mutations found in African Americans are $β^+$ mutations. For example, as discussed in *A Closer Look At...Beta-Thalassemia*, two of the most common mutations in African Americans are point mutations in the promotor region at either nucleotide −29 or −88. The mutation seen in this case is also unusual in that it results in very high levels of Hb A_2. The father in this case was actually used as a CAP survey sample. The median Hb A_2 values obtained ranged from 7.5–8.1% by various methods.

References

Steinberg MH, Adams JG, III, Hendricks R. Sickle cell beta-thalassemia: a common phenocopy of sickle cell anemia. *J Miss Med Assoc.* 1982;23:319-321.

Waye JS, Cai SP, Eng B, et al. High Hb A_2 beta zero thalassemia due to a 532 basepair deletion of the 5′ portion of the beta-globin gene region. *Blood.* 1991;77:1100-1103.

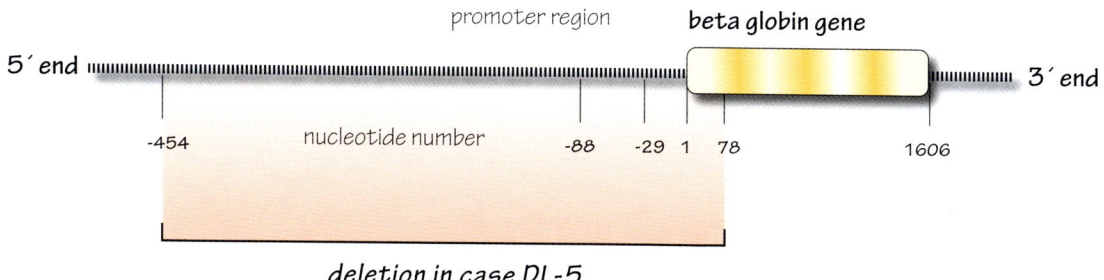

Figure DL-5.1
*Illustration of the β-thalassemia mutation in this case.
(Note: not drawn to scale due to space limitations)*

DL-6

HISTORY
This sample is from a less than one-month-old African-American girl. It was sent in follow-up of abnormal results seen on newborn screening.

BLOOD COUNT DATA
Not available.

PERIPHERAL BLOOD SMEAR
Not available.

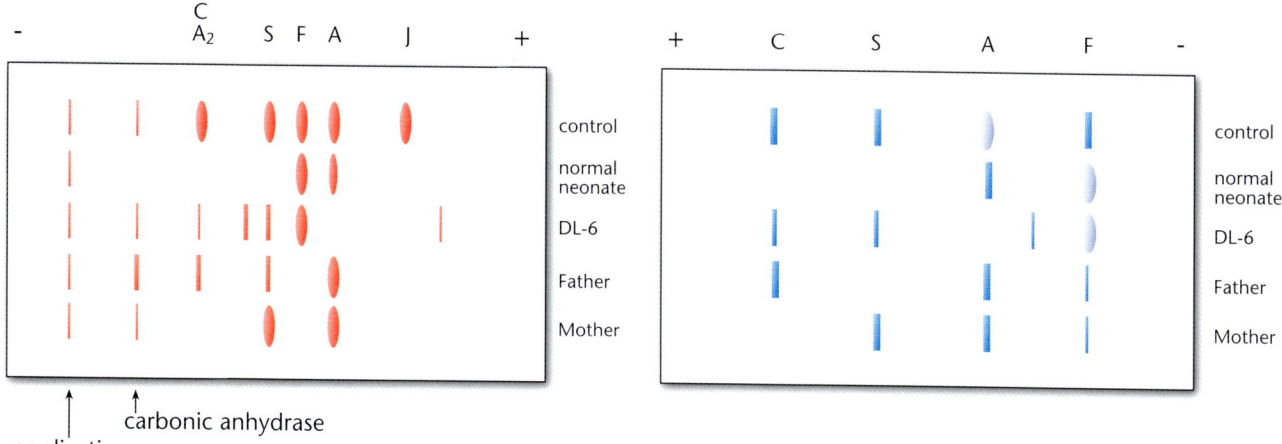

Case DL-6 Discussion

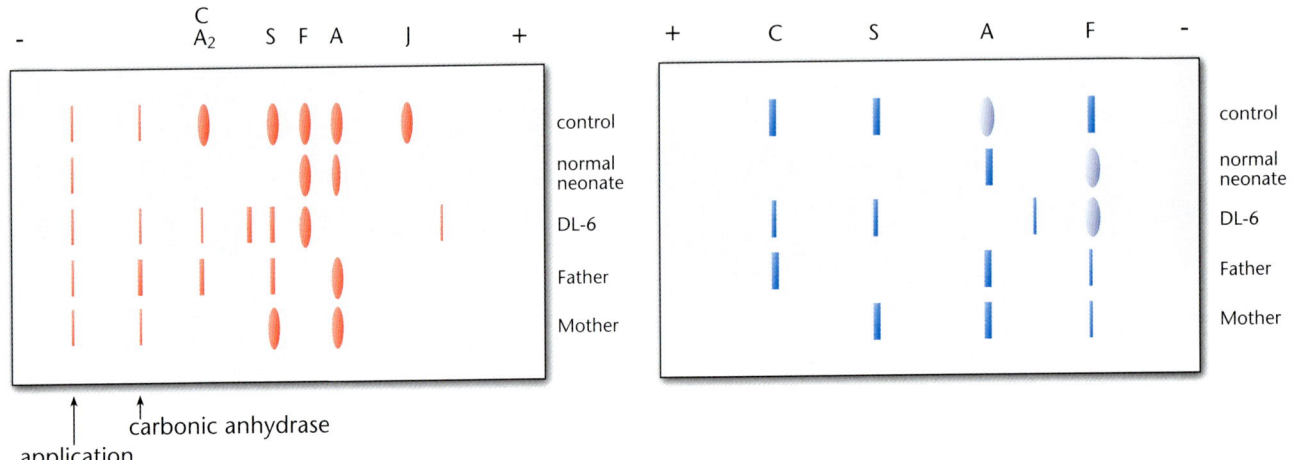

Interpretation

Examination of the alkaline gel shows no Hb A present. The amount of Hb F present is normal for age. However, there are multiple other bands present. There are bands in the S and C positions on both alkaline electrophoresis and acid electrophoresis. There are three additional bands seen on alkaline electrophoresis as well: a fast band, a band seen between the S and C position, and a band in the carbonic anhydrase position.

Diagnosis

Hb S/C/G-Philadelphia in a neonate.

Performance

The percentages of participating laboratories that correctly identified the hemoglobins present in this neonatal specimen were: Hb F, 95%; Hb S, 96%; Hb C, 91%; C/G hybrid, 55%; S/G hybrid, 48%; and F/G hybrid, 39%.

Discussion

This case presents a bewildering array of bands on alkaline electrophoresis, which may seem at first impossible to decipher. However, electrophoresis on both parents is also available for review. Examination of their electrophoretic patterns is very helpful in determining the abnormalities in the child.

The mother's alkaline and acid electrophoresis are typical for Hb S trait. The father's alkaline electrophoresis has four major bands. The presence of Hb C is confirmed by acid electrophoresis. The four bands produced are consistent with the combination of a β chain variant (Hb C) with an α chain variant. In African Americans, this is almost always Hb G-Philadelphia. The Hb C/G-Philadelphia combination is also the subject of a separate dry lab challenge (see case DL-6, page 277).

When the alkaline electrophoresis of the child is next examined, the first major abnormality noted is the absence of Hb A. Thus, there must be two β chain abnormalities present. In conjunction with the patterns seen in the parents, she must have inherited Hb C from the father and Hb S from the mother. The presence of Hb G-Philadelphia in the child is also suggested by the extra bands that are present. The bands seen in the child are (from anodal to cathodal): Hb F ($\alpha_2\gamma_2$), Hb S ($\alpha_2\beta^S_2$), and the F/G hybrid ($\alpha^G_2\gamma_2$). The A_2 position contains both Hbs C ($\alpha_2\beta^C_2$) and the S/G hybrid ($\alpha^G_2\beta^S_2$). The presence of a hemoglobin variant in this position is suggested because Hb A_2 is normally not present in a neonate. Similarly, the carbonic anhydrase is not usually seen in a neonatal specimen. The band in this position is due to the C/G hybrid ($\alpha^G_2\beta^C_2$) and the G_2 variant ($\alpha^G_2\delta_2$).

An example of S/C/G-Philadelphia in an adult is given in Figures DL-6.1 to DL-6.3.

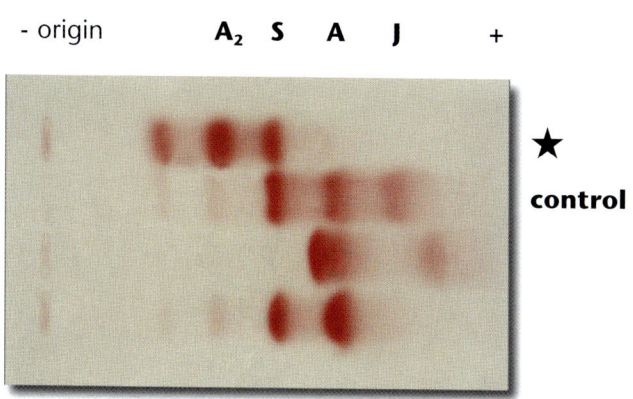

Figure DL-6.1
An example of Hb S/C/G-Philadelphia in an adult by alkaline electrophoresis (*). There are three major bands produced. This pattern is very similar in appearance to the S/G-Philadelphia combination except that all three bands are shifted by one position. There is no Hb A present. The major band in the S position is due to Hb S. The large band in the A_2 position is due to the presence of Hb C as well as the S/G hybrid. The large band in the carbonic anhydrase position is due to both the C/G hybrid as well as the G_2 variant.

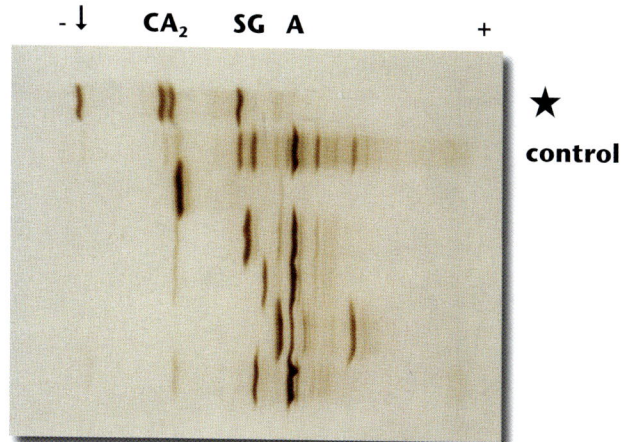

Figure DL-6.2
A case of Hb S/C/G-Philadelphia in an adult by isoelectric focusing. Four major bands are present. There is a band in the S position, corresponding to Hb S. The S/G hybrid and Hb C occur as a doublet in the approximate A_2 position. The arrow points to the combination of the C/G hybrid as well as the G_2 variant. The band normally corresponding to Hb G-Philadelphia (compare to control) is not seen. This is because there are no normal β chains present to combine with the abnormal α^G chains, which would produce the usual Hb G-Philadelphia band.

References

Rucknagel DL, Rising JA. A heterozygote for Hb β^S, Hb β^C, Hb α$^{G\text{-Philadelphia}}$ in a family presenting evidence for heterogeneity of hemoglobin alpha chain loci. *Am J Med.* 1975;59:53-60.

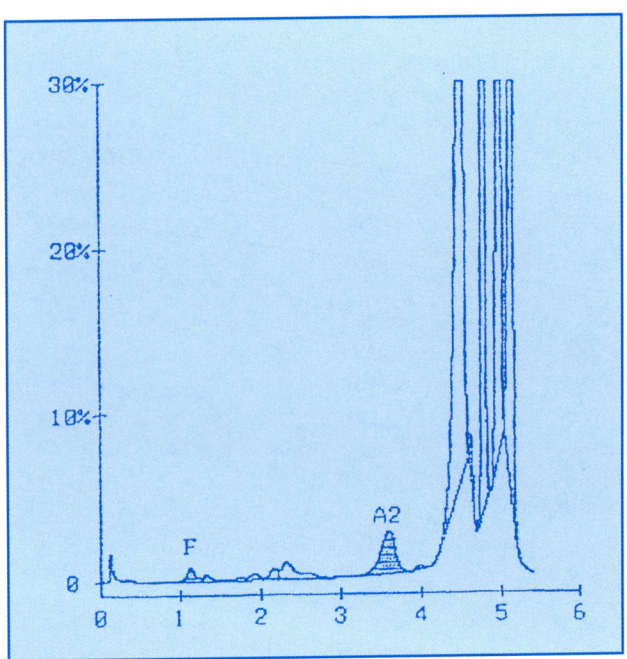

Figure DL-6.3
An example of Hb S/C/G-Philadelphia in an adult by HPLC. The four bands present are as follows: Hb S in the S window at approximately 4.5 minutes, the S/G hybrid occurring at approximately 4.8 minutes, Hb C occurring in the C window at approximately 5 minutes, and the C/G hybrid occurring at approximately 5.1 minutes. Minor bands, such as the G$_2$ variant, do not separate out as a distinct peak.

DL-7

HISTORY
The patient is a full-term baby girl, born to healthy parents of Laotian ancestry. Hemoglobin electrophoresis was performed on both parents as well as the child.

BLOOD COUNT DATA

	Baby	Father	Mother
RBC (x 10^{12}/L)	6.0	6.1	5.6
Hgb (g/dL)	17.0	15.1	13.5
MCV (fL)	85.0	76.0	72.0
WBC (x 10^9/L)	15.1	8.2	7.4
Plt (x 10^9/L)	398	293	203
Serum Ferritin (μg/L)	Not Done	198	121
Test for Unstable Hb	Not Done	Positive	Negative

PERIPHERAL BLOOD SMEAR
Baby: Target cells, polychromasia, erythroblasts.
Father: Occasional target cells.
Mother: Occasional target cells, microcytosis.

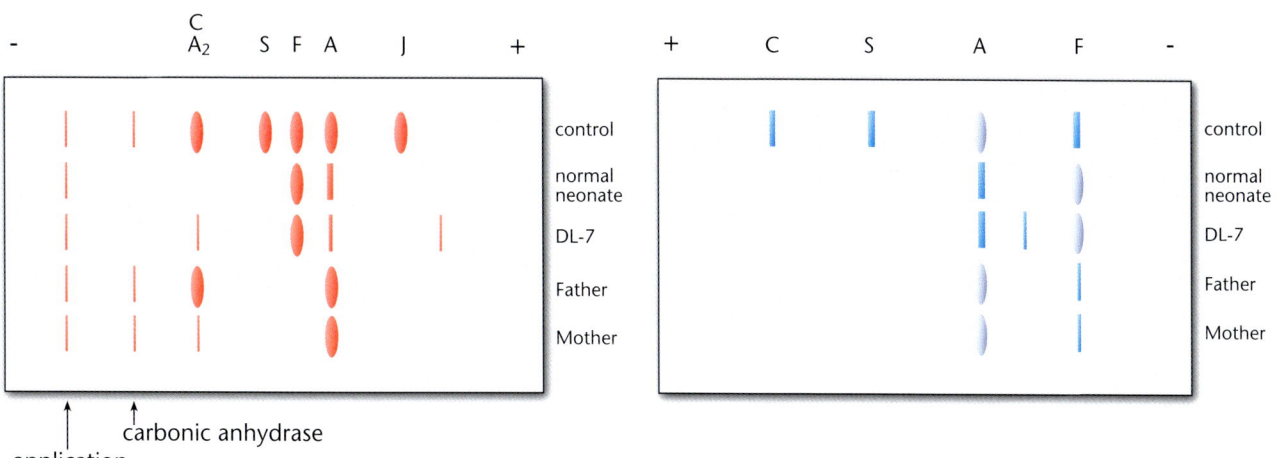

Case DL-7 Discussion

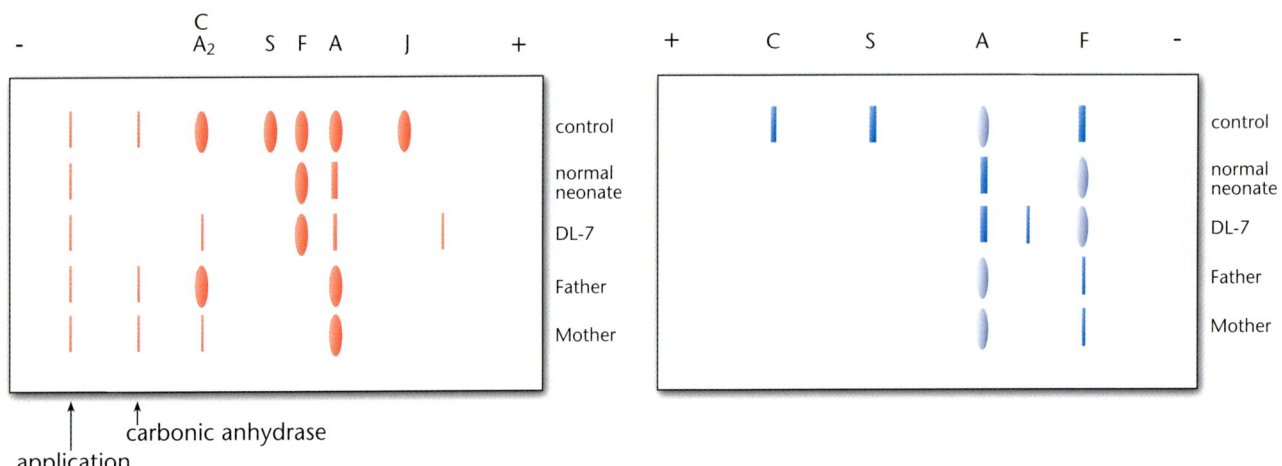

Interpretation

Examination of baby's alkaline electrophoresis gel shows, in addition to Hb A and Hb F, a small band in the A₂ position as well as a minor fast band. Acid electrophoresis shows a small band between the A and F positions.

Diagnosis

Hb E trait with α-thalassemia trait.

Performance

95% of laboratories identified the presence of Hbs A and F; 74% correctly identified Hb Bart's; and 66% identified the presence of Hb E.

Discussion

Hb E in combination with α-thalassemia has been previously discussed in a separate case (Case 34). In this neonatal specimen, two important points are emphasized:

1. In neonatal specimens, a band in the A_2 position is not typically seen and does not usually represent Hb A_2. Therefore, either the age of the child is incorrect, or a hemoglobin variant is present, such as Hb E or Hb C.

2. As discussed in other cases, the presence of Hb Bart's indicates concurrent α-thalassemia.

Examination of the patients' electrophoresis pattern helps to confirm this. Thus, the child inherited Hb E trait from his father and α-thalassemia trait from his mother.

DL-8

HISTORY
The patient is a newborn African-American female who had an abnormal hemoglobin electrophoresis by a state neonatal screening program for hemoglobinopathies. Her specimen was reexamined together with samples obtained from both parents. Neither the proband nor her parents had been recently transfused.

BLOOD COUNT DATA
Not available.

PERIPHERAL BLOOD SMEAR
Not available for review.

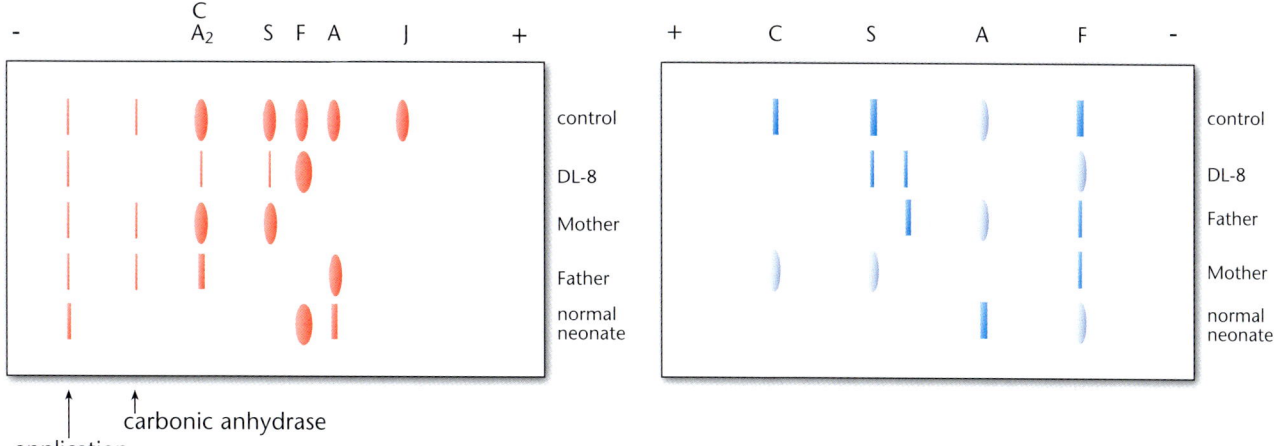

Dry Lab Challenges

Case DL-8 Discussion

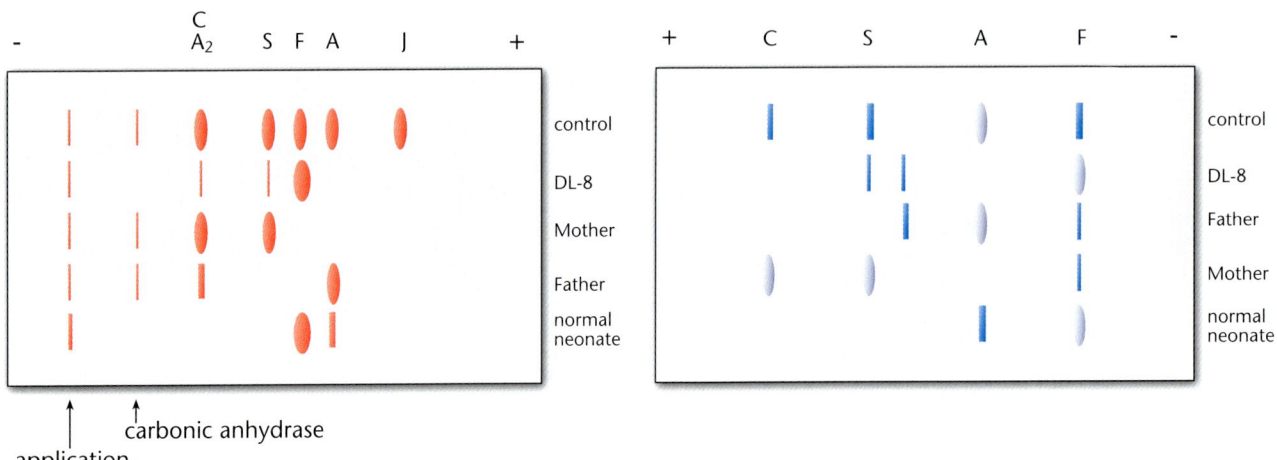

Interpretation

The alkaline electrophoresis demonstrates a predominance of Hb F in the neonate, with additional bands migrating in the S and A_2 regions. There is no detectable Hb A. The mother's electrophoresis pattern demonstrates bands in the S and A_2 positions with absence of Hb A. The father has bands in the A and A_2 positions. On acid electrophoresis, the infant has bands in the F and S positions, and a band that migrates between S and A. The mother has bands in the S and A_2 positions. The father has a band in the A position and a band that migrates between S and A, in the same position as that observed in the child.

Diagnosis

Hb S/O-Arab in a neonate.

Performance

Of respondents, 98% correctly identified the presence of Hb F, 92% correctly identified the presence of Hb S, and 71% correctly identified the presence of Hb O-Arab in the infant.

Discussion

This case represents compound heterozygosity for Hb S and Hb O-Arab in a neonate. The mother has Hb S/C disease. The father has Hb O-Arab trait. Therefore, the offspring inherited the Hb S mutation from her mother and the Hb O-Arab mutation from her father. Hb O-Arab ($\alpha_2\beta_2$121Glu→Lys) results from the replacement of glutamic acid by lysine at the amino acid 121 position in the β chain. Hb O-Arab has a wide geographic distribution, but the compound heterozygous condition, Hb S/Hb O-Arab occurs most commonly in this country in African Americans.

Hb S/O-Arab is a severe sickling disorder. Like Hb D-Los Angeles, Hb O-Arab copolymerizes with Hb S because the β121 position is an important contact site in the formation of sickle fibers. Affected individuals are anemic with normal red cell indices. Blood smears typically demonstrate the presence of sickle forms and target cells. Children with Hb S/O-Arab may develop hand-foot syndrome and acute splenic sequestration crises. A recent review (Zimmerman, et al) summarizes one institution's experience with this disorder.

This dry lab exercise asked participants to evaluate the utility of performing sickle solubility tests on the parents to predict the possibility of a sickling disorder in their offspring. A positive sickle solubility result would be expected for the mother, but not for the father. However, this does not preclude the possibility of a serious sickling disorder in their offspring, since Hb S/O-Arab is a sickling disorder. Therefore, the sickle solubility test in the parents has no predictive value for the offspring. A sickle solubility test performed on the neonate would probably be negative, because of the high proportion of Hb F and the low proportion of Hb S that are present at birth.

Another interesting aspect of this family study is that the mother also has a sickling disorder, but it is different from that of her daughter! The mother has Hb S/C disease. On alkaline electrophoresis, Hb C and Hb O-Arab have the same mobilities. Acid electrophoresis is necessary to distinguish Hb C from Hb O-Arab. Hb O-Arab has a characteristic mobility on acid electrophoresis that typically falls somewhere between S and A, although variability in the exact distance from Hb S has been observed. In some electrophoretic media, the O-Arab band displays a distinctive crescent-like pattern. This finding is a helpful clue to the presence of Hb O-Arab. On isoelectric focusing, Hb O-Arab, Hb E, and Hb C-Harlem are inseparable. An example of Hb S/O-Arab in a child is shown on HPLC (Figure DL-8.1) and isoelectric focusing (Figure DL-8.2).

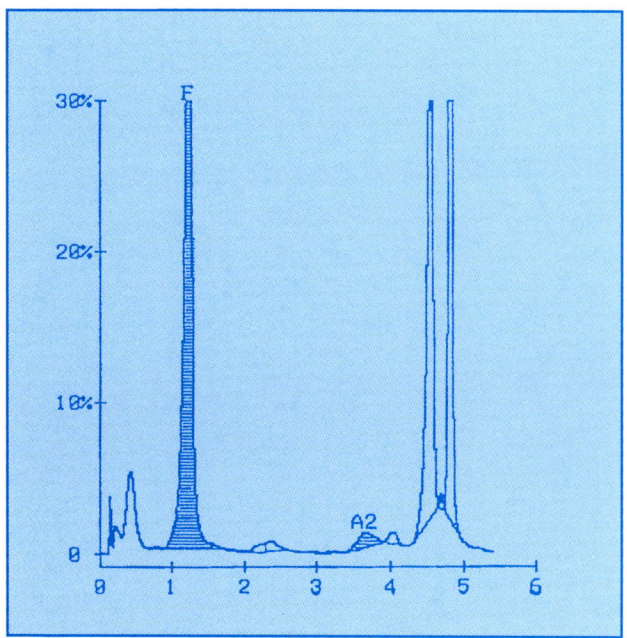

Figure DL-8.1
An example of Hb S/Hb O-Arab in a young child by HPLC. There are three major peaks present: the Hb F peak, Hb S in the S window, and Hb O-Arab in between the S and C windows at approximately 4.8 minutes.

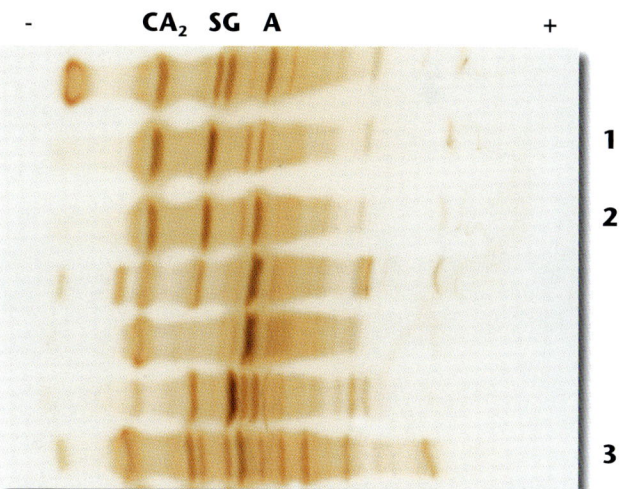

Figure DL-8.2
An example of Hb S/Hb O-Arab in a young child by isoelectric focusing. There are major bands in the S and A_2 positions (lanes 1 and 2). There is also Hb A present in this case, due to previous transfusion. Lane 3-control specimen.

References

Bunn HF, Forget BG. *Hemoglobin: Molecular, Genetic and Clinical Aspects.* Philadelphia, PA: WB Saunders Co; 1986:538.

Milner PF, Miller C, Grey R, et al. Hemoglobin O-Arab in four Negro families and its interaction with hemoglobin S and hemoglobin C. *New Engl J Med.* 1970;283:1417-1425.

Rachmilewitz EA, Tamari H, Liff F, et al. The interaction of hemoglobin O-Arab with Hb S and β^+-thalassemia among Israeli Arabs. *Hum Genet.* 1985;70:119-125.

Zimmerman SA, O'Branski EE, Rosse WF, Ware RE. Hemoglobin S/O-Arab: thirteen new cases and a review of the literature. *Am J Hematol.* 1999;60:279-284.

DL-9

HISTORY
A 22-year-old African-American woman was examined because of anemia. She was three months pregnant. She had experienced repeated episodes of pain in her extremities, and during childhood she had sometimes had painful, swollen hands and fingers. On physical examination, there was moderate pallor of conjunctivae and mucous membranes and slight scleral icterus. There was no splenomegaly on physical examination.

BLOOD COUNT DATA
RBC .... $1.91 \times 10^{12}/L$
Hb .... 6.3 g/dL
MCV .... 96.5 fL
WBC .... $11.8 \times 10^9/L$
Plt .... $194 \times 10^9/L$

OTHER LABORATORY TESTS
The solubility test for sickling hemoglobin is positive.

PERIPHERAL BLOOD SMEAR
Crescentic erythrocytes, target cells, and occasional Howell-Jolly bodies.

Hb electrophoresis alkaline (pH 8.6)

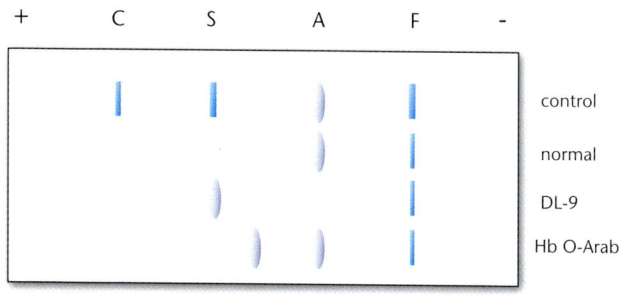

Hb electrophoresis acid (pH 6.2)

Isoelectric Focusing

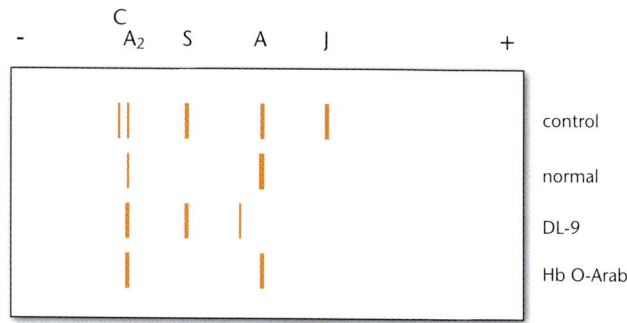

Dry Lab Challenges

Case DL-9 Discussion

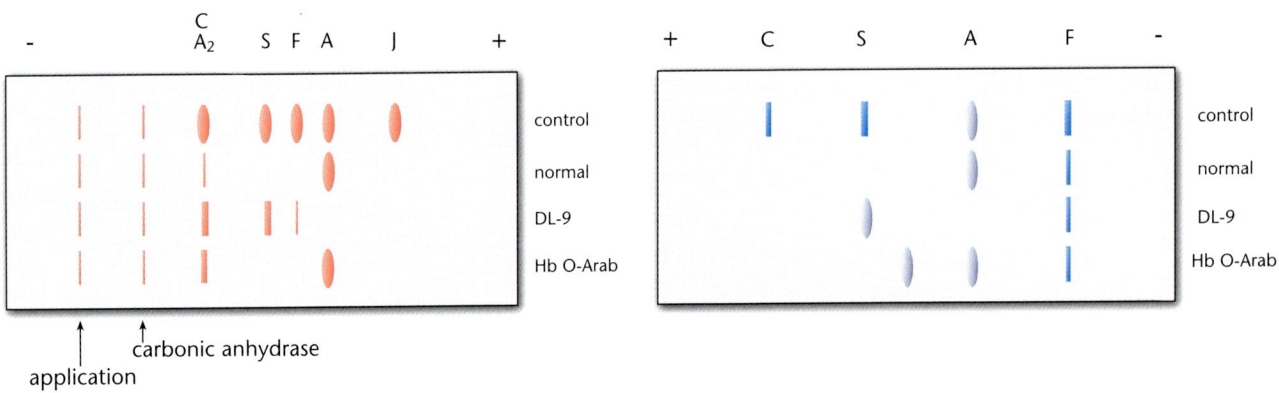

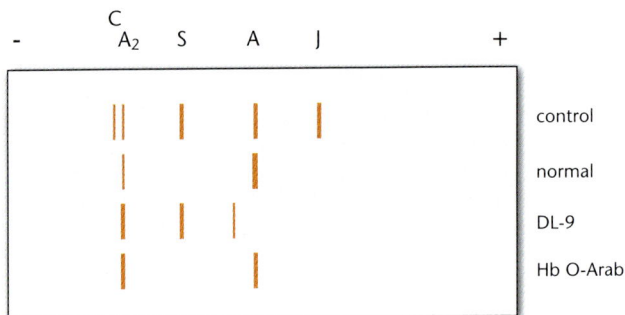

Interpretation

The alkaline electrophoresis demonstrates two major bands of approximately equal density in the S and C positions. On acid electrophoresis, both Hb variants migrate in the S position. On isoelectric focusing, there is a band in the S position and a band in the A_2 position that is distinct from Hb C.

Diagnosis

Hb S/Hb C-Harlem.

Performance

74.5% of participants identified Hb S, and 54.1% also identified the presence of Hb C-Harlem.

Discussion

Hb C-Harlem (β6Val,73Asn) is a β globin chain variant that results from two amino acid substitutions. The substitution of valine for glutamine at the amino acid 6 position is identical to the mutation for Hb S. The substitution at the amino acid 73 position of asparagine for aspartic acid is identical to the mutation for Hb Korle-Bu. It is likely that a crossover event in the distant past placed these two mutations in the same β globin gene. The presence of two mutations in the β globin gene with the resultant amino acid substitutions accounts for the characteristic migration patterns of this rare hemoglobin variant under alkaline and acid conditions.

Hb C-Harlem has very unique electrophoretic properties. Although it migrates like Hb C on alkaline electrophoresis, on acid electrophoresis it migrates in the S position (due to the S mutation that is present). On isoelectric focusing it migrates in the A_2 position (Figure DL-9.2). On HPLC it elutes between the S and C windows (Figure DL-9.1).

Hb C-Harlem is a very rare hemoglobin variant and has only been described in about 10-15 Black families. It is important to recognize this variant because it gives rise to a sickling disorder in the homozygous state and in combination with Hb S, which is more likely due to the higher gene frequency of Hb S. The property of sickling is conferred by the presence of the β6Val mutation, which results in co-polymerization with Hb S. Hb C-Harlem will result in a positive sickle solubility test, provided the hemoglobin variant is present in sufficient proportion to be detected. Immunologic assays have been developed for the detection of Hb S that are based on antibodies with specificity directed against the portion of the β chain region that includes the amino acid 6 position occupied by valine. These antibody tests will also give a positive reaction in the presence of Hb C-Harlem.

The dry lab exercise asked participants to consider the risk to the mother's unborn child of inheriting a sickling disorder. If the biological father were tested and found not to carry a hemoglobin variant, the child would not be at risk for a sickling disorder. Since the child can inherit either the $β^S$ gene or the $β^{C\text{-Harlem}}$ gene from the mother, but not both, the child will either have Hb S trait or Hb C-Harlem trait. At birth, there might not be enough Hb S or Hb C-Harlem to result in a positive sickle solubility test. An immunologic assay for Hb S is more sensitive for detecting low levels of Hb S or Hb C Harlem. A small amount of either variant hemoglobin should be detectable on both alkaline and acid electrophoreses and on isoelectric focusing at birth.

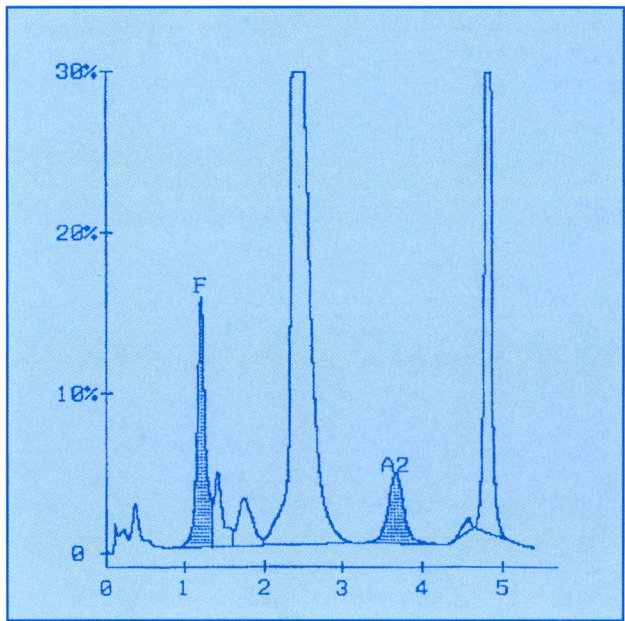

Figure DL-9.1
An example of Hb C-Harlem trait by HPLC. Hb C-Harlem elutes between the S and C windows at approximately 4.8 minutes.

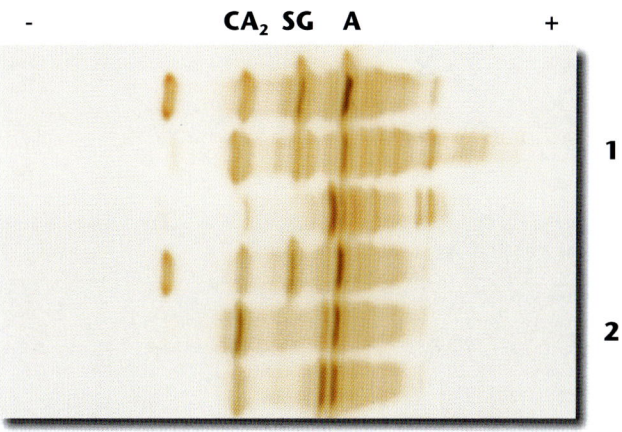

Figure DL-9.2
An example of Hb C-Harlem trait by isoelectric focusing (lane 2). In contrast to Hb C, Hb C-Harlem migrates in the A_2 position on isoelectric focusing. Lane 1-control specimen.

The differential diagnosis of Hb S/C-Harlem includes other hemoglobin variants that migrate in the A_2 position on alkaline electrophoresis, such as Hb S/C, Hb S/E and Hb S/O-Arab. The differentiation of these is usually straightforward using a combination of alkaline and acid electrophoresis. The differentiation of Hb S/O-Arab and Hb S/C-Harlem can sometimes be difficult because of the variability in position of Hb O-Arab on acid electrophoresis. It is possible that Hb O-Arab could migrate almost in the S position. However, clinically the distinction between these two possibilities is not critical as they are both sickling disorders.

Homozygous Hb S with Hb G-Philadelphia could also possibly be confused with Hb S/C-Harlem as the S/G hybrid migrates in the A_2 position on alkaline electrophoresis. Key to the differentiation of these two possibilities is the presence or absence of the G_2 variant (seen particularly well on isoelectric focusing). The S/G hybrid also accounts for a much smaller percentage of the total hemoglobin than Hb C-Harlem. Globin chain electrophoresis can also be very useful in this situation.

References

Bookchin RM, Nagel RL, Ranney HM. Structure and properties of hemoglobin C-Harlem: a human hemoglobin variant with amino acid substitutions in two residues of the beta polypeptide chain. *J Biol Chem.* 1967;242:248-255.

Garver FA, Baker MM, Grenett HE. Immunochemical properties of abnormal hemoglobins C-Harlem, S, Korle Bu, Vancouver, and Mobile. *Biochim Biophys Acta.* 1980;624:286-92.

Huisman THT, Carver MFH, Efremov D. *A Syllabus of Human Hemoglobin Variants.* Augusta, GA: The Sickle Cell Anemia Foundation; 1996.

Moo-Penn W, Bechtel K, Jue D, et al. The presence of hemoglobin S and C-Harlem in an individual in the United States. *Blood.* 1975;46:363-7.

DL-10

HISTORY
A 29-year-old woman of Chinese origin was evaluated for anemia. She stated that she had been anemic most of her life and had been given iron pills for this, but always remained anemic. The physical examination revealed slight scleral icterus. The spleen was barely palpable.

BLOOD COUNT DATA
RBC .... $4.4 \times 10^{12}/L$
Hgb .... 10.5 g/dL
MCV .... 59.6 fL
WBC .... $8.3 \times 10^9/L$
Plt .... $331 \times 10^9/L$

OTHER LABORATORY TESTS
A test for unstable hemoglobin was positive.

PERIPHERAL BLOOD SMEAR
Blood film confirmed hypochromia and microcytosis. In addition, there was a slight polychromasia and basophilic stippling, and many target erythrocytes.

Hb electrophoresis alkaline (pH 8.6)

Hb electrophoresis acid (pH 6.2)

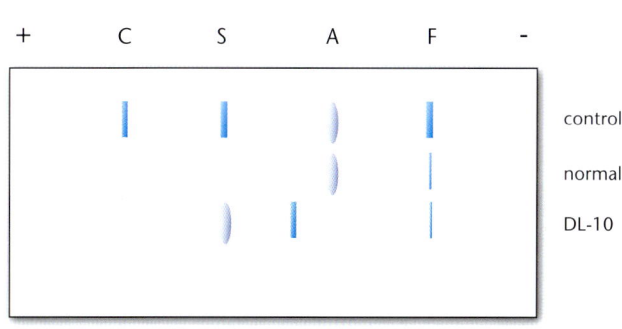

Isoelectric Focusing

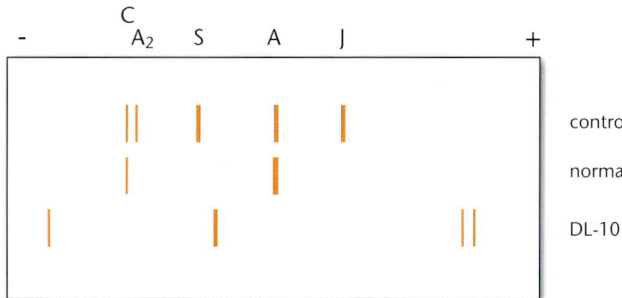

Case DL-10 Discussion

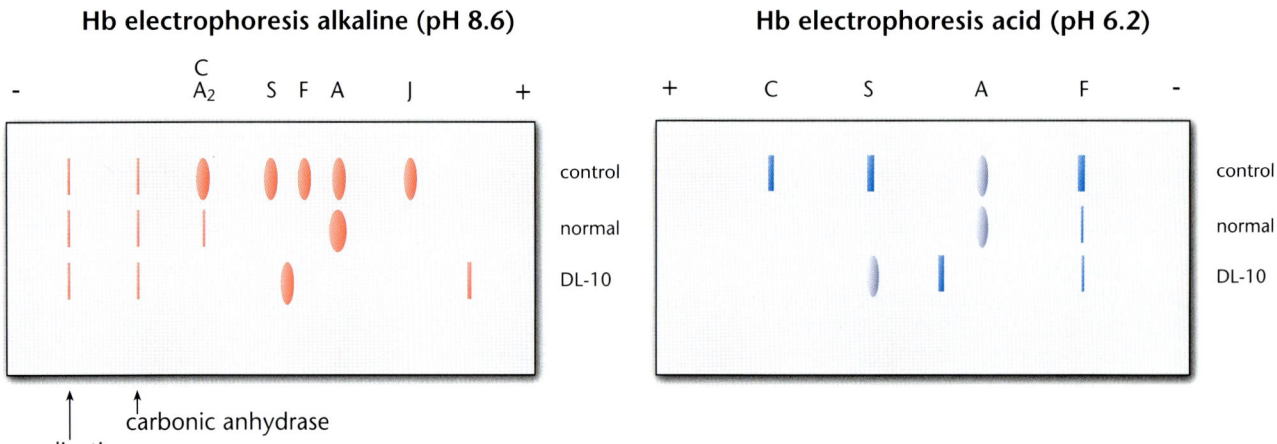

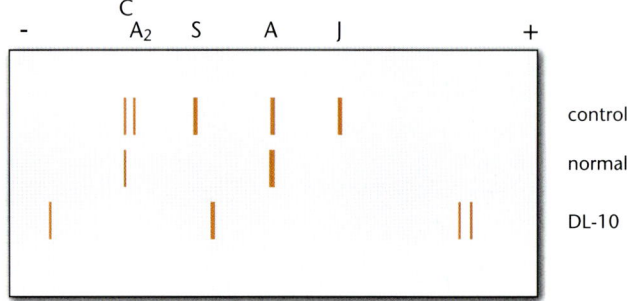

Interpretation

On alkaline electrophoresis, there is no Hb A present. There is a major band that migrates slightly anodal to the Hb S position, as well as a small fast band that is as far in front of the A position as Hb C is behind Hb A. On acid electrophoresis, there is a band in the S position and a small band between Hb A and Hb S. Isoelectric focusing shows a similar pattern as alkaline electrophoresis, except that the fast band appears as a doublet, and there is a slow minor band seen cathodal to the A_2 position.

Diagnosis

Hb Q-Thailand/Hb H disease.

Performance

78.5% of laboratories recognized the presence of Hb H, and 54.8% of laboratories correctly identified the presence of Hb Q-Thailand.

Discussion

This represents a case of Hb Q-Thailand/H disease. Hb Q-Thailand (also called Mahidol, Q-Chinese, G-Taichung, Hb Kurashiki, or Hb Asabara) is a rare α chain variant found only in those of Asian descent. The variant results from the substitution of histidine for aspartic acid at position 74 of the alpha chain (α74 [EF3] Asp→His). This variant is interesting in that it is always associated with a deletion of the contiguous upstream α2 globin gene locus ("leftward deletion"), giving the patient with the heterozygous condition a mild thalassemic blood picture. When the patient also inherits, on the other chromosome 16, the α-thalassemia-1 trait (deletion of both α globin loci), which is also common in those of Asian ancestry, Hb Q-H disease results, as in this case. In such a case, there is only one α chain present and this carries the Q-Thailand mutation. Therefore, there is neither Hb A nor F nor A_2. Excess β chains are produced, accounting for the presence of Hb H ($β_4$). On isoelectric focusing, there is an additional band seen close to Hb H, which likely represents a small amount of Hb Bart's ($γ_4$). This band was not seen in any of the other media. Additional faint bands would be Hb Q-F and Hb Q-A_2, each containing $α^Q$ globin chains. An example of Hb Q/H disease on HPLC is shown in Figure DL-10.1.

Clinically, cases of Hb Q/H disease are similar to other types of Hb H disease. These are classified as a thalassemia intermedia, with a moderate microcytic anemia and usually some degree of splenomegaly. Hb Q-Thailand is also notable historically. Cases of Hb Q-Thailand trait and Q-H disease were used as evidence to deduce that there must be four alpha chains in the normal person instead of two, as with the beta chains.

References

Beris P, Huber P, Miescher PA, et al. Hb Q-Thailand-Hb H disease in a Chinese living in Geneva, Switzerland: characterization of the variant and identification of the two α-thalassemia chromosomes. *Am J Hematol.* 1987;24:395-400.

Dormandy KM, Luck SP. Hemoglobin Q-alpha-thalassemia. *Br Med J.* 1961;1:1582-1585.

Lie-Injo LE, Pillay RP, Thuraisingham V, et al. Further cases of Hb Q-H disease (Hb Q-α thalassemia). *Blood.* 1966;28(6):830-839.

Lie-Injo LE, Dozy AM, Kan YW, et al. The α-globin gene adjacent to the gene for Hb Q-α 74 Asp-His is deleted, but not that adjacent to the gene for Hb G-α-30 Glu→Gln; three-fourths of the α-globin genes are deleted in Hb Q-α-thalassemia. *Blood.* 1979;54(6):1407-1416.

Vella F, et al. A hemoglobinopathy involving hemoglobin H and a new (Q) hemoglobin. *Br Med J.* 1958;1:752-755.

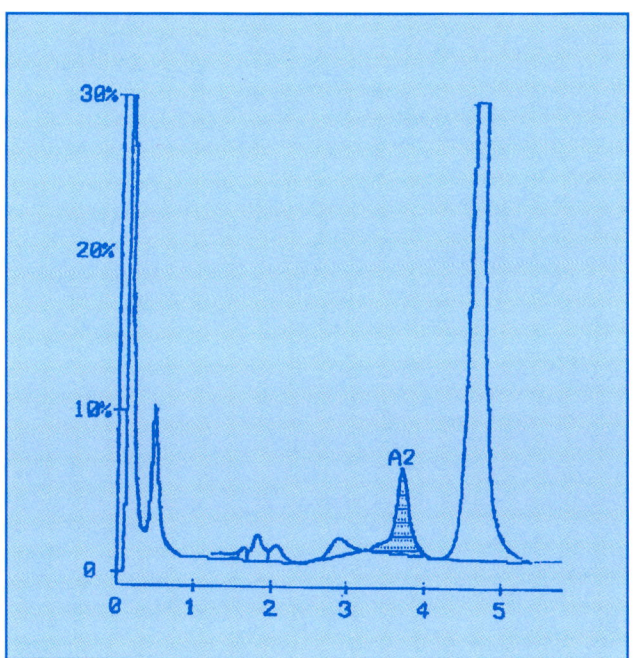

Figure DL-10.1
An example of Hb Q/Hb H disease by HPLC. There is a very fast peak at 0.5 minutes representing Hb H. There is no Hb A present but a major peak in the S window at 4.6-4.7 minutes representing Hb Q Thailand ($α^Q_2β^A_2$). The peak seen in the A_2 window cannot represent normal Hb A_2, as there are no normal α chains present. This peak likely represents the delta variant of Hb Q Thailand ($α^Q_2δ_2$). The very fast peak at 0.2 minutes in this case is unlikely to be Hb Bart's and is probably due to increased bilirubin in the specimen.

DL-11

HISTORY
The patient is a 33-year-old male from Kuwait seen for evaluation of recurrent pain in extremities and abdomen. He had never received transfusions or other therapy for anemia. The physical examination revealed only that he walked with a slight limp and that there was limitation in range of passive motion of the hip joints bilaterally. The X-ray examination of the hips showed patchy sclerosis of the femoral heads suggestive of partial asceptic necrosis.

BLOOD COUNT DATA
RBC .... 5.1×10^{12}/L
Hgb .... 9.8 g/dL
MCV .... 59 fL
WBC .... 7.6×10^9/L
Plt .... 196×10^9/L

PERIPHERAL BLOOD SMEAR
Revealed only mild anisocytosis, ovalocytosis and microcytosis. There were no target cells and no Howell-Jolly bodies.

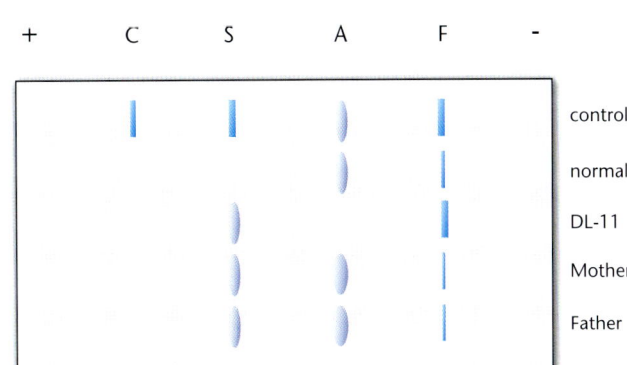

Dry Lab Challenges

Case DL-11 Discussion

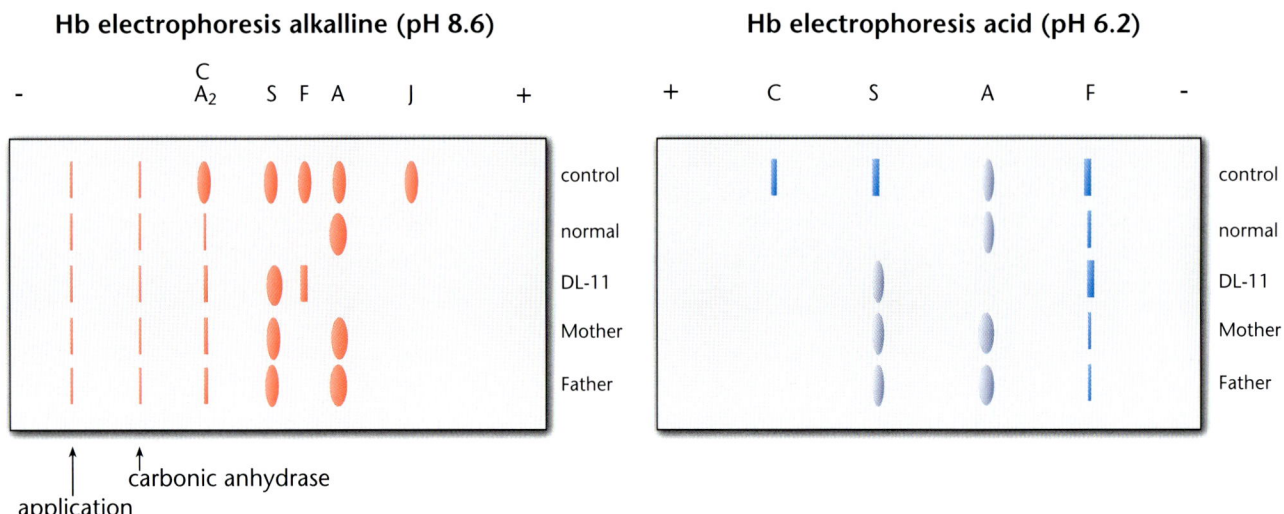

Interpretation

Both alkaline and acid electrophoresis show the absence of Hb A in the patient. There is a major band in the S position and an increase in Hb F. Both parents have bands in the A and S positions on alkaline and acid electrophoresis.

Diagnosis

Homozygous Hb S with high Hb F levels.

Performance

Of laboratories responding, 31% identified this as a case of homozygous Hb S, 31% identified this as representing homozygous Hb S with α-thalassemia, 3% as homozygous Hb S with high Hb F, and 13% as homozygous S with HPFH.

Discussion

This dry lab challenge case was based on an actual patient, with the laboratory findings as stated. He had homozygous Hb S disease, with history of pain crises, bone infarctions, and aseptic necrosis, although he suffered a milder form of sickle cell disease than we usually encounter in African Americans. He had the elevated Hb F that is typical of Saudi Arabian (and Kuwaiti) homozygous Hb S disease. The diagrams of the electrophoretic patterns of his parents' specimens illustrated Hb S trait in each, with about 25-30% Hb S, and their laboratory data indicated microcytosis, both features typical of Hb S trait with α-thalassemia trait.

A Southern blot α globin gene study of the patient's leukocyte DNA indicated that he was a compound heterozygote for the −3.7 Kb ("rightward") deletion α-thalassemia and also for the − 4.2 kb ("leftward") deletion α-thalassemia. Therefore, he has two functioning α globin genes, one on each chromosome 16.

It has long been recognized that homozygous Hb S disease in Arabs is often milder than that seen in African people, and that an elevation in Hb F is also typical. The cause of this "high Hb F determinant" appears to be a C→T mutation 158 nucleotides upstream (5′) to the $^G\gamma$ gene. This −158 position appears to be part of a $^G\gamma$ gene promoter sequence, so that associated with the Sen (Saudi/Asian) haplotype is an approximately 3- to 11-fold increase in $^G\gamma$ globin synthesis resulting in an elevated proportion of Hb F that persists into childhood and adult life. The same C→T change at position -158 of the $^G\gamma$ gene appears to be responsible for "Swiss type HPFH." It is not known whether the elevation in Hb F is responsible for the milder clinical disease. There has also been speculation that α-thalassemia, which is also prevalent in the Middle East, may be the ameliorating factor, as it is in African Americans with sickle cell disease. Studies conducted in Saudi Arabia have indicated that it is the concurrence of α-thalassemia that improves sickle cell disease in the Middle East, that having only two functioning α globin genes effects the most improvement, but some improvement occurs with a single α globin gene deletion. There seems to be little effect from the elevation in the proportion of Hb F. The reduction in severity of sickle cell disease is most evident in the lessening of the severity of anemia. However, other manifestations of sickle cell disease are also milder when homozygous Hb S occurs in the background of the Sen/Sen or Saudi/Saudi restriction endonuclease pattern, as described below.

Several types of α-thalassemia occur in the Middle East, including both the −3.7 Kb deletion and the −4.2 Kb deletion, which were demonstrated in this case. In addition, there is a Saudi Arabian type of α-thalassemia that is non-deletional, which is the result of a single nucleotide mutation (AATA<u>A</u>AA→AATA<u>G</u>) near the 3′ end of the α2 globin gene, in a nucleotide sequence that normally specifies polyadenylation of the 3′ end of the α globin gene mRNA. This mutation, which is quite common in Saudi Arabia and contiguous areas, cannot be detected by DNA probes that are sensitive only to large deletions.

The εγδβ gene cluster has been studied using a variety of restriction endonucleases. These studies have shown that there is variability within the gene cluster as to the presence or absence of DNA cleavage sites for a particular restriction enzyme. These specific polymorphism patterns have been called haplotypes. Five different haplotypes associated with the Hb S mutation have been defined and have provided evidence that the Hb S mutation has probably arisen independently at least four times. These haplotypes are named for the area in which they were first identified. The Sen (Senegal) haplotype is found most frequently on the northwest coast of Africa (Senegal, Gambia, Sierra Leone, Liberia, and Gold Coast). The Ben (Benin) haplotype is most frequent in Ghana and Nigeria. The CAR (Bantu) haplotype is most frequent in the Central African Republic, Gabon, Zaire, Angola and Kenya, and the Cam haplotype is found in Camaroon. The Saudi/Asian haplotype is found associated with the Hb S mutation in eastern Saudi Arabia, Kuwait, Pakistan, and India. This haplotype closely resembles the Sen haplotype and is probably derived from it. In African Americans and blacks from the Caribbean, the most common haplotypes are Sen, CAR, or Ben haplotypes. Mediterranean people with the β^S gene have the Ben or CAR haplotype.

The haplotypes present also influence the clinical manifestations and the severity of sickle cell anemia. For example, patients with sickle cell anemia who are homozygous Sen/Sen or Saudi/Saudi have a higher proportion of Hb F and less severe anemia than those who have the CAR or Ben haplotypes (CAR/CAR, Ben/Ben, or CAR/Ben). Those who are homozygous Sen/Sen or Saudi/Saudi also live longer and have a lower risk of renal disease or skin ulcers compared with those who have the CAR or Ben haplotypes.

References

Antonarakis SE, Boehm CD, Serjeant G, et al. Origin of the β^S-globin gene in blacks: the contribution of recurrent mutation or gene conversion or both. *Proc Natl Acad Sci USA.* 1984;81:853.

el-Hazmi MA. Clinical manifestation and laboratory findings of sickle cell anaemia in association with α-thalassaemia in Saudi Arabia. *Acta Haematol.* 1985;74:155-160.

el-Hazmi MA. Heterogeneity and variation of clinical and haematological expression of haemoglobin S in Saudi Arabs. *Acta Haematol.* 1992;88:67-71.

el-Hazmi MA, al-Swailem AR, Bahakim HM, et al. Effect of α-thalassaemia, G-6-PD deficiency and Hb F on the nature of sickle cell anaemia in southwestern Saudi Arabia. *Trop Geogr Med.* 1990;42:241-247.

Gilman JG, Huisman THJ. DNA sequence variation associated with elevated fetal $^G\gamma$ globin production. *Blood.* 1985;66:783-787.

Mears JG, Beldjord C, Benabadji M, et al. The sickle gene polymorphism in Africa. *Blood.* 1981;58:599-601.

Pagnier J, Mears JG, Dundabel O, et al. Evidence for the multicentric origin of the sickle hemoglobin gene in Africa. *Proc Natl Acad Sci USA.* 1984;81:1771-1773.

Powars DR. β^S gene cluster haplotypes in sickle cell anemia: clinical and hematologic features. *Hematol Oncol Clin North Am.* 1991;5:475-493.

DL-12

HISTORY
The patient is a 36-year-old woman of Southeast Asian ancestry. She has a life-long history of anemia for which she has received several blood transfusions. The physical examination showed mild to moderate splenomegaly.

BLOOD COUNT DATA
RBC.................4.9 x 10^{12}/L
Hgb.................8.7 g/dL
MCV.................59 fL
WBC.................12.9 x 10^9/L
Plt.................208 x 10^9/L

OTHER LABORATORY TESTS
A test for unstable hemoglobin was positive.

PERIPHERAL BLOOD SMEAR
Increased polychromasia and moderately severe anisopoikilocytosis, including many target cells, elliptocytes, and microcytes.

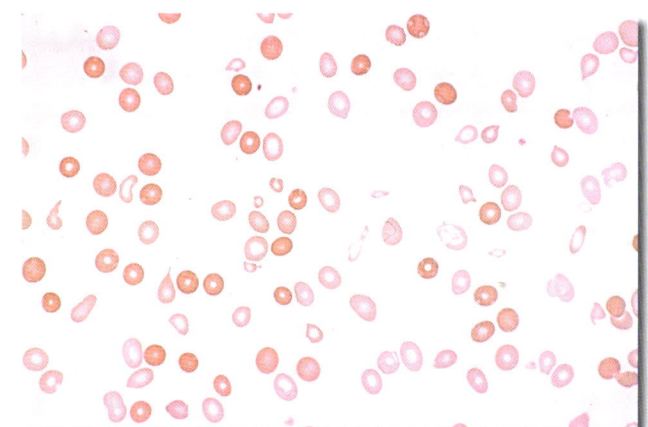

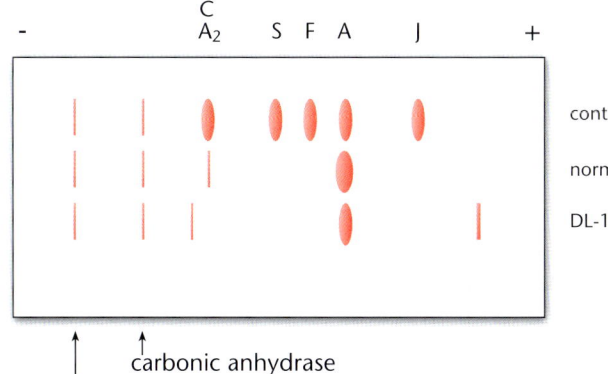

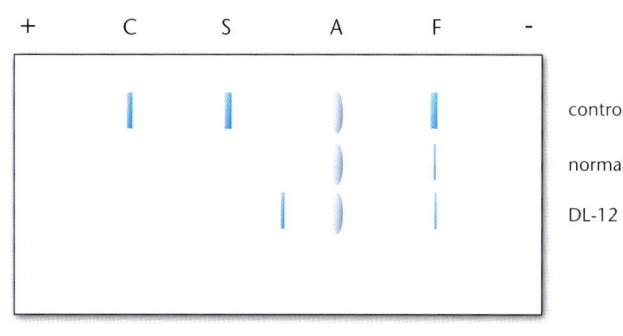

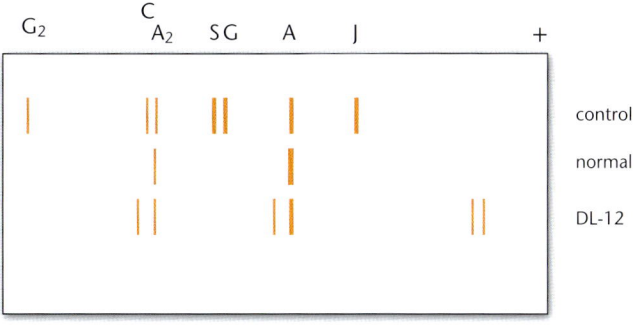

Dry Lab Challenges

Case DL-12 Discussion

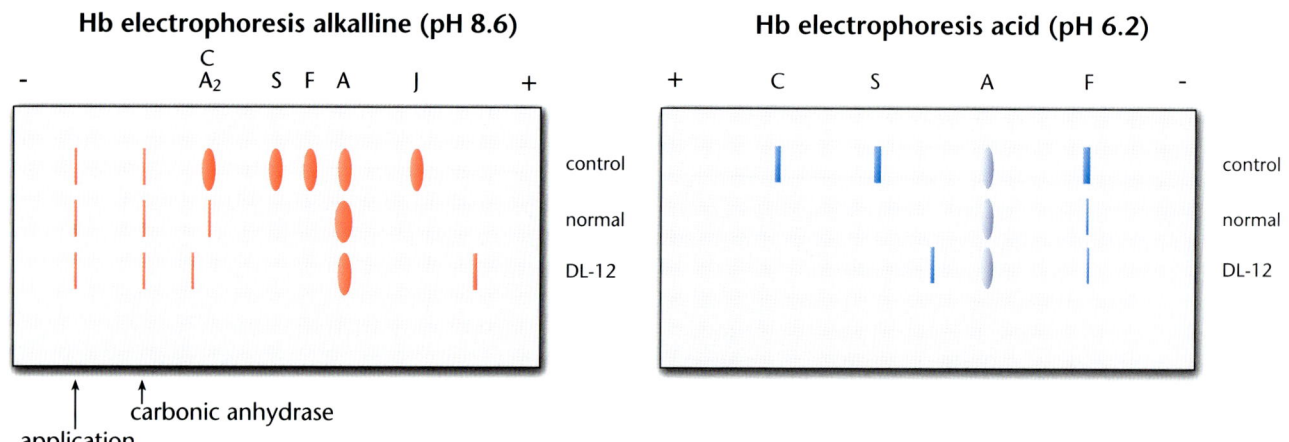

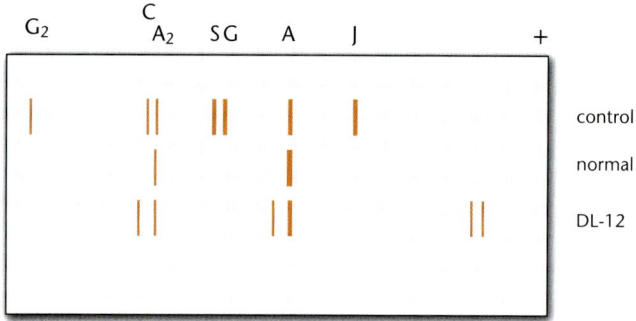

Interpretation

The alkaline electrophoresis demonstrates a single abnormal fast moving band that is located approximately twice as far from Hb A as the Hb J control. In addition, there is a faint slow moving band between the A₂ and carbonic anhydrase positions. Acid electrophoresis demonstrates an abnormal band between the A and S positions. Isoelectric focusing demonstrates a pair of fast moving bands as well as a slow moving band.

Diagnosis

Hb H/Hb Constant Spring.

Performance

Hb H/Hb Constant Spring has been used as a dry lab challenge twice. More than 90% of laboratories correctly identified the presence of Hb H disease, and 70-85% also correctly identified the presence of Hb Constant Spring.

Discussion

As discussed in case DL-1, approximately half of the cases of Hb H disease in Southeast Asian patients result from co-inheritance of α-thalassemia-1 and Hb Constant Spring (--/$\alpha^{CS}\alpha$). Hb Constant Spring is a structurally abnormal hemoglobin that results from a base substitution that eliminates the normal stop codon (codon 142, TAA→CAA) in the mRNA of the α_2 gene. This results in an abnormally long α chain (172 instead of 141 amino acids), which migrates very slowly on alkaline electrophoresis. Only very small amounts of Hb Constant Spring are produced, due to mRNA instability. Heterozygotes and homozygotes for $\alpha^{CS}\alpha$ have 1% and 3-5% Hb Constant Spring, respectively. Because the α^{CS} allele essentially functions as an α chain deletion, inheritance of both α-thalassemia-1 and Hb Constant Spring is equivalent to a three α gene deletion. Hb Constant Spring is seen in 3% of Southeast Asians.

Patients with Hb H/Hb Constant Spring have a similar syndrome as uncomplicated Hb H disease (see case DL-1). It is said that patients with the --/$\alpha^{CS}\alpha$ form of Hb H disease have a more severe anemia, perhaps because the affected upstream α allele is normally the dominant producer of α chains. The peripheral blood findings are also more pronounced, with a greater degree of anisopoikilocytosis and hypochromasia (Figure DL-12.1). Homozygous Hb Constant Spring produces a mild to moderate hemolytic anemia with splenomegaly (Figures DL-12.2 and DL-12.3).

The identification of Hb H was discussed in case DL-1. The Hb Constant Spring band may be easily overlooked in patient specimens due to its position and small size. If suspected, application of double the normal amount of hemolysate to the gel may help to visualize the minor Constant Spring band. The only slow-moving hemoglobins seen with significant frequency are A_2' and Constant Spring. Hb A_2' is seen in approximately 1-2% of African Americans and migrates between carbonic anhydrase and the application point, and thus does not correspond to the band seen in the current case. Furthermore, as discussed above, Hb Constant Spring is commonly seen in Hb H disease. In regard to the absence of a Hb A_2 band in the alkaline

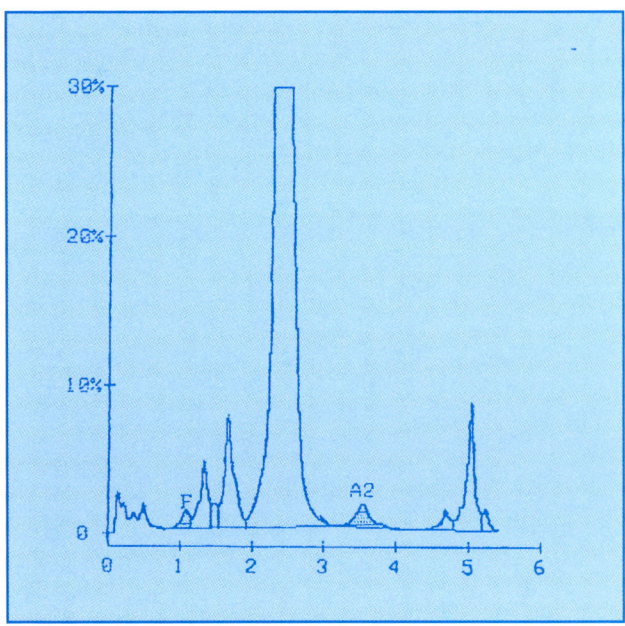

Figure DL-12.2
An example of homozygous Hb Constant Spring by HPLC. There is a prominent peak seen in the C window at 5.0 minutes representing Hb Constant Spring. The amount of this peak (5.3%) is consistent with homozygous Hb Constant Spring.

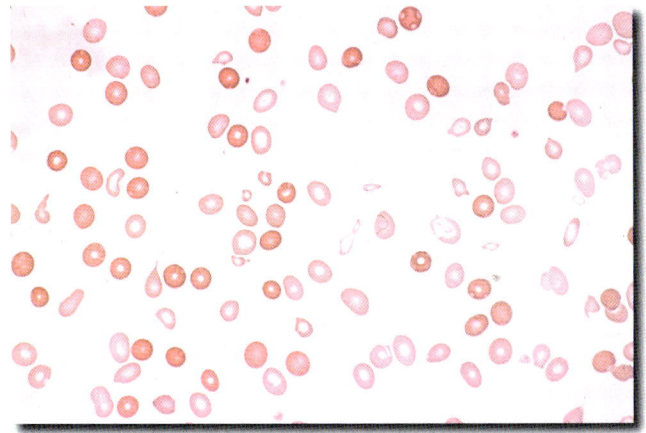

Figure DL-12.1 (Wright-Giemsa, 160x and 400x)
The peripheral blood smear in a patient with Hb H/Hb Constant Spring. This case shows a greater degree of anisopoikilocytosis

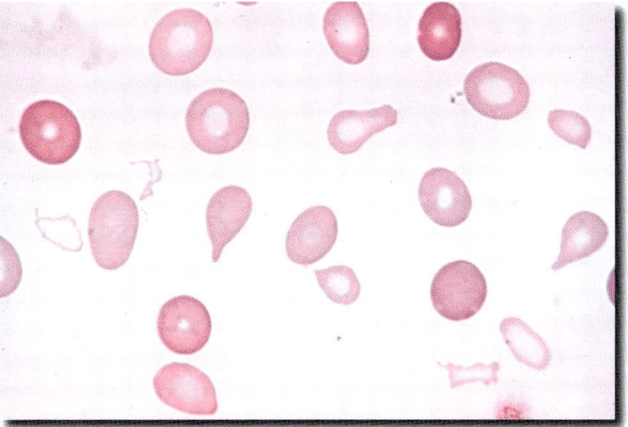

than the case shown in figure DL-1.1. This includes dacrocytes, elliptocytes, and markedly microcytic hypochromic cells.

Dry Lab Challenges

gel, for unknown reasons this band is so faint in cases of Hb H/Hb Constant Spring that it is generally not visualized. However, it is seen in the isoelectric focusing gel in the current case. An example of Hb H/Hb Constant Spring on HPLC is shown in Figure DL-12.4.

References

Bunn HF, Forget BG. *Hemoglobin: Molecular, Genetic and Clinical Aspects.* Philadelphia, PA: WB Saunders Co; 1986:299-301.

Fairbanks VF. *Hemoglobinopathies and Thalassemias. Laboratory Methods and Case Studies.* New York, NY: Brian C. Decker; 1980:231-233,188-191.

Luken JN. The thalassemias and related disorders: quantitative disorders of hemoglobin synthesis. In: Lee GR, Foerster J, Lukens J, et al, eds. *Wintrobe's Clinical Hematology.* 10th ed. Baltimore, MD: Williams and Wilkins; 1999:1405-1448.

Orkin SH, Nathan DG. The thalassemias. In: Nathan DG, Orkin SH, eds. *Hematology of infancy and childhood.* 5th ed. Philadelphia, PA: WB Saunders Co; 1998:811-886.

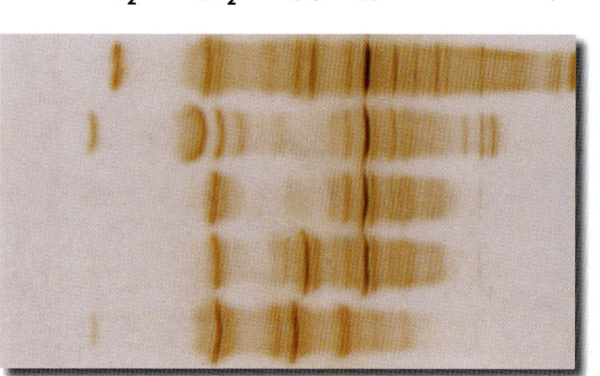

Figure DL-12.3
An example of homozygous Hb Constant Spring by isoelectric focusing (lane 2). As seen previously, there is a band cathodal to Hb A_2. There is also a band seen cathodal to the Hb Constant Spring band which appears to represent the δ chain variant (Hb $\alpha^{CS}_2\ \delta_2$). Interestingly, although not seen on alkaline electrophoresis, there is a small amount of Hb Bart's and Hb H seen on isoelectric focusing. 1-control specimen.

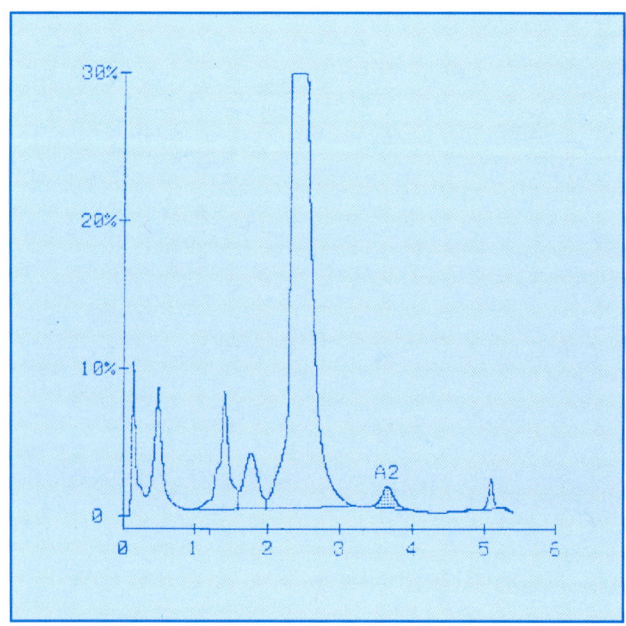

Figure DL-12.4
An example of Hb H/Hb Constant Spring trait by HPLC. In contrast to Figure DL-12.2, the Constant Spring peak accounts for only 1% of the total hemoglobin.

DL-13

HISTORY
The patient is a three-year-old African-American child seen for anemia. Since early infancy she had had recurrent, painful swelling of hands or feet. On physical examination, she had pallor of mucous membranes, scleral icterus, and splenomegaly. Specimens from both parents were also available for evaluation.

BLOOD COUNT DATA

	DL-13	Father	Mother
RBC (x 10^{12}/L)	1.9	4.9	4.4
Hgb (g/dL)	6.8	13.7	11.9
MCV (fL)	108.4	84.7	82.0
WBC (x 10^9/L)	12.9	6.4	8.1
Plt (x 10^9/L)	361	196	169
Reticulocytes (x 10^9/L)	225.0	49.0	36.0
Sickling Test	Positive	Positive	Positive

PERIPHERAL BLOOD SMEAR
The blood smear showed polychromasia and occasional elongated red cells with sharply pointed ends. The blood smears of both parents were unremarkable.

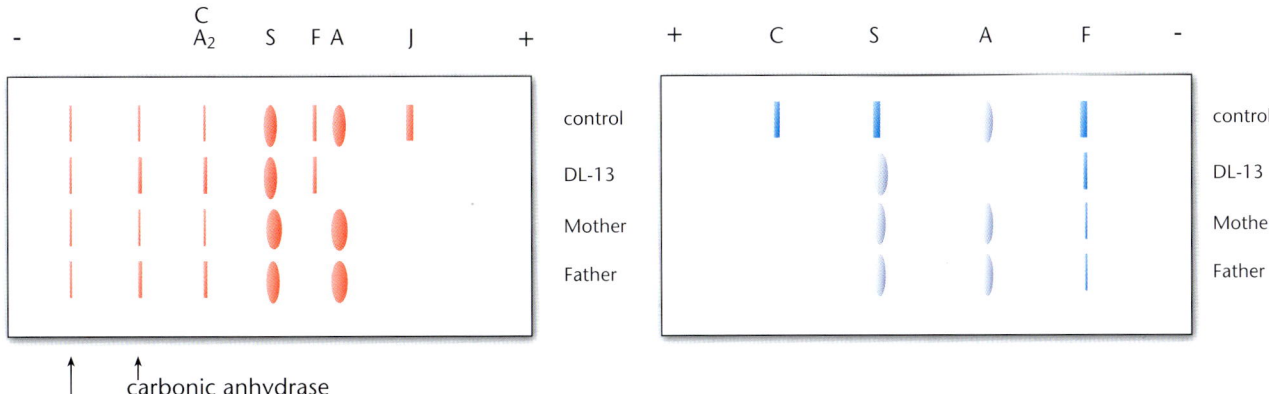

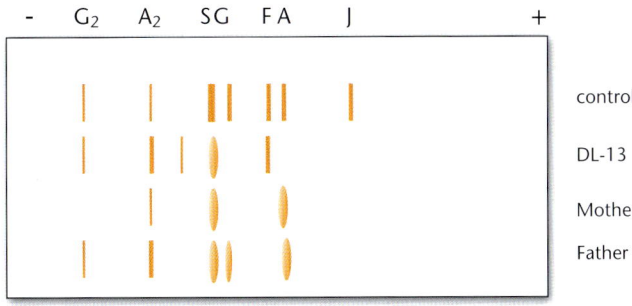

Case DL-13 Discussion

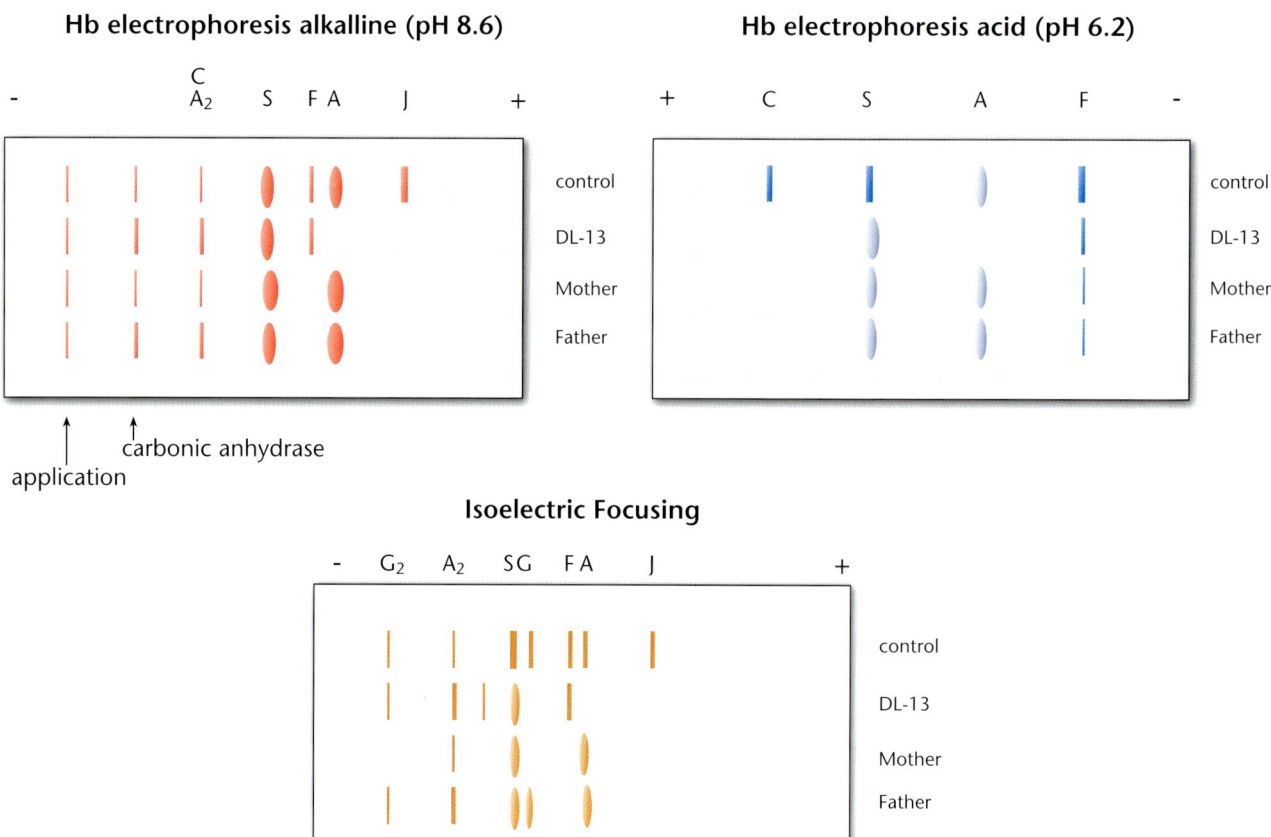

Interpretation

Examination of the child's alkaline electrophoresis shows no Hb A is present. There is a large band in the S position as well as slightly increased bands in the A_2 and carbonic anhydrase positions. There is a mild increase in Hb F. A similar pattern is seen on isoelectric focusing. Acid electrophoresis shows only bands in the A and F positions.

Diagnosis

Homozygous Hb S with Hb G-Philadelphia.

Performance

This combination has appeared as a dry lab challenge twice, but identification was only required for one of the exercises. Of laboratories reporting, 96.8% recognized the presence of Hb S, while 18.2% recognized the presence of Hb G-Philadelphia. 45.4% of laboratories identified the S/G hybrid, and 30.8% recognized the G_2 variant. However, 24.7% of laboratories misinterpreted the band in the A_2 position as Hb C-Harlem.

Discussion

This case represents another example where family studies are useful in solving difficult electrophoretic patterns. The clinical history and blood count data are consistent with a severe sickling disorder. However, the denser than usual bands in the A_2 and carbonic anhydrase positions are not consistent with simple homozygous Hb S. The mother's electrophoretic patterns are consistent with Hb S trait. The father has three major bands, which is the classic pattern obtained for Hb S/G-Philadelphia. This is readily apparent on isoelectric focusing, where a doublet is seen in the S position. Thus, the child inherited Hb S trait from the mother and both Hb S and Hb G-Philadelphia from the father. This combination is clinically equivalent to homozygous Hb S.

Hb G-Philadephia trait is expected to occur in the African population with a prevalence of about 1:5000, corresponding to a gene frequency of 1:10000. Since the inheritance of Hb G-Philadelphia is independent of the inheritance of Hb S, the frequency of the combination illustrated in this case would be expected to be 1/5000 x 1/400 (the frequency of homozygous Hb S in African Americans), or approximately one case among every two million African Americans. As mentioned in other discussions, Hb G-Philadelphia in African Americans is almost always accompanied by α-thalassemia-2 trait. This is due to a 3.7 Kb deletion that results from a crossover event.

Some may wonder why, in the child, the Hb G-Philadelphia band is not seen on isoelectric focusing or a band in the A position on acid electrophoresis, as it is in the father. The reason is that the band seen on isoelectric focusing is $\alpha^G_2\beta^A_2$. Because this child has no normal β chains, only β^S chains, the G-Philadelphia band is not seen. However, the S/G hybrid and the G_2 band are still present. Globin chain electrophoresis is also helpful for such cases as it clearly shows the presence of both an alpha and a beta chain variant (Figure DL-13-1). An example of Hb S/S/G-Philadelphia by HPLC is also shown (Figure DL-13.2).

As has been discussed in previous dry lab exercises, the differential diagnosis of Hb S/S/G-Philadelphia includes Hb S/C, Hb S/O-Arab, and Hb S/C-Harlem. One key to differentiating S/S/G-Philadelphia from these other disorders is that the A_2 band should be much denser when it is due to a β chain variant (as opposed to the lighter band produced by the S/G hybrid). Also helpful is recognition of the G_2 variant (particularly when seen on isoelectric focusing). If the G_2 variant is not recognized, and the increased band in the A_2 position is interpreted simply as an increase in A_2, a misdiagnosis of Hb S/β^o-thalassemia is possible. Clinically the distinction is not critical as both of these possibilities are sickling disorders.

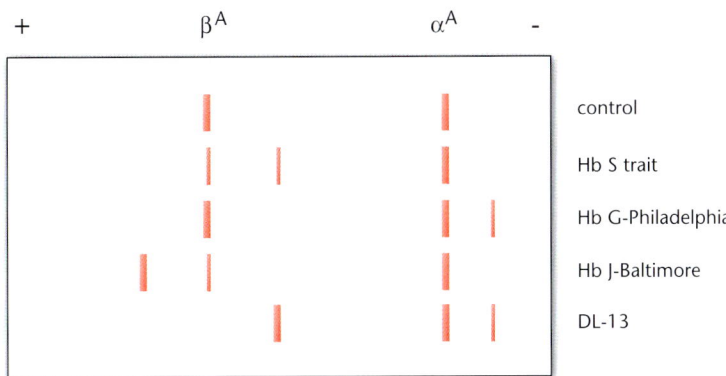

Figure DL-13.1
Alkaline globin chain electrophoresis on case DL-13. This clearly shows the absence of normal beta chains and only β^S chains. The α^G chains are also seen.

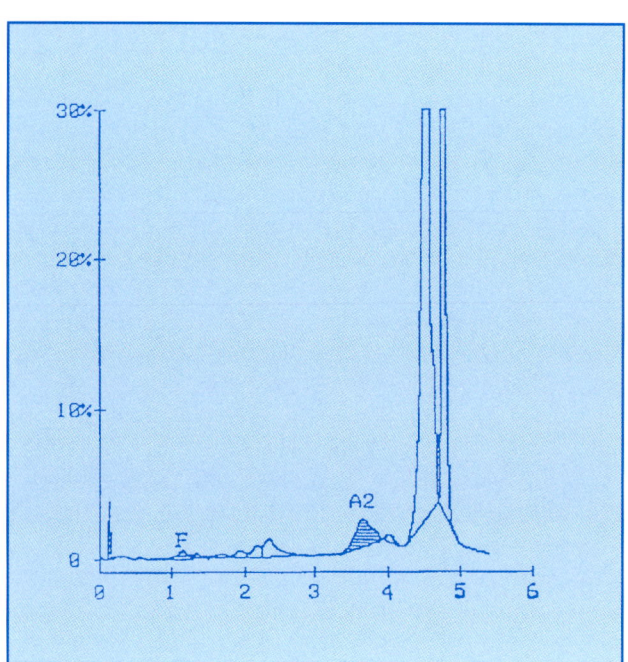

Figure DL-13.2
An example of homozygous Hb S/G-Philadelphia by HPLC. The only peaks seen are Hb S (4.5 minutes) and the S/G hybrid (4.8 minutes).

References

Milner PF, Huisman TJH. Studies on the proportion and synthesis of haemoglobin G-Philadelphia in red cells of heterozytgotes, a homozygote, and a heterozygote for both haemoglobin G and α-thalassemia. *Br J Haematol.* 1976;34:207-220.

Sciaratta GV, Sansome G, Ivaldi G, Felice AE, Huisman TJH. Alternate organization of α G-Philadelphia globin genes among U.S. black and Italian caucasian heterozygotes. *Hemoglobin.* 1984;8(6): 537-547.

DL-14

THIS CHALLENGE ILLUSTRATES FOUR UNUSUAL SITUATIONS SOMETIMES ENCOUNTERED BY LABORATORIES.

HISTORY

DL-14.1 The specimen was received for hemoglobin electrophoresis because, at another laboratory, an unusual band had been found, as in panel 1, on alkaline electrophoresis of a hemolysate prepared from whole blood. There were no clinical details or CBC data available at the time of these studies.

DL-14.2 The specimen was shipped in August from a Caribbean medical center, and initial studies were performed in another mainland U.S.A. laboratory before it was sent to a reference laboratory, several weeks later, for explanation of an unusual Hb band. No other clinical or laboratory information was available. Proportions of Hb A_2 and F were 3% and 0.7% respectively. This specimen was somewhat brownish in color and did not become the normal red color of blood upon mixing with room air.

DL-14.3 The specimen was received in the course of investigation of polycythemia. The patient was a 65-year-old white male who had marked facial rubor and a palpable mass in the left upper quadrant of the abdomen. His pertinent CBC data were: Hgb = 22.0 g/dL, Hct = 68.8%, RBC = 8.46×10^{12}/L, WBC = 17×10^9/L, and PLT = 820×10^9/L. The blood smear showed red cell crowding, neutrophilia, and thrombocytosis. Initial alkaline electrophoresis employed hemolysate prepared from whole blood, as reproduced in the first panel.

DL-14.4 The specimen was a 19-year-old Taiwanese male who was seen because of chronic pallor and fatigue. He exhibited slight scleral icterus, pallor of mucous membranes, and the tip of the spleen was palpable in the left upper quadrant of the abdomen. Pertinent CBC data were: Hb = 9.0 g/dL, Hct = 32%, RBC = 5.6×10^{12}/L, and MCV = 57 fL. Leukocytes and platelets were normal. The blood smear disclosed marked microcytosis, target cells, and polychromasia.

The first panel shows what was found on alkaline electrophoresis of whole blood hemolysate, with Ponceau-S (or Coomassie Blue) stain. The second panel, using the same hemolysate, was stained with dimethoxybenzidine (o-dianisidine). To clarify what the problems were, we obtained fresh blood specimens from each case and prepared washed, packed red cells, from which we prepared hemolysates for alkaline electrophoresis and Ponceau-S (or Coomassie Blue) stain in panel 3. The fourth and fifth panels show isoelectric focusing (IEF) patterns. Panel 4 shows IEF patterns for the original whole hemolysates, and panel 5 shows IEF patterns for washed, packed red cell lysates obtained from the original specimens (not from fresh specimens). In the fourth and fifth panels (IEF), to avoid confusion, glycosylated Hb bands, such as Hb A_{1c}, S_{1c}, etc., were not illustrated. The IEF gels were stained with dimethoxybenzidine.

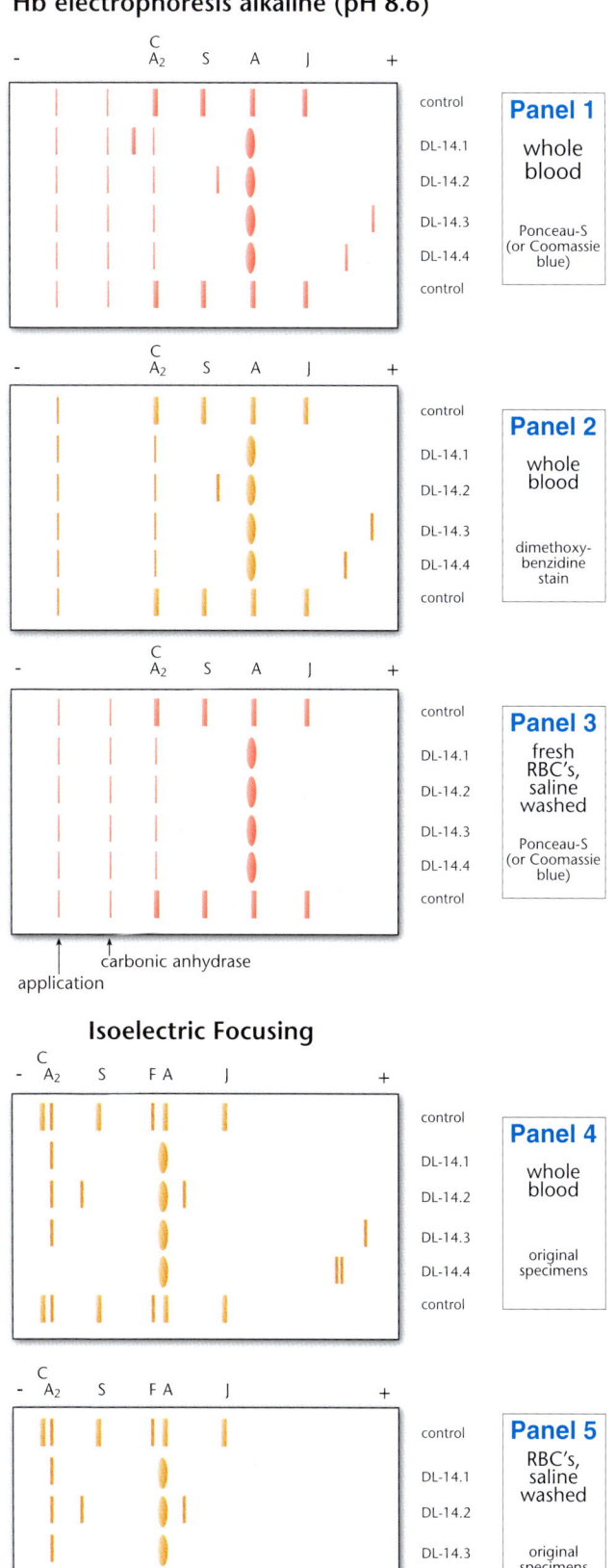

Dry Lab Challenges

Case DL-14 Discussion

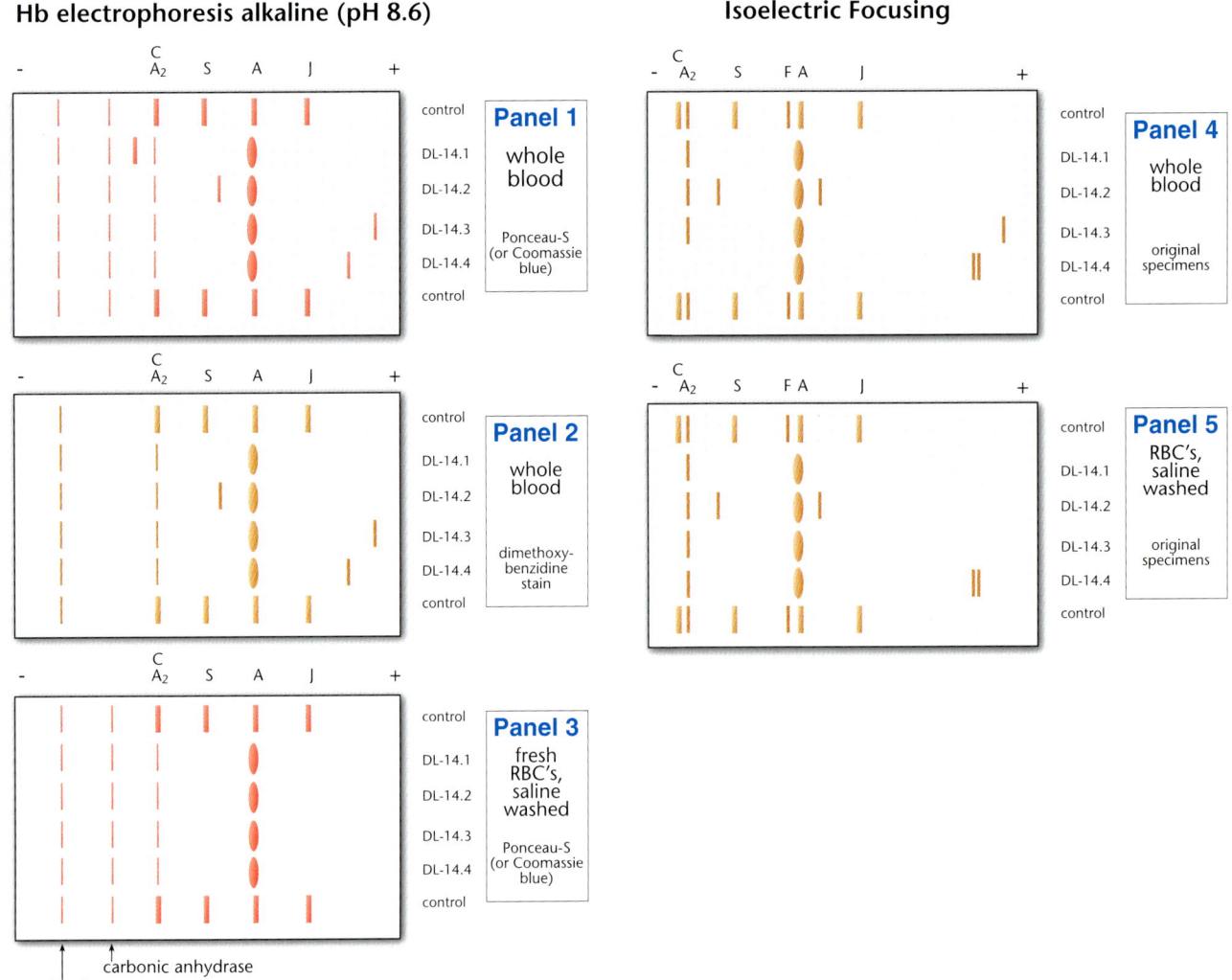

Interpretation

DL-14.1 There is an anomalous slow band seen on alkaline electrophoresis using whole blood with a Ponceau-S stain. This band is not seen using a dimethoxybenzidine stain (either on alkaline electrophoresis or IEF). It is also not seen using washed red blood cells.

DL-14.2 There is an abnormal band seen on alkaline electrophoresis between A and S using both stains. This band is not seen using fresh washed red cells. On IEF, there are two abnormal bands seen, one between the S and A_2 positions and one slightly faster than Hb A.

DL-14.3 On alkaline electrophoresis and IEF, there is a fast band present which is not present using washed packed cells.

DL-14.4 On alkaline electrophoresis, there is a fast band seen which is not present using fresh packed red blood cells. This band is seen as a fast doublet on IEF.

Diagnosis

DL-14.1 Monoclonal paraprotein in a patient with multiple myeloma.

DL-14.2 Methemoglobin in an old specimen.

DL-14.3 Peroxidase due to high WBC or PLT count.

DL-14.4 Hb H disease.

Performance

DL-14.1 64% of laboratories correctly indicated the anomalous band was likely a plasma protein.

DL-14.2 56.5% of laboratories correctly indicated that this band was likely methemoglobin.

DL-14.3 49.1% of laboratories correctly indicated that the analogous band was due either to myeloperoxidase or platelet peroxidase.

DL-14.4 77.7% of laboratories correctly indicated the fast band is likely Hb H.

Discussion

These specimens portrayed some of the technical artifacts that may lead to difficulty in interpretation of electrophoresis or isoelectric focusing patterns.

The anomalous band in DL-14.1 was present in hemolysate prepared from whole blood, but not in hemolysate prepared from washed, packed erythrocytes. When electrophoresis was performed with whole blood hemolysate and stained with dimethoxybenzidine, the band was not seen. These results indicated that it was something in the plasma, and that it was not a heme protein. The patient returned for further tests and was found to have a large monoclonal IgG peak on serum protein electrophoresis, as would be seen in multiple myeloma.

The history should have given case DL-14.2 away. Specimens that have been poorly handled, as being kept overnight at room temperature, or are more than a week old, commonly exhibit increased amounts of methemoglobin. If a drop of KCN solution (5 g/dL) is added to a small amount of the blood, and the mixture is incubated for 30 minutes before hemolysate is prepared, methemoglobin is converted to cyanmethemoglobin, which does not separate from Hb A on electrophoresis. The slightly fast band seen on isoelectric focusing is due to glycerated hemoglobin. This is another aging band that is often seen in older specimens.

Portrayed in specimen DL-14.3 is the "buffy coat" artifact that is not infrequently seen when hemolysate is prepared from whole blood that has an elevated leukocyte or platelet count. That this is not derived from erythrocytes or plasma can be shown by preparing buffy coat by centrifugation, lysing the buffy coat, and performing electrophoresis or isoelectric focusing. Then, if the buffy coat is largely free of erythrocytes, one observes only the very anodic (very fast) buffy coat band, and no Hb A. The buffy coat band is a peroxidase, i.e., a heme protein, and therefore gives a positive stain with dimethoxybenzidine.

Portrayed in DL-14.4 is a typical case of Hb H disease. The third illustration is to remind participants that "fast" bands, such as Hb H and the buffy coat band, may move right off the end of the membrane, into the wick and the buffer chamber, if electrophoresis is too prolonged. Of course, with IEF, "fast bands" do not run off the gel; they move to their isoelectric points and stay put. As portrayed on IEF, Hb H seems typically to exhibit two bands close together. The explanation for this is not totally clear; however, such "doublets" have been observed with other applications of IEF in protein separation.

DL-15

HISTORY
The patient is a 34-year-old asymptomatic, pregnant, African-American female.

BLOOD COUNT DATA
RBC..................................4.09 x 10^{12}/L
Hgb.................................14.0 g/dL
MCV ....97.3 fL
WBC................................6.6 x 10^9/L
Plt.....................................201 x 10^9/L

OTHER LABORATORY TESTS
The solubility test for sickling hemoglobin is positive.

PERIPHERAL BLOOD SMEAR
The peripheral blood smear showed no abnormalities.

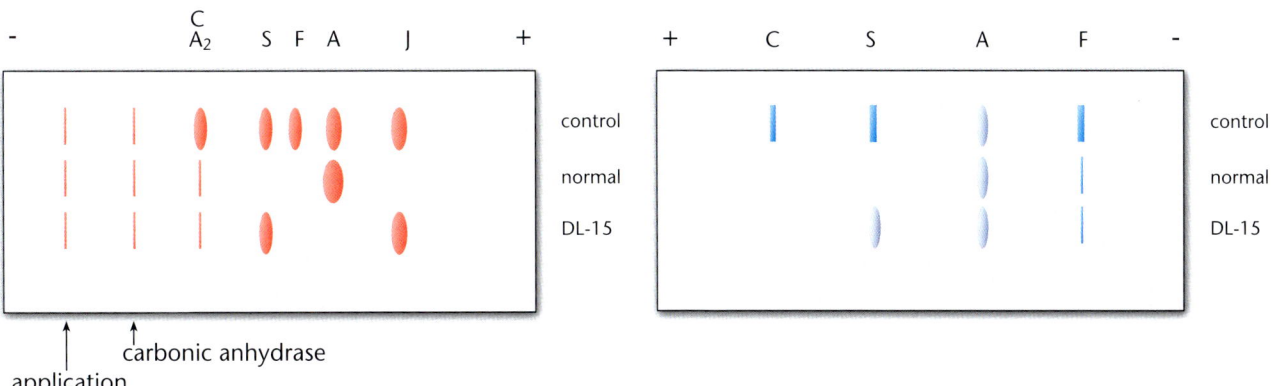

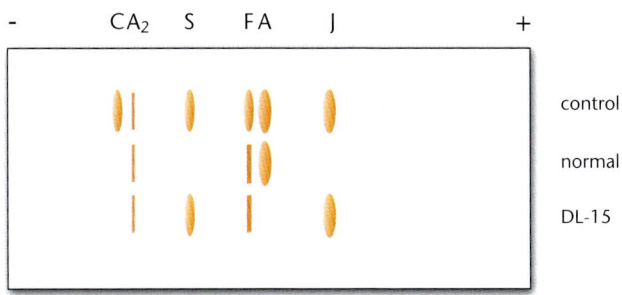

Case DL-15 Discussion

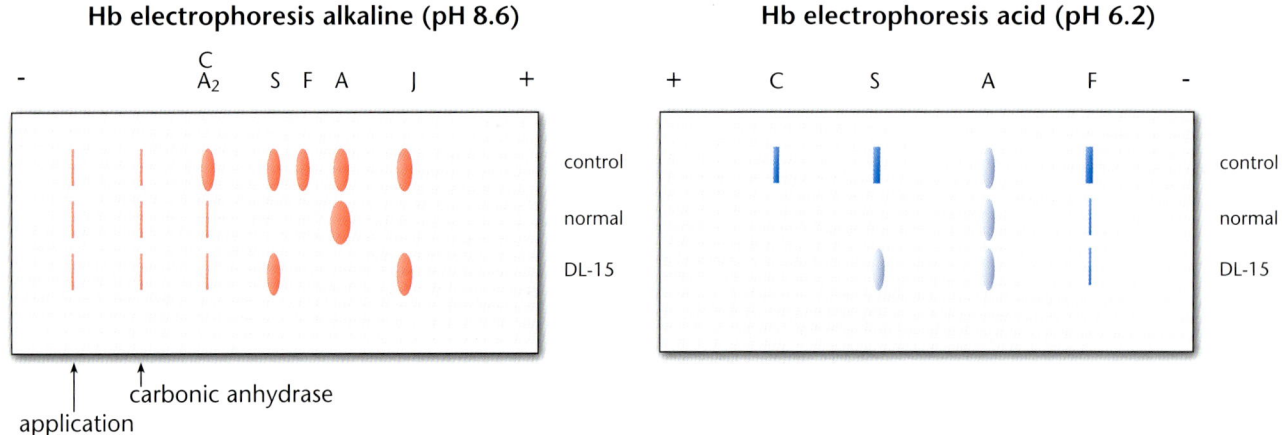

Interpretation

On alkaline electrophoresis, there is no Hb A present. There is a band in the S position and a fast band that is as far ahead of Hb A as Hb S is behind it. Acid electrophoresis shows bands in the S and A positions. The fast variant accounts for approximately 60% of the total hemoglobin.

Diagnosis

Hb S/Hb J-Baltimore.

Performance

80.7% of laboratories correctly identified this case as Hb S in combination with a Jβ variant.

Discussion

This represents a case of Hb S in combination with Hb J-Baltimore. Hb J-Baltimore [β16 (A13)Gly$\rightarrow$Asp] is the most common of the "fast" β chain hemoglobin variants migrating in the "J" position. This variant has been reported in persons of northern European ancestry as well as in African Americans. The combination of Hb S and Hb J-Baltimore has been previously reported. These two variants do not co-polymerize, so the clinical effects that are seen are equivalent to that of Hb S trait alone (i.e., clinically benign).

A number of laboratories identified this as a combination of Hb S with a Jα variant. Two aspects of the case are inconsistent with an α chain variant. First, the percentage of the variant (60%) is too high for a typical α chain variant, in which the percentage would be expected to be approximately 25%. Additionally, the fact that there was no Hb A present is strong evidence that there are two β chain variants present. As with any α chain variant, the presence of a Hb A_2 variant (the variant in combination with normal δ chains) is a helpful feature. However, in Jα variants (such as J-Oxford), this variant has been shown to migrate in the approximate Hb S position and so would be masked by the Hb S that is present in this case. There should be a major band present corresponding to the S/J hybrid ($\alpha^J_2\beta^S_2$) similar to that seen in the S/G-Philadelphia combination. This hybrid hemoglobin band, which might be seen in or near the Hb A position, was not seen in this case, and this observation is consistent with the combination Hb S/Hb J-Baltimore.

References

Baglioni C, Weatherall DJ. Abnormal human hemoglobins, IX: chemistry of hemoglobin J-Baltimore. *Biochim Biophys Acta.* 1963;78:637-643.

Fairbanks VF. *Hemoglobinopathies and Thalassemias.* New York, NY: Brian C. Decker; 1980:196-199.

Weatherall DJ. Hemoglobin J (Baltimore) coexisting in a family with hemoglobin S. *Bull Johns Hopkins Hosp.* 1964;114:1-12.

DL-16

HISTORY
The patient is a 27-year-old African-American male who is asymptomatic. The physical examination was normal.

BLOOD COUNT DATA
RBC.................................4.98 x 10^{12}/L
Hgb..................................13.3 g/dL
MCV..................................85.9 fL
WBC..................................6.6 x 10^9/L
Plt....................................143 x 10^9/L

PERIPHERAL BLOOD SMEAR
Increased target cells were present.

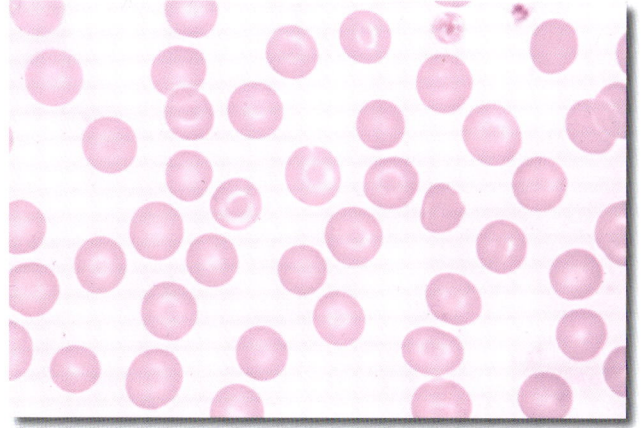

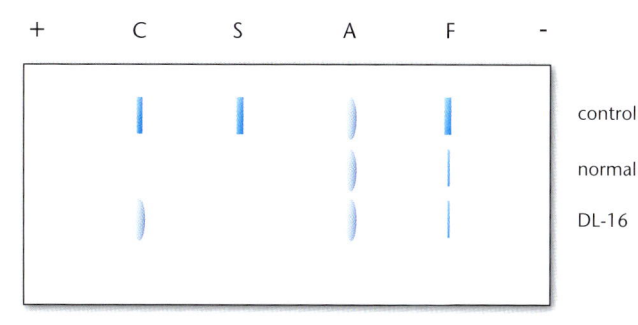

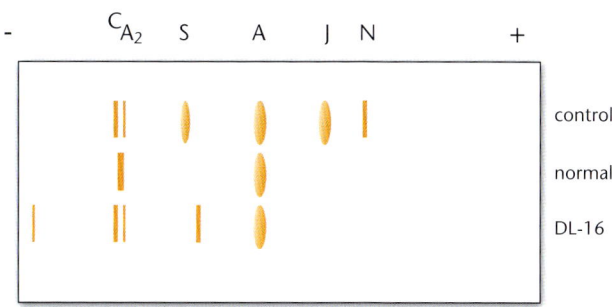

Case DL-16 Discussion

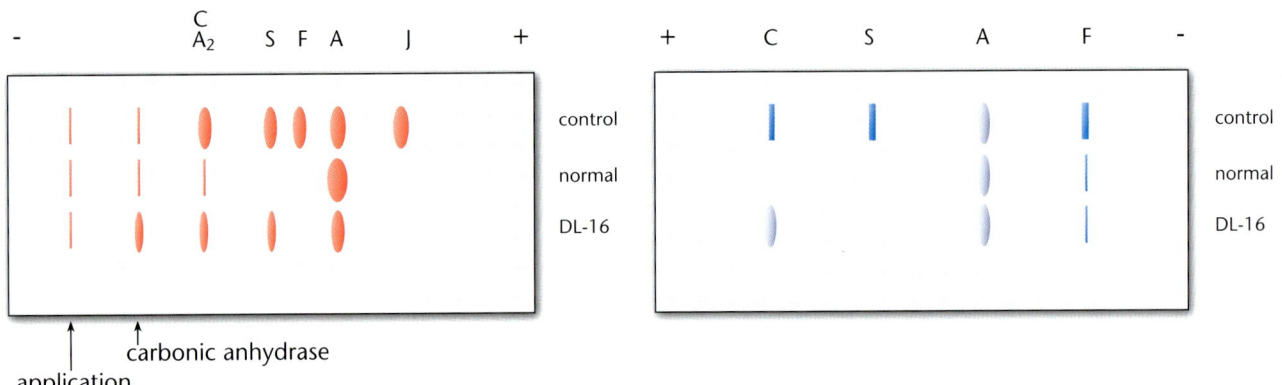

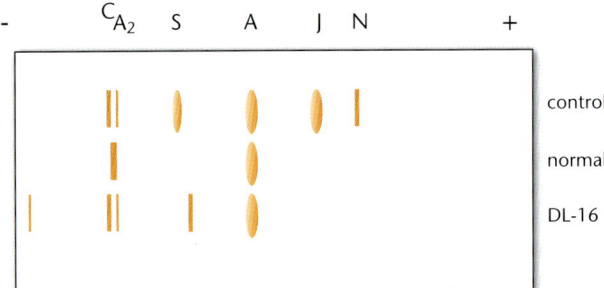

Interpretation

Alkaline electrophoresis and isoelectric focusing show four bands to be present: a band in the A position, a band in the S position, a band in the C position, and an increased band in the carbonic anhydrase position. Acid electrophoresis shows bands in the A position and in the C position.

Diagnosis

Hb C/G-Philadelphia.

Performance

97.7% of laboratories correctly identified the presence of Hb C and an additional variant either described as a Gα variant (52.9%) or, more specifically, as Hb G-Philadelphia (55.4%). Since the addition of these two responses add up to >100%, some laboratories entered both responses.

Discussion

This case represents a case of Hb C/G-Philadelphia; in other words, the patient is a double heterozygote for both Hb C (a beta chain variant) and Hb G-Philadelphia (an alpha chain variant). Both of these variants have been discussed in detail in other cases. The four bands that are seen in this case represent Hb A, Hb G-Philadelphia, Hb C, and Hb C/G hybrid (i.e., $\alpha^{G-Philadelphia}$ with β^C). The combination of Hb C plus a Gβ variant would produce only two bands in the S and C positions, and no Hb A. As illustrated, isoelectric focusing is particularly helpful in this case, as by this method, Hb G-Philadelphia migrates slightly anodal to Hb S, and Hb C distinctly separates from Hb A_2. Additionally, the C-G hybrid is well visualized. An example of Hb C/G-Philadelphia on HPLC is shown in Figure DL-16.1. Globin chain electrophoresis is also helpful in this case; this will show the presence of both a beta chain and an alpha chain variant (Figure DL-16.3).

The presence of multiple bands on cellulose acetate usually indicates the presence of both an alpha chain and a beta chain variant. Of course, the most notable and most frequently encountered of these would be the S/G-Philadelphia combination, which has been included in this survey before. The frequency of Hb C and Hb G in the African-American population is about 3% and 0.2% respectively. Therefore, a double heterozygote should be found in 0.0003% (3/1 million) in this population group. This combination is clinically benign. The peripheral blood smear is similar to Hb C trait alone (Figure DL-16.2).

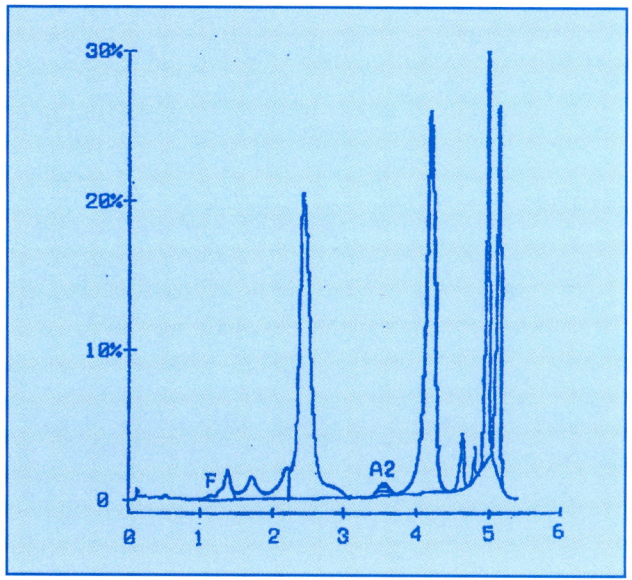

Figure DL-16.1
An example of Hb C/Hb G-Philadelphia by HPLC. In addition to the Hb A peak, there are three slower peaks seen. There is a peak in the D window (4.2 minutes), representing Hb G-Philadelphia ($\alpha^G_2\beta^A_2$), and a peak in the C window (5.0 minutes), representing Hb C. The final peak at 5.1 minutes, after the Hb C peak, represents the Hb C/G hybrid ($\alpha^G_2\beta^C_2$).

A second, less likely explanation for multiple bands on cellulose acetate are those hemoglobin variants that form asymmetric hybrids *in vitro*. An example of this is Hb Richmond, in which the three bands seen are Hb A; the hybrid band containing α_2^A, β^A and $\beta^{Richmond}$; and a slower band with α_2^A and $\beta_2^{Richmond}$.

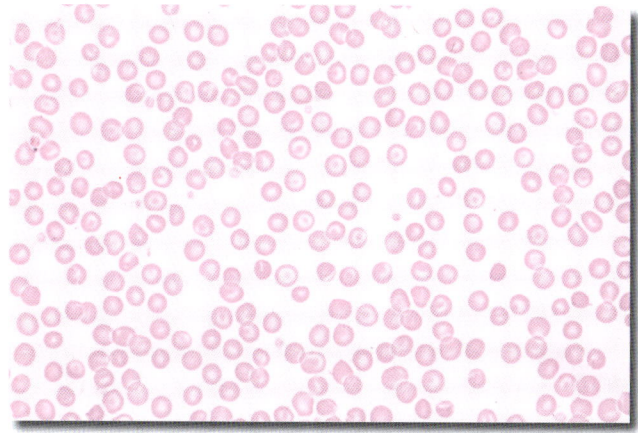

Figure DL-16.2 (Wright-Giemsa, 160x, 400x)
The peripheral blood smear from a patient with Hb C/G-

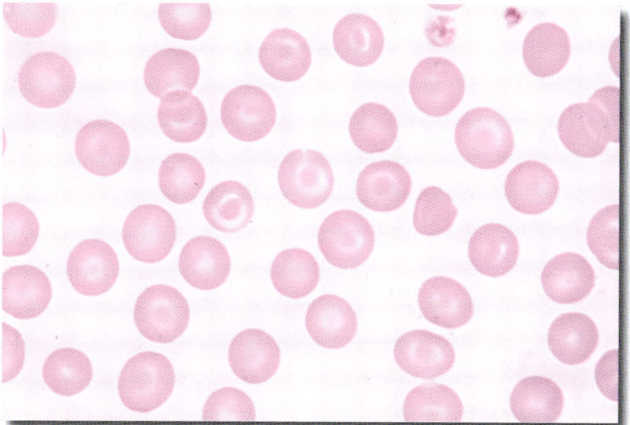

Philadelphia. There are increased target cells and mild anisocytosis, similar to the findings seen in Hb C trait.

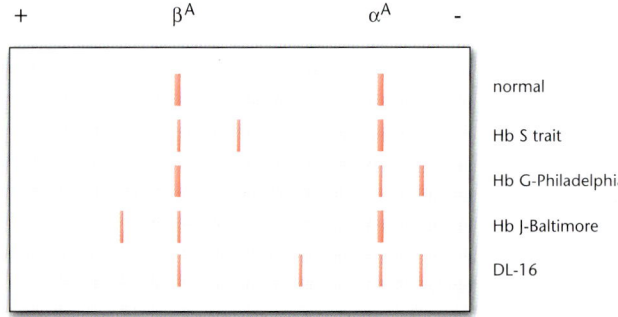

Figure DL-16.3 *Alkaline globin chain electrophoresis for Case DL-16. The presence of both a beta chain variant (Hb C) and an alpha chain variant (Hb G-Philadelphia) is clearly shown.*

References

Baglioni C, Ingram VM. Abnormal human haemoglobins, V: chemical investigation of haemoglobins A, G, C, X from one individual. *Biochim Biophys Acta.* 1961;48:253-265.

Efremov GD, Huisman THJ, Smith LC, et al. Hemoglobin Richmond, a human hemoglobin which forms asymmetric hybrids with other hemoglobins. *J Biol Chem.* 1969;244:6105-6116.

Fairbanks VF. *Hemoglobinopathies and Thalassemias.* New York, NY: Brian C. Decker; 1980:196-199.

Rucknagel DL, Rising JA. A heterozygote for Hb β^S, Hb β^C, Hb $\alpha^{G-Philadelphia}$ in a family presenting evidence for heterogeneity of hemoglobin alpha chain loci. *Am J Med.* 1975;59:53-60.

DL-17

HISTORY
The specimen in this case comes from the spontaneous abortus of a 30- to 32-weeks gestation. The fetus was pale, edematous, and appeared to have been dead for some time. Both parents were of Laotian ancestry.

BLOOD COUNT DATA

	Mother	Father
RBC	$4.9 \times 10^{12}/L$	$6.6 \times 10^{12}/L$
Hgb	8.7 g/dL	14.7 g/dL
MCV	59 fL	68 fL
WBC	$7.2 \times 10^9/L$	$5.3 \times 10^9/L$
Plt	$215 \times 10^9/L$	$310 \times 10^9/L$

PERIPHERAL BLOOD SMEAR
The mother's peripheral blood smear showed hypochromia, microcytosis, target cells, coarse basophilic stippling, and polychromasia. The father's peripheral blood smear showed microcytosis and occasional target cells. The fetus' peripheral blood showed marked anisopoikilocytosis with many nucleated RBC's.

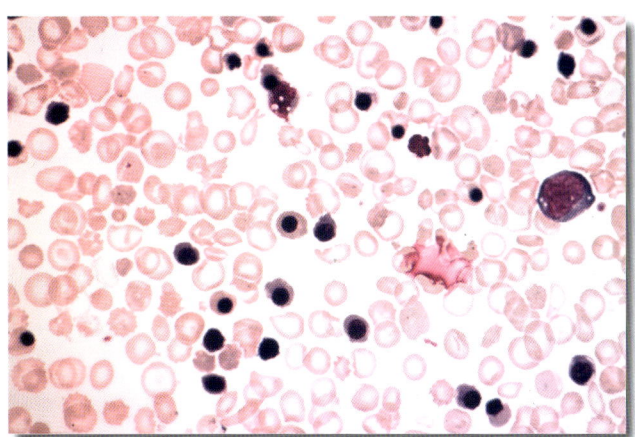

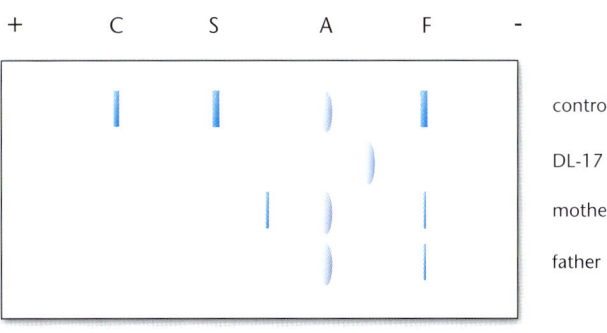

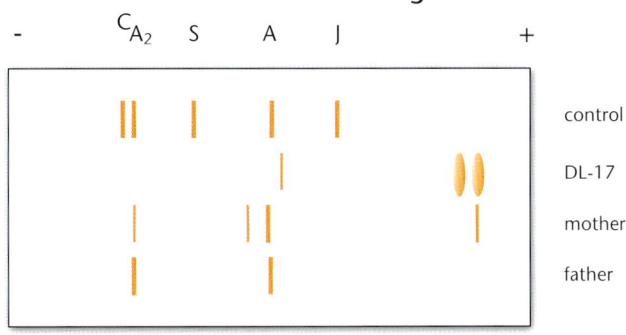

Dry Lab Challenges

Case DL-17 Discussion

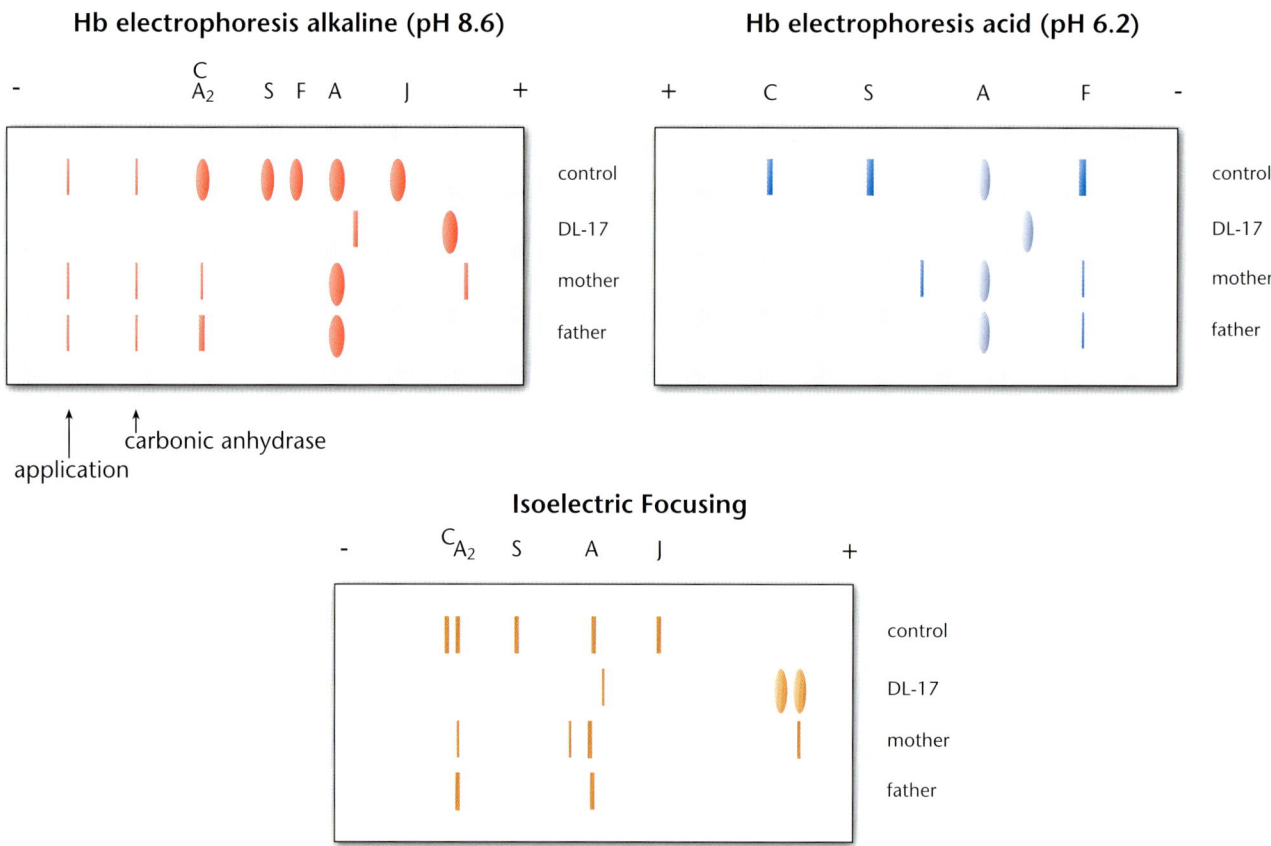

Interpretation

Fetus Alkaline electrophoresis demonstrates no Hb A, Hb F, or Hb A_2. Instead, there are two fast moving bands: A major band anodal to the Hb J position and a minor band slightly anodal to the Hb A position. On acid electrophoresis, there is a single band between the A and F positions. Isoelectric focusing demonstrates a pair of very fast moving bands and a minor band that migrates slightly faster than Hb A.

Mother On alkaline electrophoresis, there is an abnormal fast moving band that is approximately twice as far from Hb A as the Hb J control; this band is anodal to the one seen in the fetus. On acid electrophoresis, there is a minor abnormal band between A and S. On isoelectric focusing, there is a single abnormal fast band.

Father Alkaline electrophoresis demonstrates an accentuation of the "Hb A_2" band (quantified at 20% of total hemoglobin). Acid electrophoresis demonstrates a normal pattern.

Diagnosis

Hb Bart's hydrops fetalis (4 gene deletion α-thalassemia).

Performance

78% of laboratories recognized this as an example of homozygous α-thalassemia-1 (4 alpha gene deletion).

Discussion

Hb Bart's hydrops fetalis is the most severe form of α-thalassemia, resulting from homozygous inheritance of the α-thalassemia-1 mutation (--/--) (see *A Closer Look At...Alpha-Thalassemia,* page 18). This disorder is lethal in fetal life because of the total absence of α globin chains. Because of the lack of α chains, the excess γ chains tetramerize to form Hb Bart's. Hb Bart's has a markedly left-shifted oxygen dissociation curve and thus does not effectively deliver oxygen to tissues. Hb Bart's hydrops fetalis is a relatively common cause of early fetal death in Southeast Asia, where the prevalence of heterozygosity for α-thalassemia-1 is approximately 20%. It is also occasionally seen in Greece but is virtually non-existent in African Americans because of the rarity of the α-thalassemia-1 mutation in this population.

Fetuses affected with Hb Bart's hydrops fetalis have severe anemia *in utero*, with hemoglobin concentrations averaging 6.2 g/dL. However, the essentially non-functional Hb Bart's represents most of this hemoglobin. The small amounts of embryonic hemoglobins present are responsible for the minimal oxygen that is delivered to the tissues. The profound lack of functional hemoglobin results in pallor, edema, cardiac failure, hepatosplenomegaly, and massive extramedullary hematopoiesis. Most infants are stillborn between 30 and 40 weeks gestation, although a few will survive for a short time after birth. Rarely, an infant with this disorder may be rescued with intrauterine transfusions. Blood smears from affected fetuses/infants demonstrate marked anisopoikilocytosis, microcytosis, and erythroblastosis (Figure DL-17.1).

Because of the absence of α chains, infants with Hb Bart's hydrops fetalis have no Hb A, Hb F, or Hb A_2. Instead, the large majority of the hemoglobin is comprised of Hb Bart's (γ tetramers). Hb Bart's is a fast hemoglobin that migrates slightly cathodal to Hb H on alkaline electrophoresis; the distance from Hb H to Hb Bart's is similar to the distance between Hb A and Hb S. On acid electrophoresis, Hb Bart's migrates between A and F, and on isoelectric focusing, it is seen as a pair of fast bands similar in position to Hb H. Approximately 5-20% of the hemoglobin is represented by the embryonic hemoglobins Gower-1 ($\zeta_2\varepsilon_2$) and Portland ($\zeta_2\gamma_2$). These migrate slightly anodal to Hb A on alkaline electrophoresis, with Hb Bart's on acid electrophoresis, and slightly faster than Hb A on isoelectric focusing. The clinical findings and electrophoretic patterns in this case are diagnostic of Hb Bart's hydrops fetalis. An example of Hb Bart's hydrops fetalis by HPLC is shown in Figure DL-17.2.

Of interest in the current case are the electrophoretic findings in the parents. As we know that the infant is homozygous for α-thalassemia-1, we can conclude that each parent carries this allele. In addition, the mother carries an additional α-thalassemia-2 allele, resulting in three deleted alpha genes and the typical hematologic and electrophoretic findings of Hb H disease (see case DL-1, page 215; and case DL-12, page 261). The father, on the other hand, has an abnormal slow hemoglobin species that represents 20% of the total hemoglobin. This variant migrates in the A_2/C position on alkaline electrophoresis and isoelectric focusing, and with Hb A on acid electrophoresis. These

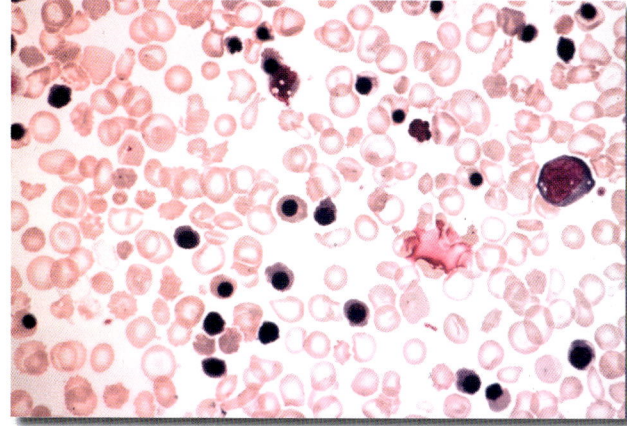

Figure DL-17.1 (Wright-Giemsa, 160x and 400x)
The peripheral blood smear from a fetus with Hb Bart's hydrops fetalis. There is marked anisopoikilocytosis, microcytosis, and hypochromia. There are many nucleated RBCs. (Source: Berkeley

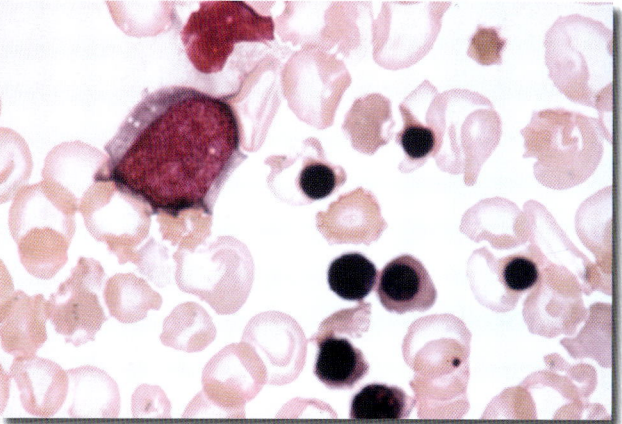

CK, Peterson LC. Hydrops fetalis with Hemoglobin Bart's: pathophysiology and prenatal detection. ASCP Checksample: Hematology. Chicago, IL: ASCP Press; 1991:33(2). Used with permission.)

findings are characteristic of Hb E (see Case 9, page 49). However, in the heterozygous state, Hb E usually accounts for 30-35% of total hemoglobin. The decreased percentage of Hb E in the father is due to the concomitant α-thalassemia-1 mutation; this combination typically results in 20-25% Hb E (see *A Closer Look At...Hb E-Associated Disorders,* page 72).

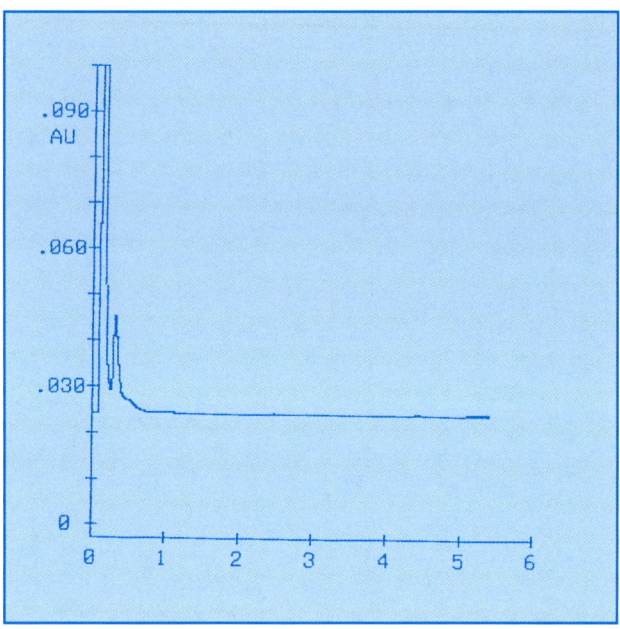

Figure DL-17.2
An example of Bart's hydrops fetalis by HPLC. There is no Hb A or Hb F present. There is a very fast peak eluting at 0.1 minutes which represents Hb Bart's. The slightly later peak may represent Hb Portland or a small amount of Hb H.

References

Kan YW, Allen A, Loewenstein L. Hydrops fetalis with alpha thalassemia. *N Engl J Med.* 1967:276:18-23.

Lie-Injo LE, Jo BH. A fast-moving hemoglobin in hydrops fetalis. *Nature.* 1960;185:698.

Lie-Injo LE. Alpha-chain thalassemia and hydrops fetalis in Malaya: report of five cases. *Blood.* 1962;20:581.

Orkin SH, Nathan DG. The thalassemias. In: Nathan DG, Orkin SH, eds. *Hematology of Infancy and Childhood.* 5th ed. Philadelphia, PA: WB Saunders Co; 1998:811-886.

Pootrakul S, Wasi P, Na-Nakorn S. Haemoglobin Bart's hydrops fetalis in Thailand. *Ann Hum Genet.* 1967;30:293-311.

Todd D, Lai MC, Beaven GH, Huehns ER. The abnormal hemoglobins in homozygous alpha-thalassemia. *Br J Haematol.* 1970;19:27-31.

DL-18

HISTORY

The patient is a 20-year-old Cambodian female. She has had a lifelong history of anemia. The physical examination reveals moderate hepatosplenomegaly. The parents of this patient were also available for evaluation. They are both asymptomatic.

BLOOD COUNT DATA

	Case DL-18	Mother	Father
RBC (x 10^{12}/L)	4.9	5.82	5.59
Hgb (g/dL)	8.8	11.9	13.8
MCV (fL)	59.8	65.1	76.3
WBC (x 10^9/L)	7.6	5.6	8.4
Plt (x 10^9/L)	200	266	250

PERIPHERAL BLOOD SMEAR

Case DL-18: The red blood cells show moderate anisopoikilocytosis with numerous target cells.
Mother: Microcytosis, target cells, basophilic stippling.
Father: Microcytosis and a few target cells.

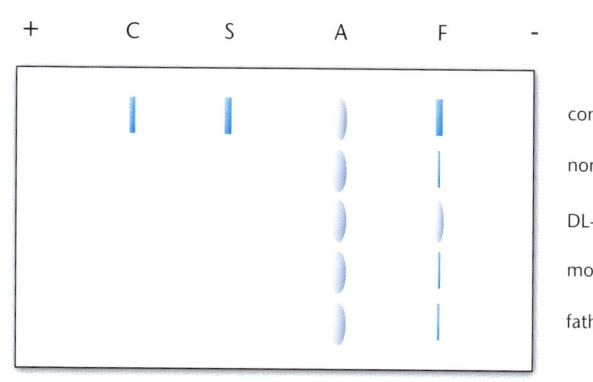

Dry Lab Challenges

Case DL-18 Discussion

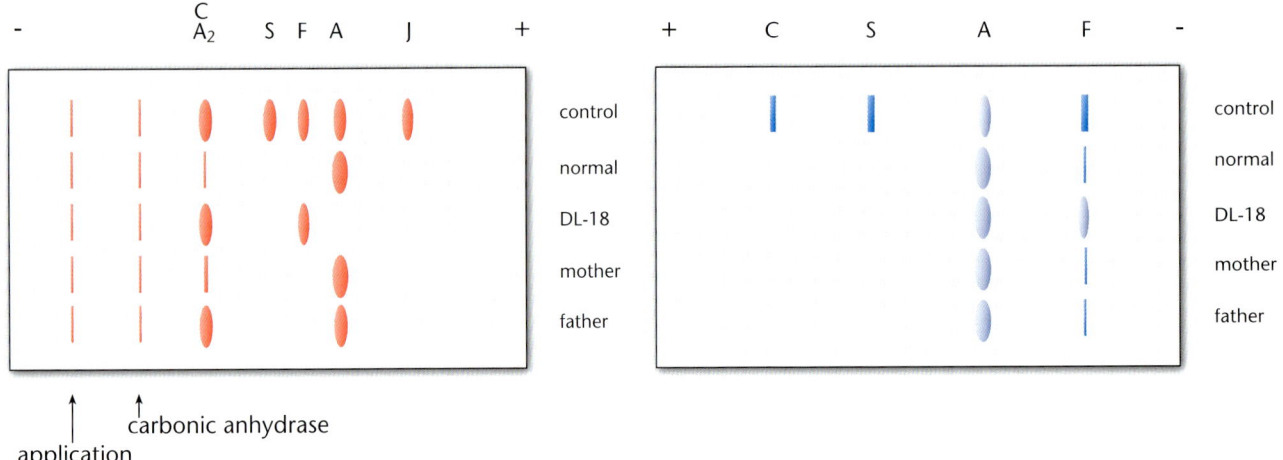

Interpretation

On alkaline electrophoresis, the patient is seen to have a large band in the A_2 position, an increased amount of Hb F, and no Hb A. On acid electrophoresis, there are bands seen only in the A and F positions. Examination of the mother's alkaline electrophoresis pattern shows a band in the A position and a mild increase in the band in the A_2 position. Acid electrophoresis is unremarkable. The father's alkaline electrophoresis pattern shows a band in the A position and a major band in the A_2 position. On acid electrophoresis, there is a band only in the A position.

Diagnosis

Hb E/β°-thalassemia.

Performance

91.4% of laboratories (487) correctly identified this as a case of Hb E/β°-thalassemia. The remaining laboratories (5.3%) identified this as a case of homozygous Hb E.

Discussion

This represents a case of Hb E/β⁰-thalassemia. Examination of the parents in this case was very useful, as the mother has findings indicative of β-thalassemia trait, whereas the father's findings are consistent with Hb E trait.

This case was included to highlight the differences in clinical severity between homozygous Hb E and Hb E/β⁰-thalassemia. Homozygous Hb E is essentially a benign condition. The patients usually have only mild microcytosis and erythrocytosis with an MCV of approximately 65 fL. Males with this condition are usually not anemic, although it has been reported that females may be mildly anemic (Hgb >11.0 g/dL). The Hb F should not be elevated. Importantly as well, there should be no splenomegaly. In contrast, Hb E/β⁰-thalassemia, as illustrated, is a thalassemic condition and can have all of the manifestations of β-thalassemia major, such as splenomegaly, severe microcytic anemia, and even extramedullary hematopoietic tumors. The Hb F level is usually elevated. The peripheral blood findings show mild to moderate anisopoikilocytosis with increased target cells, dacryocytes, spherocytes, and hypochromia. If the patient has undergone splenectomy, there are usually frequent nucleated red blood cells in addition to the usual post-splenectomy changes (figure DL-18.10).

Patients are usually severely anemic, although the severity of anemia can vary. They often require repeated blood transfusions. In fact, an accurate transfusion history is necessary in these cases so that the presence of a small amount of Hb A is not misinterpreted as a Hb E/β⁺-thalassemia disorder. Finally, as illustrated, if there is any confusion in the distinction between homozygous Hb E and Hb E/β⁰-thalassemia, family studies are very useful for further clarification. An example of Hb E/β⁰-thalassemia on HPLC and isoelectric focusing is shown in Figures DL-18.2 and DL-18.3.

As previously discussed, Hb E is very common in Southeast Asia. However, within different countries and ethnic groups, there is a wide variability in the percentages of Hb E. For example, Hb E is very common in Cambodia, Laos, and Thailand. At the junction of these three countries, the frequency of Hb E reaches percentages of 50-60% (the so-called "Hb E triangle"). Conversely, Hb E is uncommon in those persons of ethnic Chinese or Vietnamese origin. Hb E is also found on the Indian subcontinent, particularly in Bengalese, from Bangladesh or West Bengal, and in the Indian State of Assam.

In most geographic regions, there are a small number of β⁰-thalassemia mutations, which when combined, account for the majority of mutations in that area. As illustrated in Table DL-18.1, there are four mutations seen in Chinese and Southeast Asians that account for 71% of the total number of mutations in

Table DL-18.1
Common Beta-Thalassemia Mutations in Chinese and Southeast Asians*

Mutation	Type	Percentage
Frameshift 41-42	β⁰	28
IVS-2 nt 654	β⁰	20
Nonsense Codon 17	β⁰	10
-28 A→G	β⁺	13
Total		71

*Modified from Kazazian HH, Boehm CD. Molecular basis and prenatal diagnosis of ß-thalassemia. Blood. 1988;72:1107-1116.

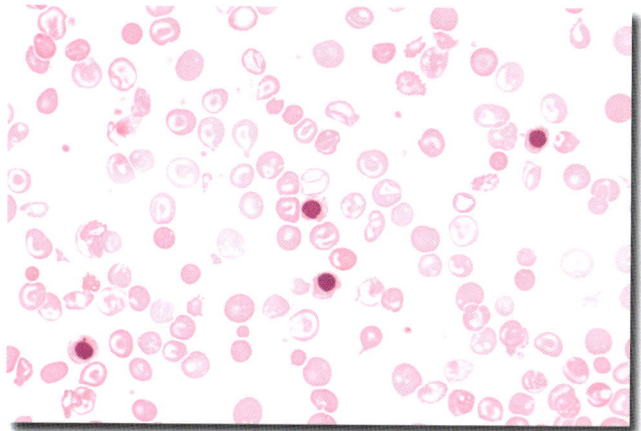

Figure DL-18.1 (Wright-Giemsa, 160x and 400x)
The peripheral blood smear from a patient with Hb E/β⁰-thalassemia post-splenectomy. In contrast to homozygous hemoglobin E, there is prominent anisopoikilocytosis, including target cells, spherocytes, dacrocytes, and nucleated red blood cells.

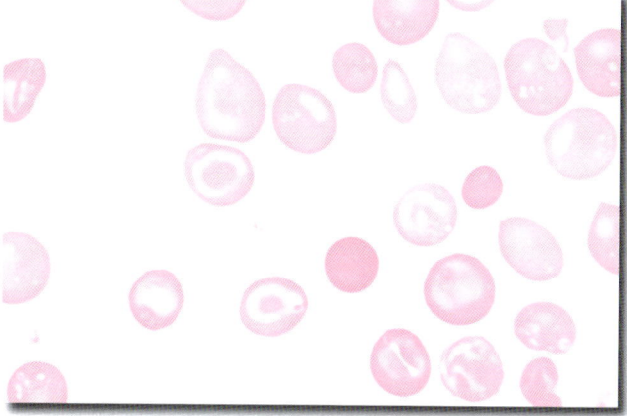

this area. Three of the four of these mutations are β^0 mutations (no production of β chains from the affected locus). Thus, it is not surprising that the most common thalassemic syndrome seen in Southeast Asia is Hb E/β^0-thalassemia and not homozygous β-thalassemia.

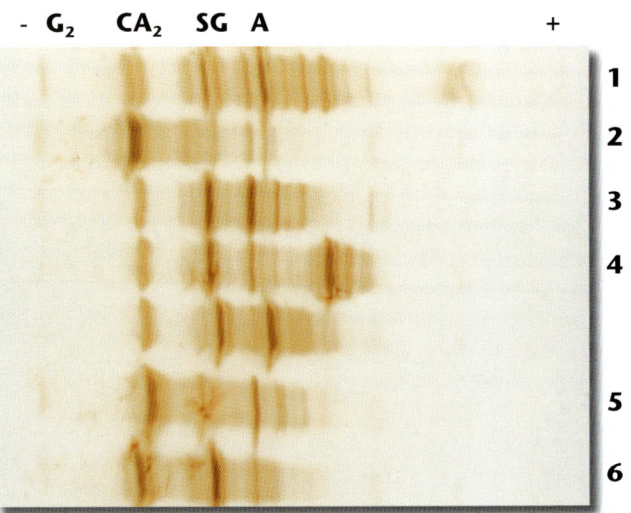

Figure DL-18.3
An example of Hb E/β^0 thalassemia by isoelectric focusing. There is no Hb A present, only a large band in the A_2 position representing Hb E and an increased amount of Hb F (lane 5). Lane 1- control specimen, Lane 2- homozygous C, 3-Hb S/HPFH, 4-Hb S/Hb N Baltimore, 6-Hb S/Hb C.

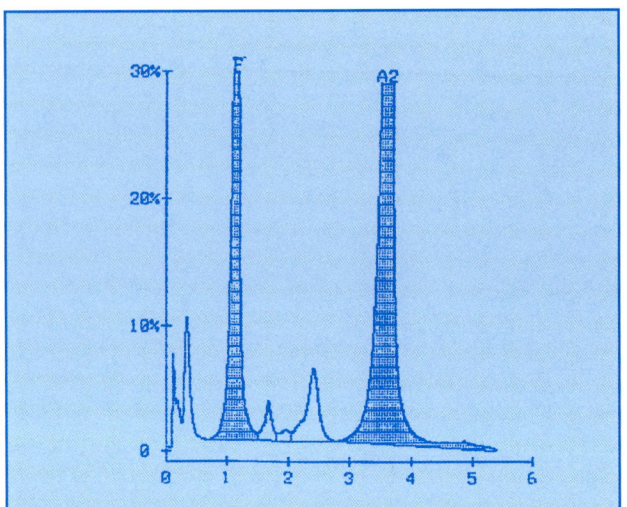

Figure DL-18.2
An example of Hb E/β^0-thalassemia by HPLC. There are two major peaks present: the Hb F peak and a prominent peak in the A_2 position representing Hb E. A small peak seen at approximately 2.3-2.4 minutes does not represent Hb A, as it was not seen on cellulose acetate electrophoresis or isoelectric focusing. The fast peak ahead of Hb F represents acetylated Hb F.

References

Bunn HF, Forget BG. *Hemoglobin: Molecular, Genetic and Clinical Aspects.* Philadelphia, PA: WB Saunders Co; 1986:420-427.

Fairbanks VF, Oliveros R, Brandabur JH, et al. Homozygous hemoglobin E mimics β-thalassemia minor without anemia or hemolysis: hematologic, functional and biosynthetic studies of first North American cases. *Am J Hematol.* 1980;8:109-121.

Fucharoen S. Hemoglobin E disorders. In: Steinberg MH, Forget BJ, Higgs DR, Nagel RL, eds. *Disorders of Hemoglobin: Genetics, Pathophysiology and Clinical Management.* Cambridge, England: Cambridge University Press; 2001:1139-1154.

Kazazian HH, Boehm CDL. Molecular basis and prenatal diagnosis of β-thalassemia. *Blood.* 1980;72:1107-1116.

Monzon CM, Fairbanks VF, Burgert EO Jr, et al. Hematologic genetic disorders among Southeast Asian refugees. *Am J Hematol.* 1985;19:27-36.

Winichagoon P, Thonglairoam V, Fucharoen S, et al. Severity differences in β-thalassemia/haemoglobin E syndromes: implication of genetic factors. *Br J Haematol.* 1993;83:633-639.

Winter, WP. *Hemoglobin Variants in Human Population.* Vol 2. Boca Raton, FL: CRC Press, Inc; 1987:111-118.

DL-19

HISTORY
The patient is a 37-year-old asymptomatic Caucasian woman who was examined because of persistent unexplained anemia. The physical examination revealed pallor and slight splenomegaly. Several members of her family were also anemic. Laboratory data are shown in the following table for the patient and her parents.

BLOOD COUNT DATA

	DL-19	Mother	Father
RBC ($\times 10^{12}$/L)	5.2	4.8	6.3
Hgb (g/dL)	7.8	12.9	9.3
MCV (fL)	58	81	59
WBC ($\times 10^9$/L)	7.3	7.5	5.9
Plt ($\times 10^9$/L)	180	210	195

OTHER LABORATORY TESTS

	DL-19	Mother	Father
Ferritin (µg/L)	245	142	498
Hb A_2 (%)	7.2	2.8	6.7
Hb F (%)	15.3	1.3	12.9

Specimens from the patient and her father exhibited reticulocytosis, ranging from 200-300 $\times 10^9$/L (or about 5%).

PERIPHERAL BLOOD SMEAR
Blood smears from the patient and her father show hypochromia, microcytosis, target cells, coarse basophilic stippling, and increased polychromasia. The blood smear from her mother was entirely normal.

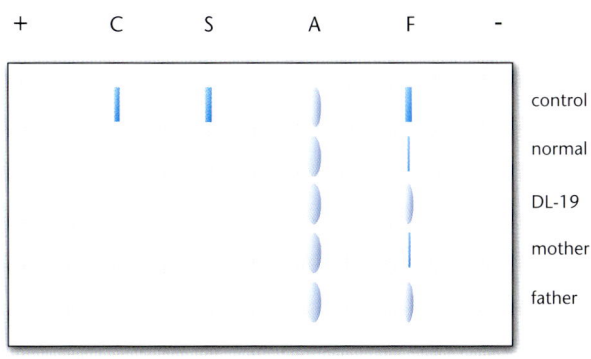

Hb electrophoresis alkaline (pH 8.6)

Hb electrophoresis acid (pH 6.2)

Case DL-19 Discussion

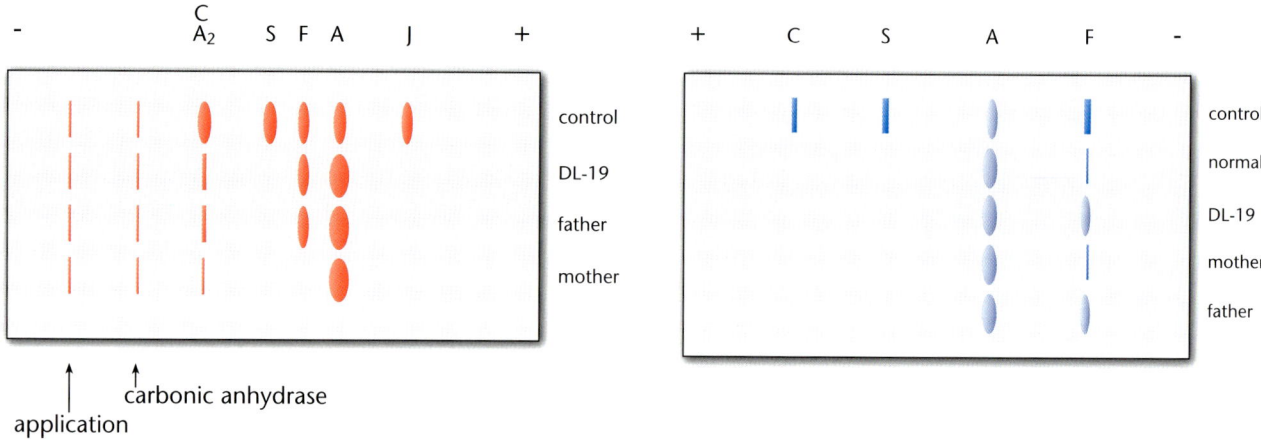

Interpretation

Alkaline electrophoresis shows no abnormal bands, only an increase in the A_2 band in both the patient and in her father, corresponding to the quantitative increase in Hb A_2. The patient and her father also show an increase in Hb F. The mother's alkaline electrophoresis is normal.

Diagnosis

Beta-thalassemia trait.

Performance

Several questions were asked of participants. The majority of participants recognized that the findings seen in this case were not typical for beta-thalassemia trait, but also did not represent the findings seen in homozygous β^+-thalassemia.

Discussion

While, for most practical purposes, it is still reasonable to rely on measurement of Hb A₂ and Hb F for identifying persons with β-thalassemia, in unusual cases like DL-19, more specific tests may be useful. In this case, a DNA specimen was submitted for analysis of the β globin gene. This showed that case DL-19 is heterozygous for a stop codon mutation at β globin gene codon 121: GAA →TAA. Instead of properly coding for Glu at this position, codon 121 TAA codes for chain termination. The result appears to be the production of β globin chains that are incomplete and are rapidly degraded within the developing erythrocyte. The mutation generally causes a microcytic anemia of moderate severity, e.g., Hgb of about 7.0 g/dL, which distinguishes it from the very mild anemia (or microcytosis without anemia) characteristic of most beta-thalassemia heterozygotes. Several families have now been reported with this mutation. They have been mostly of northern European origin, but the mutation has also been reported from Japan. This type of β-thalassemia trait is typically expressed in anemia of variable severity, splenomegaly, reticulocytosis, and hyperbilirubinemia. Heinz bodies may be demonstrated in bone marrow erythroblasts, so the β121-stop-codon mutation thalassemia has also been called "inclusion body β-thalassemia." The inclusion bodies are believed to represent precipitated α globin.

Several other mutations to stop codons (TAA, TAG, or TGA, the so-called "ochre, amber, and opal nonsense codons," respectively) have been reported as causes of β-thalassemia, including β15 TGG (Trp)→ TAG, β15 TGG→TGA, β17 AAG(Lys)→TAG, β22 GAA (Glu)→TAA, β39 CAG (Gln)→TAG. Each of these is a β° mutation, i.e., the affected gene fails to direct the synthesis of any functional β globin. By far the most common of these is the stop codon mutation at β39, especially among Italians and Italian-Americans. It is the mutation found in two-thirds of β-thalassemia genes in Italy. It is also the most common β-thalassemia gene in England, Spain, Portugal, and France. It has a lower frequency in Greece, where it comprises only about 12% of β-thalassemia genes, and its frequency is lower yet in Asia Minor, the Middle East, south Asia, and eastern Asia.

References

Fei YJ, Stoming TA, Kutlar A, Huisman THJ, Stamatoyannopoulos G. One form of inclusion body beta thalassemia is due to a GAA→TAA mutation at codon 121 of the beta chain. *Blood.* 1989;73: 1075-1077.

Kazazian HH Jr, Orkin SH, Boehm CD, et al. Characterization of a spontaneous mutation to a beta thalassemia allele. *Am J Hum Genet.* 1986;38:860-867.

Stamatoyannopoulos G, Woodson R, Papayannopoulou TH, et al. Inclusion-body beta-thalassemia trait: a form of beta thalassemia producing clinical manifestations in simple heterozygotes. *N Engl J Med.* 1974;290:939-943.

Thein SL, Hesketh C, Taylor P, et al. Molecular basis for dominantly inherited inclusion body beta-thalassemias. *Proc Natl Acad Sci USA.* 1990;87: 3924-3928.

DL-20

HISTORY
The patient is a 60-year-old African-American male evaluated for anemia.

BLOOD COUNT DATA
RBC .... $3.92 \times 10^{12}/L$
Hgb .... 10.9 g/dL
MCV .... 81.8 fL
WBC .... $8.7 \times 10^9/L$
Plt .... $310 \times 10^9/L$

PERIPHERAL BLOOD SMEAR
The peripheral blood smear showed no significant abnormalities.

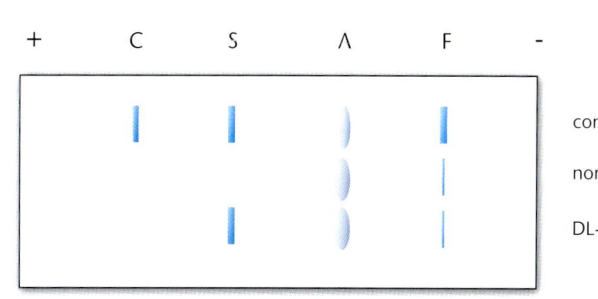

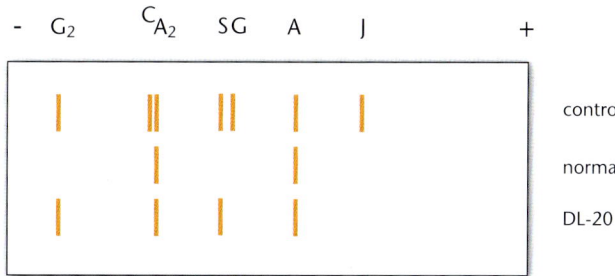

Case DL-20 Discussion

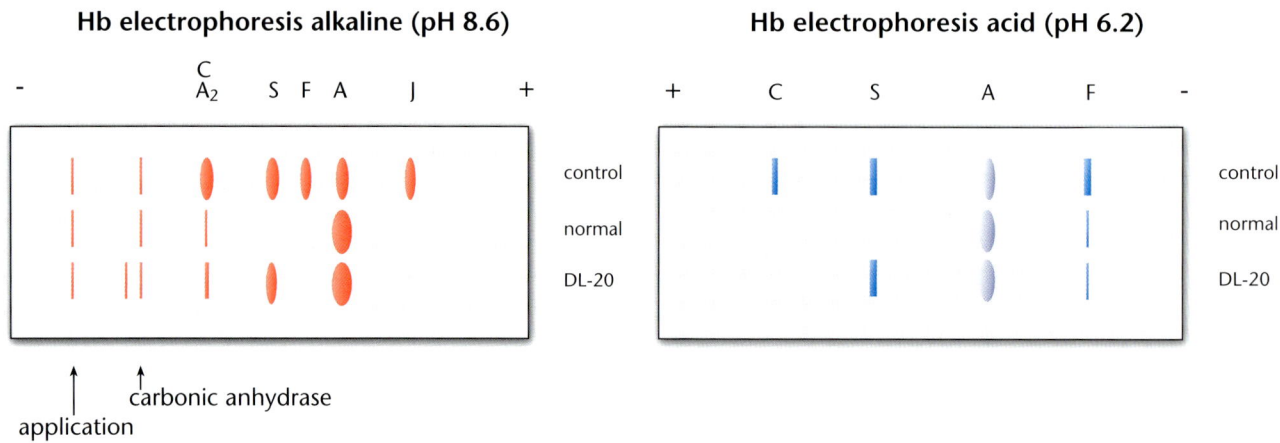

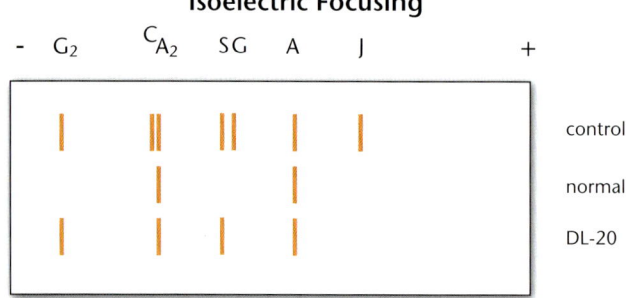

Interpretation

The alkaline electrophoresis pattern demonstrates bands in the Hb A, Hb S, and Hb A_2 positions. In addition, a faint band is detected cathodal to carbonic anhydrase, which is approximately equal in intensity to the Hb A_2 band. The acid electrophoresis confirms the presence of Hb A and Hb S. There is a faint band of Hb F, which is normal. No additional abnormal bands are observed. On isoelectric focusing, four bands are present, which correspond to Hb A, Hb S, Hb A_2, and an unknown Hb variant. This hemoglobin variant has an isoelectric point that is very close to that of Hb G_2, which is shown for comparison in the control lane.

Diagnosis

Hb S/Hb A_2'.

Performance

97.6% of participants correctly identified the presence of Hb S, and 61.4% successfully identified the presence of Hb A_2'.

Discussion

Hb A_2' is the most frequently identified δ chain variant, occurring in approximately 1-2% of African Americans. Hb A_2', also known as Hb B_2, results from the substitution of arginine for glycine at the amino acid 16 position of the δ globin chain. This single amino acid substitution results in a net positive charge change on the δ globin, which explains its slower mobility under alkaline conditions. Since the Hb A_2' mutation is an allele of the normal δ globin gene, there are approximately equal proportions of normal Hb A_2 and the variant Hb A_2 in heterozygotes (Hb A_2' trait).

This African-American man has compound heterozygosity for Hb S and Hb A_2'. Both Hb S trait and Hb A_2' trait are clinically harmless conditions, and there does not appear to be any interaction between them that would result in clinical manifestations. Therefore, it is most likely that the patient's anemia is due to some other cause, which should be investigated.

The alkaline electrophoretic pattern observed in this patient could suggest the interpretation of Hb G-Philadelphia. Hb G-Philadelphia is an α globin chain variant that co-migrates with Hb S under alkaline conditions. In addition, a G_2 band migrates near the carbonic anhydrase position, similar to A_2'. However, the acid electrophoresis pattern in this case excludes Hb G as a possibility and confirms that Hb S is the hemoglobin variant that is present. A positive sickling (solubility) test is also a helpful discriminator. Hb G_2 refers to the minor hemoglobin component that is composed of $α^G$ chains and normal δ globin chains. Hb G_2 has a mobility on alkaline electrophoresis that is as cathodal to Hb A_2 as Hb G is to Hb A, which places Hb G_2 in approximately the same position as carbonic anhydrase. On isoelectric focusing, Hb G-Philadelphia and Hb S are separated on the basis of their different isoelectric points. In this patient, the IEF pattern also confirmed the presence of Hb S and excluded Hb G-Philadelphia. Notice that the isoelectric points of Hb A_2' and Hb G_2 are very similar, yet distinct.

References

Ball EW, Meynell MJ. Hemoglobin A_2' $α_2δ_2$ glycine-arginine. *Nature.* 1966;209:121-122.

Fairbanks VF. *Hemoglobinopathies and Thalassemias: Laboratory Methods and Clinical Cases.* New York, NY; Thieme Stratton Inc; 1980:185-186.

Horton B, Payne RA, Bridges MT, Huisman HJ. Studies on an abnormal minor hemoglobin component (Hb-B_2). *Clinica Chimica Acta.* 1961;6:246-253.

Jones RT, Brimhall B. Structural characterization of two δ chain variants. *J Biol Chem.* 1967;242:5141-5145.

Vella F. Variation in hemoglobin A_2. *Hemoglobin.* 1977;1:619-650.

DL-21

HISTORY
The specimen is from a three-month-old African-American boy who was being evaluated for an abnormal newborn hemoglobin screen. The parents and a three-year-old sister were also evaluated. They were all asymptomatic and hematologically normal.

BLOOD COUNT DATA
RBC .... 3.62 x 10^{12}/L
Hgb .... 9.2 g/dL
MCV .... 73.8 fL
WBC .... 6.2 x10^9/L
Plt .... 215 x10^9/L

PERIPHERAL BLOOD SMEAR
No abnormalities.

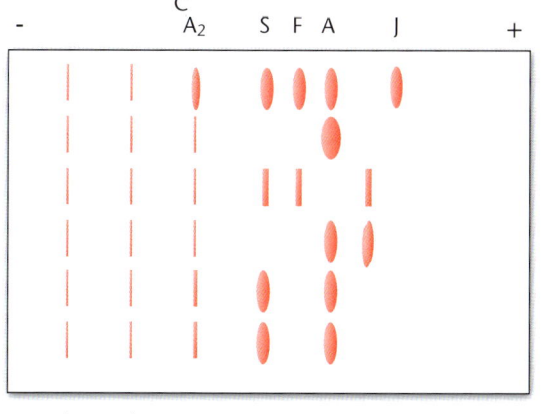

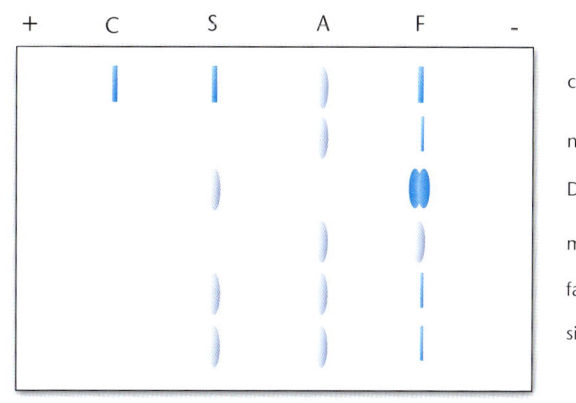

Case DL-21 Discussion

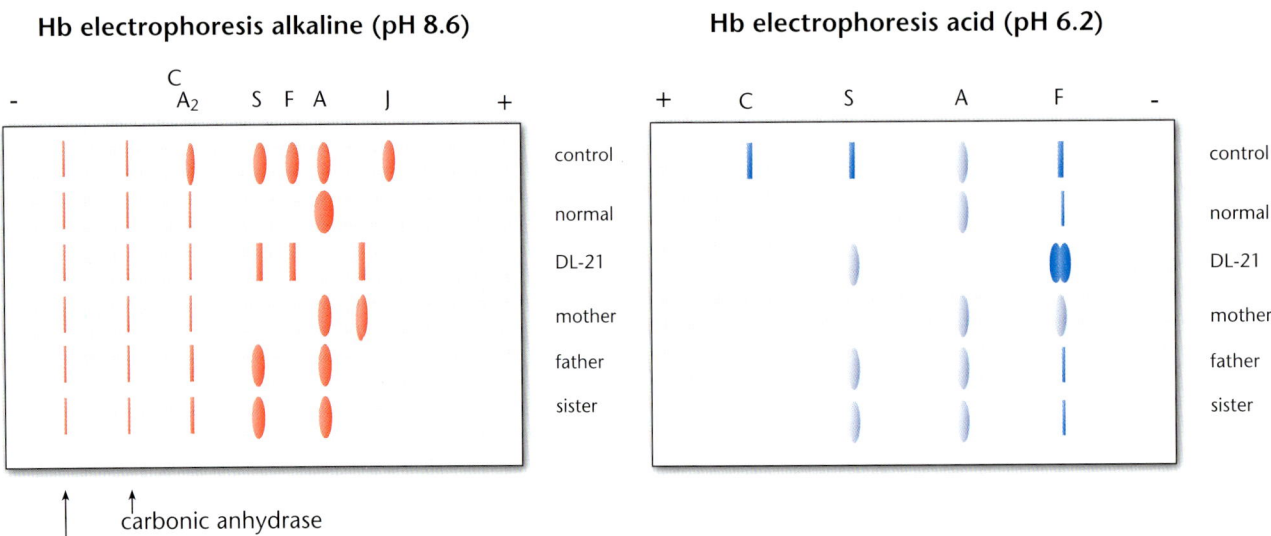

Interpretation

The alkaline electrophoresis for the infant shows a band in the region of Hb F and two variant hemoglobin bands. One variant migrates in the position of Hb S, and the other is a fast-moving Hb variant. There is no Hb A present. The acid electrophoresis confirms the presence of Hb S. The band in the Hb F region is very wide, consistent with co-migration of the Hb variant with Hb F.

Diagnosis

Hb S/Hb K-Woolwich.

Performance

97.4% of participants identified the presence of Hb S, and 69.2% identified Hb F. Hb K-Woolwich, Hb Hope, and Hb Camden were selected by 41.8%, 36.9%, and 18.3% of participants, respectively.

Discussion

Hb K-Woolwich results from a single amino acid substitution in the β globin chain. Lysine is replaced by glutamine at the amino acid 132 position. Hb K-Woolwich was first reported in a family from Jamaica. Its occurrence was subsequently reported from many African countries. Most of the Hb K carriers have originated from the Akan, an ethnic group of Ghana and the Ivory Coast. Exact prevalence data are not known. Initial studies on a single family suggested that Hb K resulted in a β-thalassemia phenotype; however, β globin synthesis studies have since demonstrated balanced globin chain synthesis in Hb K heterozygotes. The proportion of Hb K present in heterozygotes is usually in the range of 30-40%. Compound heterozygosity for Hb K and Hb S or Hb C has been reported, and these are apparently clinically harmless conditions.

The majority of laboratories correctly identified compound heterozygosity for Hb S and another β chain hemoglobin variant in this child. Based on their mobility patterns, Hb K-Woolwich, Hb Hope, or Hb Camden were selected by the majority of participants. These three hemoglobin variants have similar mobilities on alkaline and acid electrophoresis, and are difficult to distinguish with certainty by the use of these methods alone. If known controls are available, their use may facilitate distinction of these hemoglobin variants by alkaline and acid electrophoresis. Isoelectric focusing may be additionally informative (Figure DL-21.2). For this exercise, Hb K-Woolwich, Hb Hope, and Hb Camden were all considered good responses and are all reasonable possibilities in African Americans. By HPLC, Hb K-Woolwich elutes very close to Hb F (Figure DL-21.1). In this child, two discrete peaks were observed in the F region, which provided additional confirmation of Hb K-Woolwich.

The family study provides an instructive example of Mendelian inheritance of autosomal traits. The mother has Hb K-Woolwich trait. The father and sister have Hb S trait. The Survey exercise posed several questions concerning the segregation of these two traits in the family and the probabilities of the possible hemoglobinopathy conditions in the offspring. Figure DL-21.3 shows the expected probabilities of the possible genotypes for the offspring of these parents. The probability that the father will pass on a Hb S gene is 50%. Similarly, the probability that the mother will pass on a Hb K gene is 50%. The probability that a child of theirs will inherit both hemoglobin variants is 50% x 50%, or 25%. Only one out of four of their children would be expected to have a normal hemoglobin genotype, and 50% of their children will carry one or the other trait.

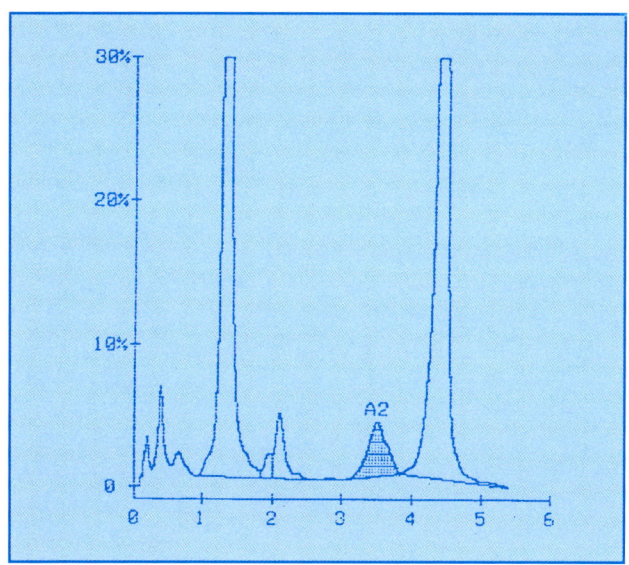

Figure DL-21.1
An example of Hb S/K-Woolwich by HPLC. In addition to a peak in the S window, representing Hb S, there is a fast peak that elutes at 1.3 minutes (P2 position), representing Hb K-Woolwich.

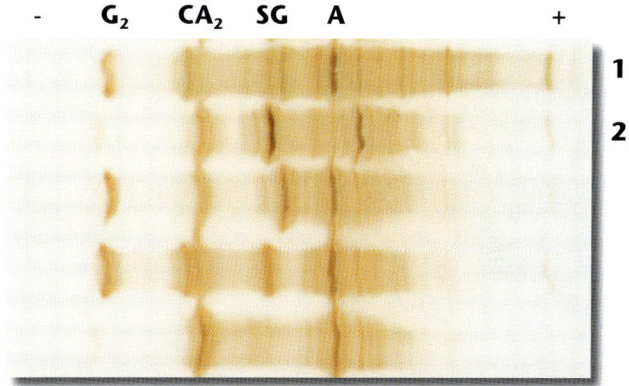

Figure DL-21.2
The same case as Hb S/Hb K-Woolwich seen in Figure DL-21.1 by isoelectric focusing. There is no Hb A present, only a band in the S position and a band anodal to Hb A. Lane 1-control specimen.

	Father	
	A	**S**
Mother **A**	AA 25%	AS 25%
Mother **K**	AK 25%	KS 25%

Figure DL-21.3
Inheritance probabilities in the family discussed in case DL-21.

Dry Lab Challenges

References

Bunn HF, Forget BG. *Hemoglobin: Molecular, Genetic and Clinical Aspects*. Philadelphia, PA: WB Saunders Co; 1986:404.

Cabannes R, Amegnizin P, Sangare A, et al. Haemoglobin K-Woolwich: a study of the family of a homozygote. *J Med Genet.* 1980;3:183-187.

Zago MA, Costa FF, Greene LJ, Bottura C. Balanced globin synthesis by Hb K-Woolwich heterozygotes. *Br J Haematol.* 1986;1:207-210.

DL-22

HISTORY
The patient is an 8-year-old male of Southeast Asian heritage who presents for a work-up due to RBC microcytosis found on a CBC. The physical examination is normal.

BLOOD COUNT DATA
RBC .... 2.87 x10^{12}/L
Hgb .... 7.6 g/dL
MCV .... 69.1 fL
WBC .... 5.5 x10^9/L
Plt .... 170 x10^9/L

OTHER LABORATORY TESTS
The solubility test for sickling hemoglobin was negative.

PERIPHERAL BLOOD SMEAR
Microcytosis, target cells.

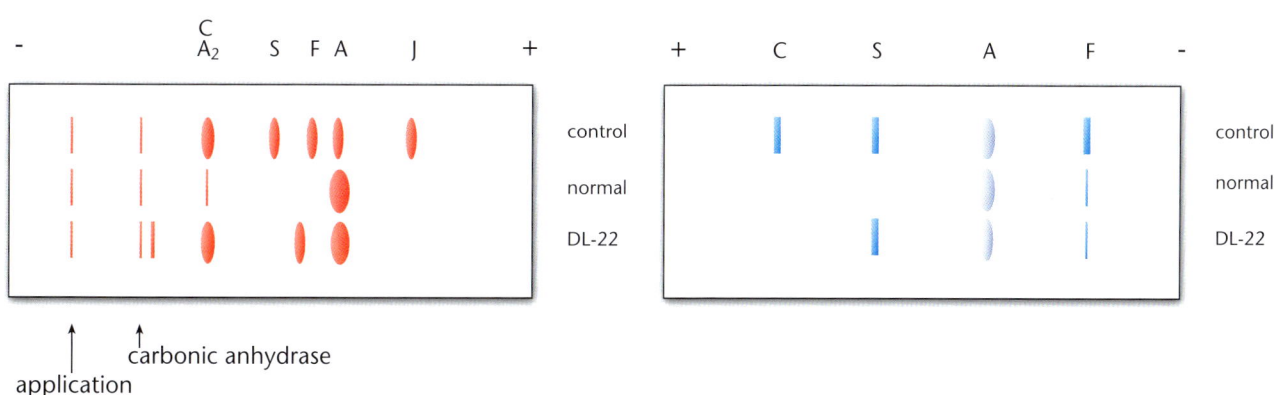

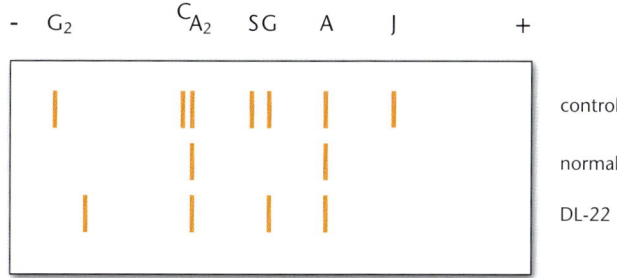

Case DL-22 Discussion

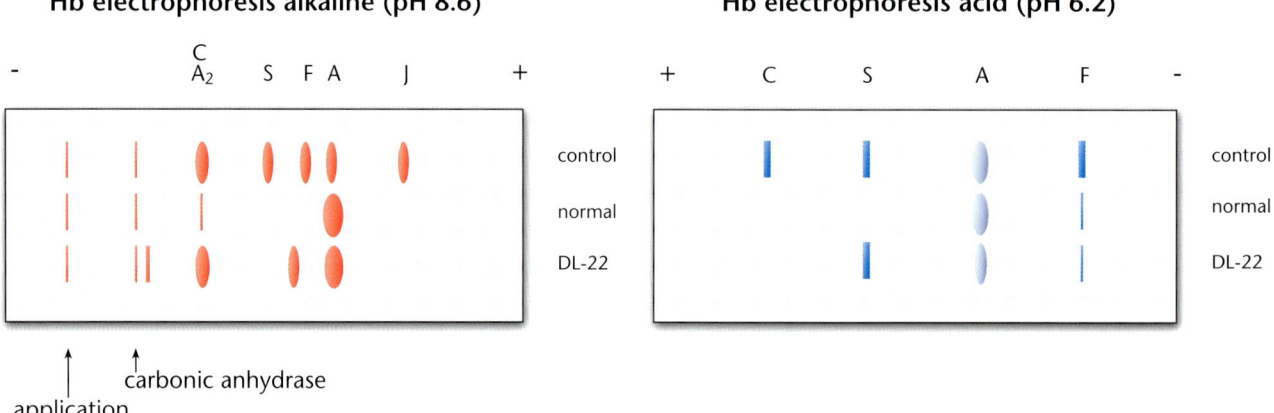

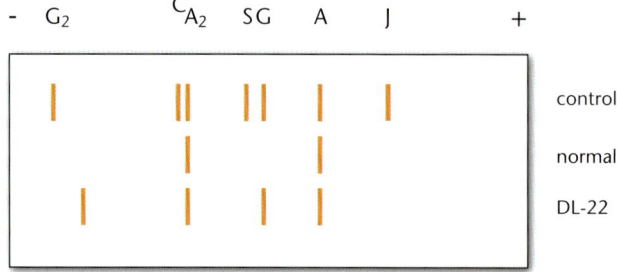

Interpretation

Examination of the alkaline electrophoresis shows there are three major bands and one minor band present. There is a band in the A position, which represents 48.7% of the total hemoglobin based on densitometry. There is also a band present between A and S (23% of total hemoglobin) and a band in the A_2 position (19.8% of the total hemoglobin). In addition, there is a small band seen just in front of the position where carbonic anhydrase migrates. This band accounts for 7.5% of the total hemoglobin. On acid electrophoresis, there are two bands seen, one in the A position and one in the S position. Similar to alkaline electrophoresis, on isoelectric focusing, there are four bands seen: one in the A position, in the position where Hb G-Philadelphia migrates, one in the A_2 position, and a further band behind the A_2 position, but not in the same position as the G_2 variant of Hb G-Philadelphia.

Diagnosis

Hb Q-Thailand/Hb E.

Performance

72.1% of laboratories correctly identified the β chain variant as Hb E. 87% of laboratories correctly deduced that the results seen were due to the combinations of an α chain variant plus a β chain variant, with 40% correctly identifying this as Hb Q-Thailand. Approximately 40% of laboratories identified the variant as Hb G-Philadelphia.

Discussion

This challenging and unusual case represents Hb E in combination with the α chain variant Hb Q-Thailand. The combination of an α and a β chain variant is not frequently seen outside of African Americans.

The bands seen on both alkaline electrophoresis and isoelectric focusing are as follows. The band in the A position represent the normal Hb A (α^A_2, β^A_2). The band between A and S represent Hb Q-Thailand (α^Q_2, β^A_2). The band in the A_2 position represents Hb E (α^A_2, β^E_2). The band near carbonic anhydrase on alkaline electrophoresis and near the G_2 position on isoelectric focusing represents both the Q/E hybrid (α^Q_2, β^E_2) and the delta variant of Hb Q-Thailand (α^Q_2, δ_2). This type of pattern is very similar to that produced when Hb G-Philadelphia is seen in combination with β chain variants also seen in African Americans, such as Hb S or Hb C. However, the α chain variant's position on alkaline electrophoresis and acid electrophoresis, and the δ variant (α^Q_2, δ_2) on isoelectric focusing are all incompatible with Hb G-Philadelphia. In cases such as this, globin chain electrophoresis can be helpful, as this demonstrates the presence of both an α and a β chain variant (Figure DL-22.2).

Hb E (β26 [B8] Glu→Lys) has appeared many times in this Atlas. As previously discussed, Hb E trait is commonly found in persons of Southeast Asian ancestry but can be seen rarely in Europeans as well as African Americans. Within Southeast Asia, it is most commonly seen in persons from Laos, Cambodia, and Thailand. At the junction of Laos, Cambodia, and Thailand, the frequency of Hb E trait approaches 50-60% of the total population. This area has been called the "Hb E triangle." Hb E is also seen in a lower frequency in other countries, such as Burma, Indonesia, and India. Interestingly, Hb E is rare in ethnic Vietnamese and is also rare in northern Asians, such as the Japanese, Chinese, and Koreans. Hb E trait results in a mild thalassemic condition accounting only for microcytosis. The alteration in the 26th codon from GAG (Glu) to AAG (Lys) creates a nucleotide sequence which activates a cryptic splicing site. If this cryptic splicing site is used, an abnormal and probably nonfunctional messenger RNA is produced. If the normal splicing site is used, a functional β chain with the Hb E mutation is produced. Thus, the Hb E mutation results in an overall decreased production of β chains, similar to other β-thalassemia mutations that affect RNA splicing.

Hb Q-Thailand (α74 [EF3] Asp→His) is a rare α chain variant that has been found in those of Asian descent, but specifically has been reported in Japanese, Thai, and, particularly, Chinese families. It has also been called Hb Mahidol, Hb Taichung, Hb Asabara, or

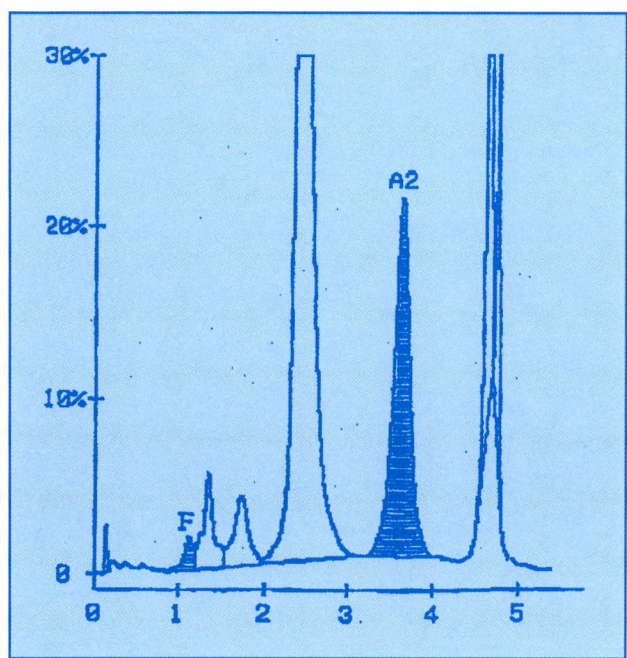

Figure DL-22.1

An example of Hb Q/Hb E by HPLC. In addition to Hb A, there is a large peak in the A_2 window, representing Hb E. There are two peaks very close together between 4.5 and 5.0 minutes. The first of these is in the S window (4.65 minutes) and represents Hb Q Thailand ($\alpha^Q_2\beta^A_2$). The second peak has a retention time of 4.75 minutes and represents the Hb Q/Hb E hybrid ($\alpha^Q_2\beta^E_2$).

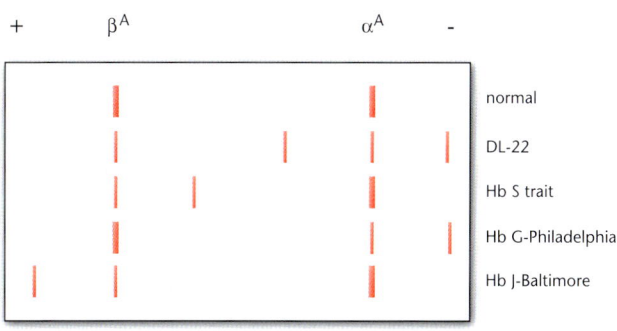

Figure DL-22.2

A diagram of alkaline globin chain electrophoresis in this case. This clearly shows the presence of both an alpha chain and beta chain variant. The alpha globin chain variant has an electrophoretic mobility very similar, but not identical, to Hb G-Philadelphia.

Hb Kurashiki. The mutation occurs on the α1 gene and is always associated with a deletion of the α2 globin gene on the same chromosome. Thus, a patient who inherited Hb Q-Thailand from one parent and a 2 α chain deletion (α-thalassemia-1 trait) would have a form of Hb H disease which has been entitled Hb Q/H disease. This combination has been discussed in case DL-10.

The combination of Hb Q and Hb E appears to be very rare. This may be due to the different ethnic groups in which the two variants are found. Hb E is rare in Chinese and Japanese, where the majority of cases of Hb Q-Thailand have been reported. Only in the Thai have both variants been reported. The hematologic manifestations of this combination are not known. It would seem reasonable to surmise that the α chain deletion associated with Hb Q-Thailand and the decreased β chain synthesis associated with Hb E trait would tend to negate each other. However, this patient is manifesting a microcytic anemia, so it is likely that there is some α/β globin chain imbalance present in this case.

References

Dormandy KM, Luck SP. Haemoglobin Q-alpha thalassemia. *Br J Med.* 1961;1:1582-1585.

Fairbanks VF. *Hemoglobinopathies and Thalassemias.* New York, NY: Brian C. Decker; 1980:174-176.

Higgs DR, et al. The genetic bases of Hb Q-H disease. *Br J Haematol.* 1980;46(3):387-400.

Lie-Injo CE, et al. The α-globin gene adjacent to the gene for Hb Q α74 asp→his is deleted, but not that adjacent to the gene for Hb G-α30 glu→gln; three-fourths of the α-globin genes are deleted in Hb Q-α-thalassemia. *Blood.* 1979;54(6):1407-1416.

Thompson MW, et al. *Genetics in Medicine.* Philadelphia, PA: WB Saunders Co; 1991:266-269.

Vella F, et al. A haemoglobinopathy involving hemoglobin H and a new (Q) haemoglobin *Br J Med.* 1958;1:752-755.

DL-23

Blood specimens from two patients were sent for hemoglobin electrophoresis.

CASE DL-23a

HISTORY
The patient is a 35-year-old male from Kuwait. He has a history of chronic anemia since childhood and has had multiple blood transfusions. He had a splenectomy 8 years previous for splenic enlargement.

BLOOD COUNT DATA
RBC .... 2.90 x10^{12}/L
Hgb .... 8.2 g/dL
MCV .... 94.0 fL
WBC .... 12.9 x10^9/L
Plt .... 775.0 x10^9/L

PERIPHERAL BLOOD SMEAR
The peripheral blood smear shows marked red blood cell anisopoikilocytosis. This includes target cells, microcytes, and acanthocytes. There are Howell-Jolly bodies and Pappenheimer bodies. There is moderate polychromasia and many nucleated RBCs.

CASE DL-23b

HISTORY
The patient is a 13-year-old African-American female. She has been healthy her entire life and has never needed a blood transfusion. The physical examination is normal.

BLOOD COUNT DATA
RBC .... 6.00 x10^{12}/L
Hgb .... 14.4 g/dL
MCV .... 76.9 fL
WBC .... 5.2 x10^9/L
Plt .... 325.0 x10^9/L

PERIPHERAL BLOOD SMEAR
The peripheral blood smear is essentially unremarkable.

The parents for both of these patients were also available for evaluation.

	DL-23a Father	DL-23a Mother	DL-23b Father	DL-23b Mother
RBC (x10^{12}/L)	5.97	5.57	5.62	4.70
Hgb (g/dL)	12.9	11.4	14.3	12.7
MCV (fL)	67.8	65.3	79.4	82.2
HbF (%)	5.1	5.2	32.0	31.8
HbA$_2$ (%)	5.6	5.9	2.2	2.0

Hb electrophoresis alkaline (pH 8.6)

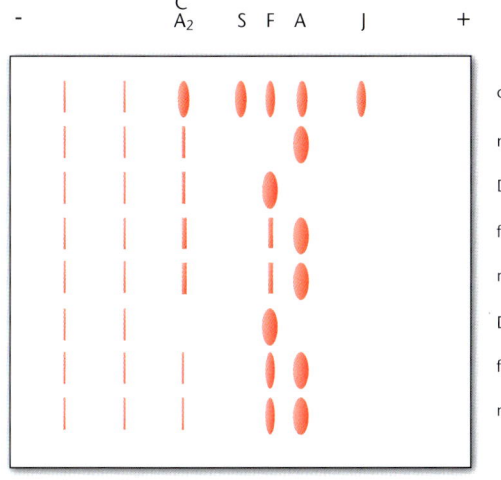

Hb electrophoresis acid (pH 6.2)

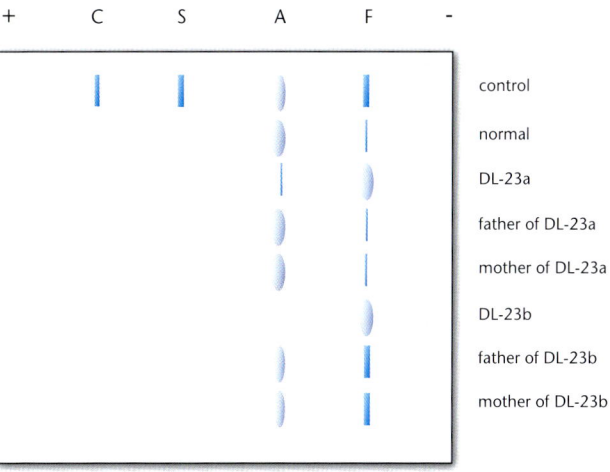

Dry Lab Challenges

Case DL-23 Discussion

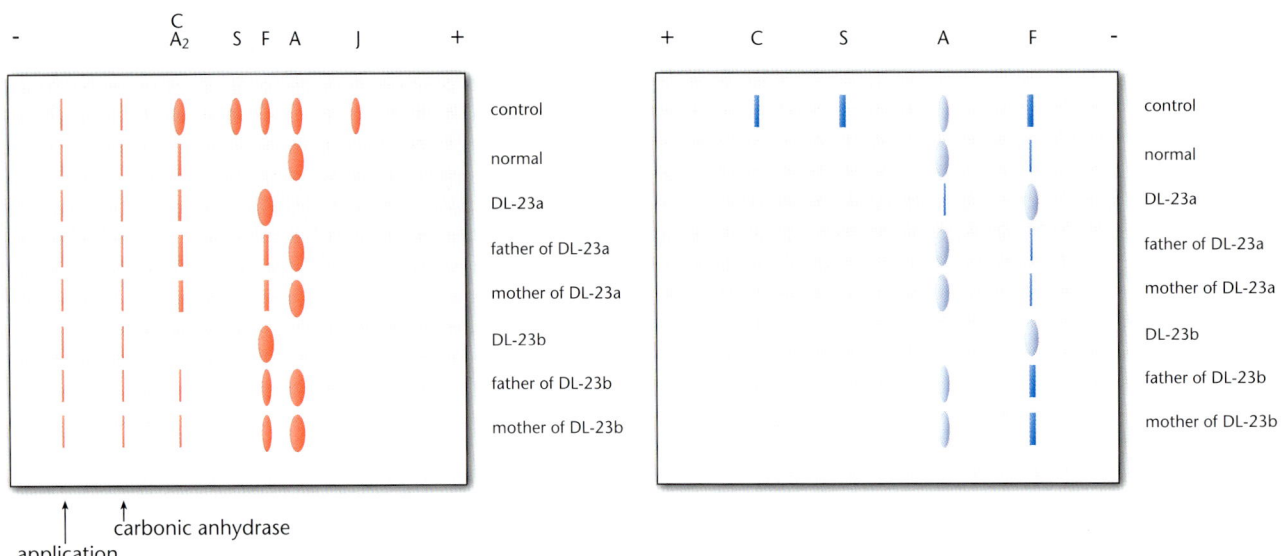

Interpretation

The alkaline and acid electrophoresis for DL-23a show no Hb A is present; only Hb F and a slight increase in Hb A_2. No other variants are present. For DL-23b, alkaline and acid electrophoresis show only Hb F to be present. There is no Hb A or Hb A_2 present. The HPLC chromatograms on these two patients are shown in Figure DL-23.1 and Figure DL-23.2.

Diagnosis

DL-23a Homozygous β°-thalassemia (β-thalassemia major).
DL-23b Homozygous hereditary persistence of fetal hemoglobin (HPFH).

Performance

For DL-23a, 93.8% of laboratories correctly identified this as a case of β-thalassemia major. For DL-23b, 98.3% of laboratories correctly identified this as representing homozygous HPFH.

Discussion

Both of these patients have similar electrophoretic patterns (i.e., mostly Hb F), but markedly different clinical histories and blood count data. Evaluation of both sets of parents is very instructive: the parents of DL-23a both have findings that are consistent with β-thalassemia trait, whereas the parents of DL-23b have elevated Hb F levels consistent with HPFH trait.

Beta-thalassemia can be due to a wide variety of genetic lesions; there are almost 200 different molecular mutations that have been described for β-thalassemia. In contrast to the alpha-thalassemias, only a minority of these mutations (17) are due to deletions, which involve either parts or all of the β globin gene. The vast majority (179 at last count) are nondeletional in nature. These are usually, but not always, point mutations that can affect the promoter regions, any of the three exons, or either intron. These mutations interfere with various aspects of DNA transcription and translation. This is discussed more fully in *A Closer Look At...Beta-Thalassemia*, page 24. The patient in DL-23a did undergo DNA analysis and was shown to be homozygous for a β-thalassemia mutation, which involves the first nucleotide of the second intron (IVS-II-1). There is a G to A substitution, which abolishes the 5′ splicing site, resulting in a β° mutation.

Hereditary persistence of fetal hemoglobin is characterized by elevation of Hb F into adulthood. At the molecular level, there are a wide variety of mutations seen which are found in many different ethnic groups. There are seven different deletional mutations that have been described in blacks, Indians, Italians, and Vietnamese. These are all due to large deletions that span both the δ and β genes. In the heterozygous (trait) form of these types of HPFH, Hb F accounts for 15-30% of the total hemoglobin. Hb A_2 is normal to slightly decreased. There are also 14 nondeletional HPFH mutations that have been described. These involve nucleotide substitutions in the $^G\gamma$ or $^A\gamma$ globin genes. For example, one type found in blacks is due to a C to G substitution at position –202 of the $^G\gamma$ gene (in the promoter region). This appears to cause a change in the binding sites of two proteins, which causes persistent overexpression of the $^G\gamma$ chains. Because this is not a deletional mutation, there is still some production of normal β chains (and thus Hb A) from the affected chromosome. The combination of Hb S with HPFH was discussed in Case 22.

It is interesting to contrast homozygous β-thalassemia (β-thalassemia major) and homozygous HPFH. In β-thalassemia major, the patients are usually moderately to severely anemic and will require lifelong transfusions. There is often splenomegaly and other signs

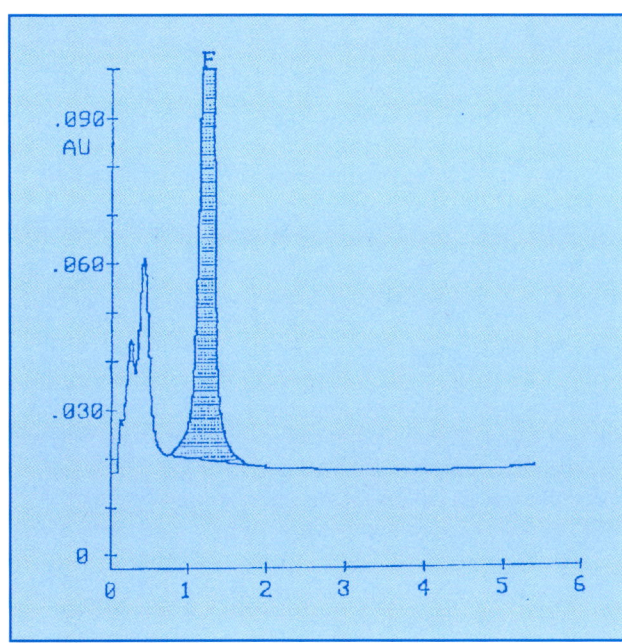

Figure DL-23.1
An example of homozygous HPFH by HPLC. There is no Hb A present. There is a prominent Hb F peak. The small peak eluting before Hb F at approximately 0.5-0.6 minutes represents acetylated Hb F.

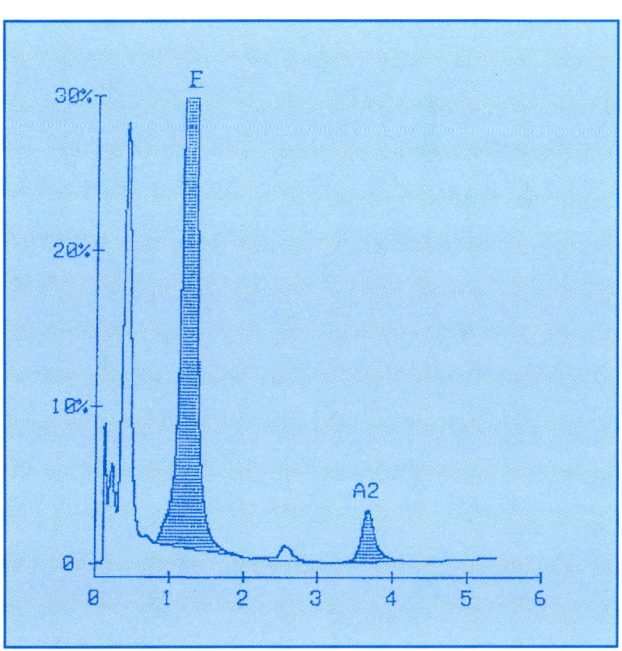

Figure DL-23.2
An example of homozygous beta-thalassemia by HPLC. This chromatogram looks very similar to that seen in Figure DL-23.1. However, there is an A_2 peak present, which was not seen in this previous example.

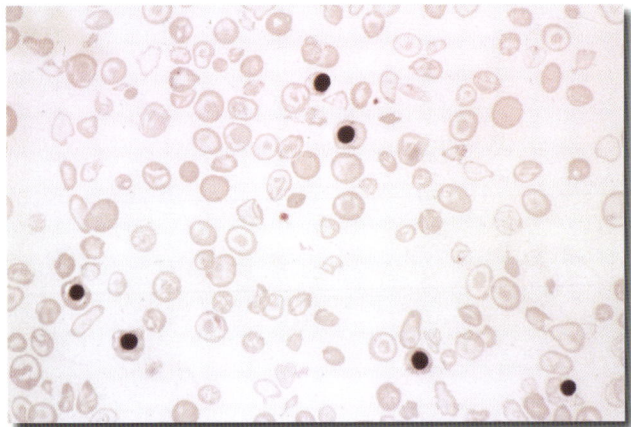 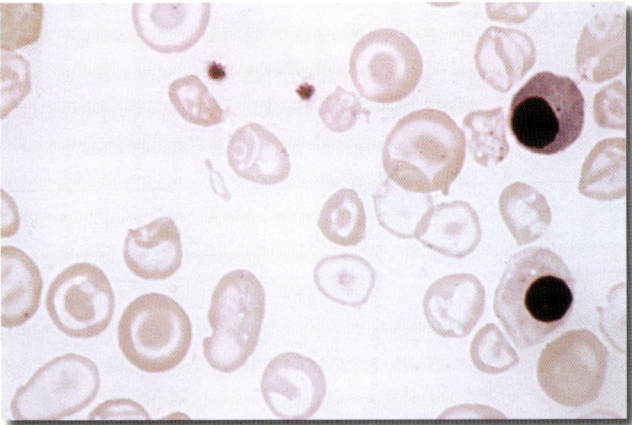

Figure DL-23.3 (Wright-Giemsa, 160x and 400x)
The peripheral blood smear from a case similar to DL-23a. There is prominent anisopoikilocytosis with many target cells and nucleated RBCs. Howell-Jolly bodies are present, indicating a previous splenectomy.

of increased bone marrow expansion, such as frontal bossing or extramedullary tumors. Because many HPFH deletions span large DNA segments that delete both the δ and β globin genes, it may be assumed that homozygous HPFH patients would also be moderately to severely anemic. However, these patients are not anemic and, in fact, usually have a mild erythrocytosis. This is due to Hb F being somewhat of a high oxygen affinity variant (due to its physiologic function *in utero*). The reason that patients with homozygous HPFH do not show the moderate to severe anemia of β-thalassemia major is likely due to the fact that the regulatory sequences for the β globin gene are also removed in deletional HPFH mutations, whereas they remain in β-thalassemia mutations. Thus, in HPFH, there can be no switch over to adult β chains, and the affected chromosome remains "locked" into production of Hb F. The α to β globin chain imbalance that is characteristic in β-thalassemia major is not present in homozygous HPFH, as the persistent production of γ chains abolishes much of this globin chain imbalance.

Some laboratories questioned the MCV value listed for DL-23a (94 fL), stating that this must be an error. These were in fact the actual CBC results from this patient at the time of his evaluation in our laboratory. The reasons for this normal MCV value are given in the case history. Most importantly, there is a previous history of splenectomy. The description of the peripheral blood mentions increased polychromasia and many nucleated red blood cells (in fact, 228/100 WBCs!). Both of these are results of the splenectomy, as the spleen is no longer able to trap the abnormal nucleated and non-nucleated RBCs. Both of these factors will act to elevate the MCV in this patient (Figure DL-23.3).

References

Bollekens JA, Forget BG. Delta beta thalassemia and hereditary persistence of fetal hemoglobin. *Hematol Oncol Clin North Am.* 1991;5:399-422.

Collins FS, Cole JL, Lockwood WK, Ianuzzi MC. The deletion in both common types of hereditary persistence of fetal hemoglobin is approximately 105 kilobases. *Blood.* 1987;70:1797-1803.

Huisman THJ, Carver MFH, Baysal E. *A Syllabus of Thalassemia Mutations.* Augusta, GA: Sickle Cell Anemia Foundation; 1997.

DL-24

HISTORY
The patient was a 10-month-old Hispanic male who presented to the emergency room with complaints of fever. The physical examination was remarkable only for pallor of mucous membranes; the spleen was not palpable. There were no prior hospitalizations or emergency room visits. The mother and father were both hematologically normal.

BLOOD COUNT DATA
RBC .... $4.9 \times 10^{12}/L$
Hgb .... 8.1 g/dL
MCV .... 79.6 fL
WBC .... $31.4 \times 10^{9}/L$
Plt .... $604 \times 10^{9}/L$

PERIPHERAL BLOOD SMEAR
Moderate sickle cells, moderate ovalocytes, and moderate target cells.

OTHER LABORATORY DATA
A solubility test for sickling hemoglobin was positive.

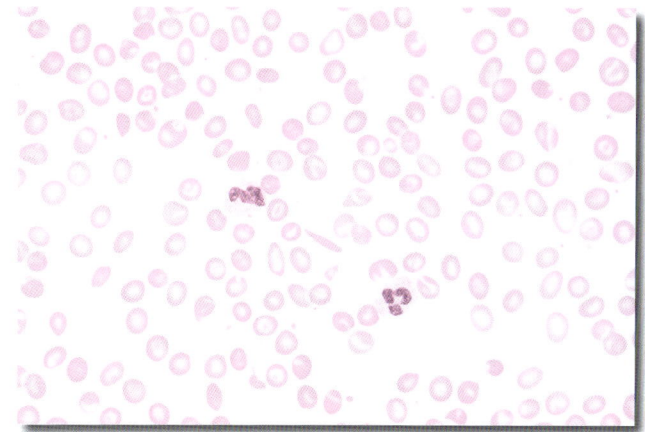

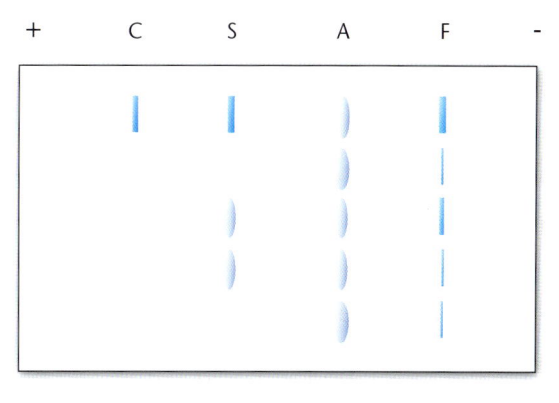

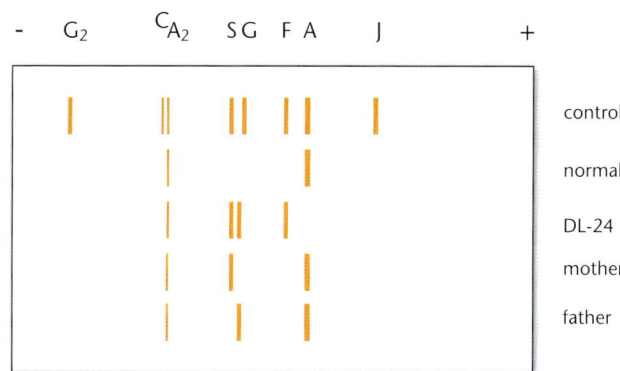

Dry Lab Challenges

Case DL-24 Discussion

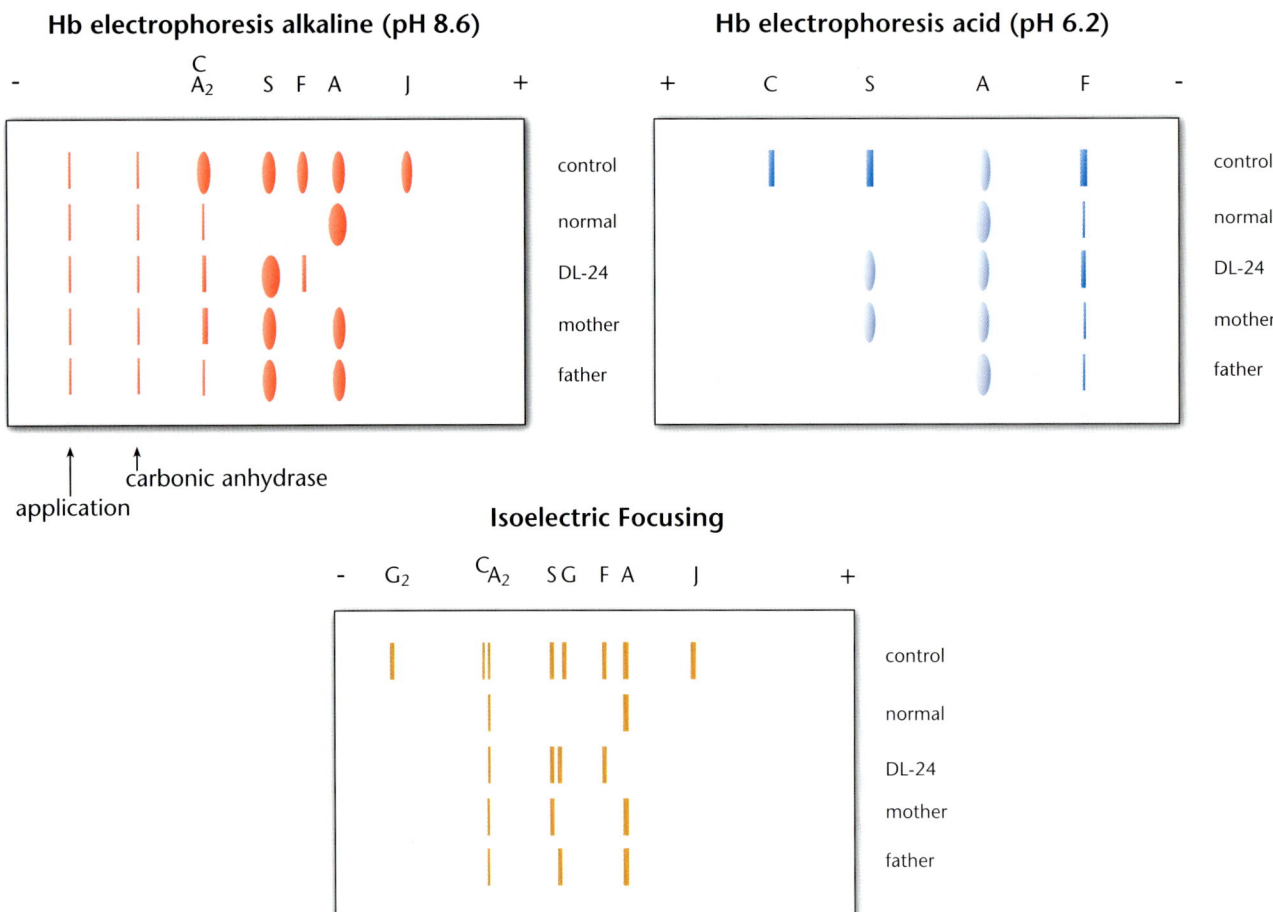

Interpretation

DL-24 Alkaline electrophoresis demonstrates a single major band in the S position and an enhanced F band. On acid electrophoresis, there are two major bands in the A and S positions. Isoelectric focusing demonstrates an abnormal band in the S position, and one that is slightly anodal to S but cathodal to the G control.

Mother On alkaline and acid electrophoresis and isolectric focusing, there are major bands in the A and S positions.

Father Alkaline electrophoresis demonstrates major bands in the A and S positions, but acid electrophoresis shows a major band only in the A position. Isoelectric focusing demonstrates Hb A and an abnormal band slightly anodal to the S position and slightly cathodal to the G control, corresponding to the one seen in the patient.

Diagnosis

Hb S/D-Los Angeles.

Performance

73.5% of participants correctly identified the presence of Hb S, and 43.8% recognized Hb D-Los Angeles. In addition, 17.8%, 34.5%, and 6.0% of participants reported the presence of Hb G-Philadelphia, HbS/G-Philadelphia, and Hb Gα, respectively.

Discussion

This case represents a case of double heterozygosity for Hb S [β6 (A3) Glu→Val] and Hb D-Los Angeles (β121 Glu→Gln). Both variants have been discussed previously (see Cases 7 and 11). Hemoglobin D-Los Angeles by itself is an innocuous variant; even in the homozygous state, it results in no hematologic abnormalities. However, despite this, when Hb D-Los Angeles is present in the double heterozygous state with Hb S, it produces a sickling disorder. This is thought to be due to the amino acid substitution at the 121st amino acid of the β chain, a critical contact site for Hb S polymerization. Therefore, while Hb D-Los Angeles is not itself a sickling hemoglobin, it participates in the polymerization of Hb S. These characteristics are shared by Hb O-Arab, another variant with a substitution at the 121st amino acid of the β chain. Both Hb S and Hb D are rare in Latino populations, although isolated areas in Mexico with a prevalence of S-trait as high as 6% have been described. The combination of Hb S and Hb D has been previously reported from Mexico.

Clinically, Hb S/D disease is a moderately severe hemolytic disorder with hemoglobin levels typically in the range of 7-10 g/dL. Some individuals have a debilitating disease with frequent pain crises, similar to SS disease. However, more commonly, pain crises are infrequent or absent. In addition, splenomegaly may be seen, in contrast to the uniform finding of splenic auto-infarction in SS disease. Blood smears from patients with S/D disease will demonstrate sickled cells, target cells, and increased polychromasia (Figure DL-24.1).

On alkaline electrophoresis, in Hb S/D disease one sees a single major band in the S position, mimicking SS disease. However, on acid electrophoresis, there are two major bands in the S and A positions. In the current case, the infant inherited Hb S from his mother and Hb D-Los Angeles from his father. The major differential diagnoses for a hemoglobin migrating in the S position on alkaline electrophoresis and the A position on acid electrophoresis are Hb G-Philadelphia and Hb Lepore. However, Hb G-Philadelphia is an α chain variant and will represent a smaller proportion of the total hemoglobin than Hb D-Los Angeles. Furthermore, the combination of Hb S and Hb G-Philadelphia produces a complex and virtually diagnostic pattern on alkaline electrophoresis (see Case 17, page 85). Finally, Hb S/G-Philadelphia is a benign combination that produces no clinical or hematologic abnormalities. Isoelectric focusing may be helpful to confirm Hb D (as in the current case), as it has a different isoelectric point from Hb S and Hb G-Philadelphia. Hb Lepore is an underproduced δ/β hybrid hemoglobin which represents only 7-15% of total hemoglobin in the heterozygous state. The rare variant Hb Korle-Bu may be very difficult to distinguish from Hb D-Los Angeles. However, when there is no Hb A present (as in the current case), Hb Korle-Bu can be seen to migrate slightly anodal to Hb A on acid electrophoresis (see Case 20, page 97). HPLC can be very helpful in distinguishing these two hemoglobin variants. Hb D-Los Angeles elutes in the D window (approximately 4.20 minutes), whereas Hb Korle-Bu elutes in the A_2 window (approximately 3.80 minutes). (Compare Figure DL-24.2 with Figure 20.1, page 99.)

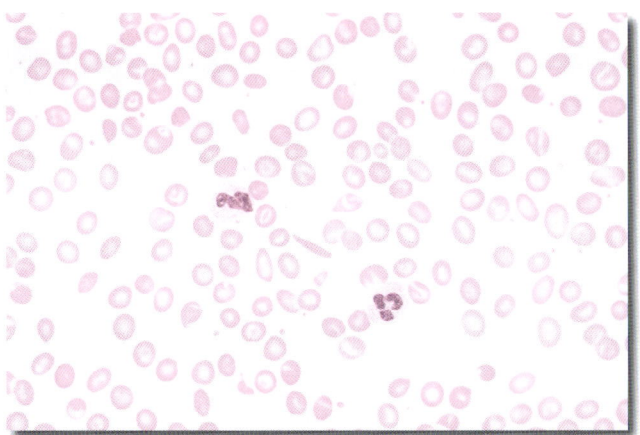
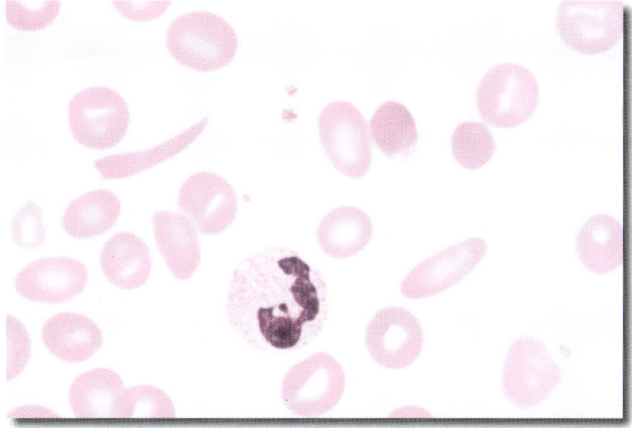

Figure DL-24.1 (Wright-Giemsa, 160x and 400x)
The peripheral blood smear from a patient with Hb S/D-Los Angeles. In addition to occasional sickle cells, there are target cells, elliptocytes, and spherocytes.

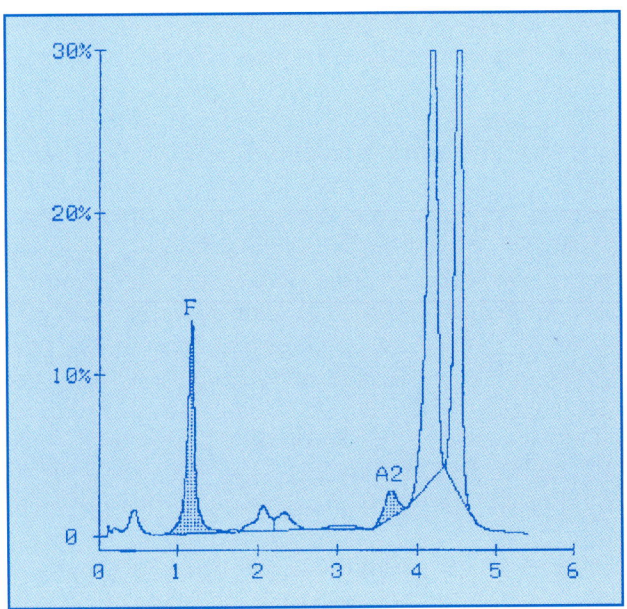

Figure DL-24.2
An example of Hb S/D-Los Angeles by HPLC. There is no Hb A present. Hb S elutes in the S window at approximately 4.5 minutes, and Hb D-Los Angeles elutes in the D window at approximately 4.2 minutes.

References

Cawein MJ, Lappat EJ, Brangle RW, et al. Hemoglobin S-D disease. *Ann Intern Med.* 1965;64:62-70.

Dover GJ, Platt OS. Sickle cell disease. In: Nathan DG, Orkin SH, eds. *Hematology of Infancy and Childhood.* 5th ed. Philadelphia, PA: WB Saunders Co; 1998:762-809.

Itano HA. A third abnormal hemoglobin associated with hereditary hemolytic anemia. *Proc Nat Acad Sci USA.* 1951;37:775-784.

Kelleher JF Jr, Park JO, Kim HC, et al. Life-threatening complications in a child with hemoglobin SD-Los Angeles disease. *Hemoglobin.* 1984;8:203-213.

Perea FJ, Casas-Castaneda M, Villalobos-Arambula AR, et al. Hb D-Los Angeles associated with Hb S or beta-thalassemia in four Mexican Mestizo families. *Hemoglobin.* 1999;23:231-237.

Reyes Cruz G, Hernandez Acasiete M, Ruiz Reyes G. Identification of a focus of beta-thalassemia in Tamiahua, Veracruz. *Rev Invest Clin.* 1990;42:189-192.

Schneider RG, Ueda S, Alperin JB, et al. Hemoglobin D Los Angeles in two Caucasian families: hemoglobin SD disease and hemoglobin D thalassemia. *Blood.* 1968;32:250-259.

Sturgeon P, Itano HA, Bergren WR. Clinical manifestations of inherited abnormal hemoglobins, I: the interaction of hemoglobin-S with hemoglobin-D. *Blood.* 1955;10:389-404.

Wang WC, Lukens JNL. Sickle cell anemia and other sickling syndromes. In: Lee GR, Foerster J, Lukens J, et al, eds. *Wintrobe's Clinical Hematology.* 10th ed. Baltimore, MD: Williams and Wilkins; 1999:1346-1397.

Section IV: Appendix

Year	Survey Number	Result
1986	HG-01	δβ-Thalassemia Trait
	HG-02	Hb S Trait
	HG-03	Iron Deficiency in a Southeast Asian
	HG-04	Hb Lepore Trait
	HG-05	β-Thalassemia Trait
	HG-06	Hb E Trait
	HG-07	Hereditary Persistence of Fetal Hemoglobin (HPFH)
	HG-08	Hb Malmö Trait
1987	HG-01	Hb S/C Disease
	HG-02	Hb D-Los Angeles Trait
	HG-03	Hb Köln Trait
	HG-04	Hb J-Baltimore Trait
	HG-05	β-Thalassemia Trait
	HG-06	Hb S Trait/G-Philadelphia Trait
	HG-07	E Trait with Iron Deficiency
	HG-08	Hb C Trait
1988	HG-01	Homozygous Hb E
	HG-02	Hb Lepore Trait
	HG-03	Hb D-Los Angeles Trait
	HG-04	Hb S/G-Philadelphia
	HG-05	Hb S/α-Thalassemia-2/Hb A_2'
	HG-06	Hb O-Arab Trait
	HG-07	Hb S/HPFH
	HG-08	β-Thalassemia Trait/ Hb A_2' Trait
	HG-09	Hb H Disease (DL)
1989	HG-01	Hb S/β⁰-Thalassemia
	HG-02	Hb Hasharon Trait
	HG-03	Hb Q-Thailand Trait/α-Thalassemia-2 Trait
	HG-04	G-6-PD Deficiency
	HG-05	Hb G-Philadelphia trait/α-Thalassemia-2 Trait (neonate) (DL)
	HG-06	Hb C/β⁰-Thalassemia
	HG-07	β-Thalassemia Trait
	HG-08	Hb E Trait/α-Thalassemia
	HG-09	Pyruvate Kinase Deficiency
	HG-10	Hb F-Texas I Trait (DL)

Appendix A

General References Pertaining to Hemoglobinopathies and Thalassemias

Many participants in the CAP Hemoglobinopathy Survey have asked about general references that pertain to hemoglobin disorders. Previously, the choices were few, as many texts were out of print and not available. Fortunately, in the past year, several new texts have become available. The following is a list of books that we have found very useful.

Fairbanks VF. *Hemoglobinopathies and Thalassemias.* New York, NY: Brian C. Decker; 1980.

Bunn HT, Forget BG. *Hemoglobin: Molecular, Genetic and Clinical Aspects.* Philadelphia, PA: WB Saunders Co; 1986.

Winter WP (Ed). *Hemoglobin Variants in Human Populations.* Vols. I and II. Boca Raton, FL: CRC Press Inc; 1986.

The preceding three books are now out of print. However, these still contain much useful information if a copy can be found. The Winter text is a epidemiologic study of hemoglobin variants in many ethnic groups throughout the world.

Steinberg MH, Forget BG, Higgs DR, Nagel RC. *Disorders of Hemoglobin. Genetics, Pathophysiology and Clinical Management.* Cambridge, England: Cambridge University Press; 2001.

This is a new, very comprehensive text, which covers both hemoglobinopathies and thalassemias. It largely replaces the Bunn and Forget text that is cited above.

Weatherall DJ, Clegg JB. *The Thalassemia Syndromes.* 4th ed. Oxford, England: Blackwell Science Ltd; 2001.

This authoritative text is now in its fourth edition. This is the best review of thalassemic disorders that is available.

Bain B. *Haemoglobinopathy Diagnosis.* Oxford, England: Blackwell Science Ltd; 2001.

This new book is a good general review of hemoglobinopathies and thalassemias. It is well illustrated and contains a series of case studies at the back of the book.

Huismann THJ, Carver MFH, Efremov CD. *A Syllabus of Human Hemoglobin Variants.* 2nd ed. Atlanta, GA: Sickle Cell Anemia Foundation; 1998.

Huisman THJ, Carver MFH, Baysal E. *A Syllabus of Thalassemia Mutations.* Atlanta, GA: Sickle Cell Anemia Foundation; 1997.

These two texts list every known hemoglobin variant and thalassemic mutation that has been reported in the literature up to the date of publication. These two volumes will be too detailed for those seeking a general overview. However, they are a good source of information for those seeking details about a specific hemoglobin variant or thalassemia mutation, particularly rare ones.

Appendix B

A Listing of Samples Used in the CAP Hemoglobinopathy Survey by Year

Year	Survey Number	Result
1986	HG-01	δβ-Thalassemia Trait
	HG-02	Hb S Trait
	HG-03	Iron Deficiency in a Southeast Asian
	HG-04	Hb Lepore Trait
	HG-05	β-Thalassemia Trait
	HG-06	Hb E Trait
	HG-07	Hereditary Persistence of Fetal Hemoglobin (HPFH)
	HG-08	Hb Malmö Trait
1987	HG-01	Hb S/C Disease
	HG-02	Hb D-Los Angeles Trait
	HG-03	Hb Köln Trait
	HG-04	Hb J-Baltimore Trait
	HG-05	β-Thalassemia Trait
	HG-06	Hb S Trait/G-Philadelphia Trait
	HG-07	E Trait with Iron Deficiency
	HG-08	Hb C Trait
1988	HG-01	Homozygous Hb E
	HG-02	Hb Lepore Trait
	HG-03	Hb D-Los Angeles Trait
	HG-04	Hb S/G-Philadelphia
	HG-05	Hb S/α-Thalassemia-2/Hb A_2'
	HG-06	Hb O-Arab Trait
	HG-07	Hb S Trait/HPFH Trait
	HG-08	β-Thalassemia Trait/ Hb A_2' Trait
	HG-09	Hb H Disease (DL)
1989	HG-01	Hb S/$β^+$-Thalassemia
	HG-02	Hb Hasharon Trait
	HG-03	Hb Q-Thailand Trait/α-Thalassemia-2 Trait
	HG-04	G-6-PD Deficiency
	HG-05	Hb G-Philadelphia Trait/α-Thalassemia-2 Trait (neonate) (DL)
	HG-06	Hb C/$β^+$-Thalassemia
	HG-07	β-Thalassemia Trait
	HG-08	Hb E Trait/α-Thalassemia
	HG-09	Pyruvate Kinase Deficiency
	HG-10	Hb F-Texas I Trait (DL)

Note: DL= Dry Lab Challenges

Year	Survey Number	Result
1990	HG-01	Hb S-Trait
	HG-02	Homozygous Hb A_2'
	HG-03	Hb British Columbia Trait
	HG-04	High Hb A_2 and Hb F
	HG-05	Hb D-Los Angeles Trait
	HG-06	Hb S/Hb Hope
	HG-07	Hb AE-Bart's Disease (DL)
	HG-08	Hb S Trait
	HG-09	Hb C/β^o-Thalassemia
	HG-10	Hb I Trait
	HG-11	Hb S Trait
	HG-12	Hb D-Los Angeles Trait
	HG-13	β-Thalassemia Trait
	HG-14	Hb S/β^o-Thalassemia (neonate) (DL)
1991	HG-01	Hb S Trait
	HG-02	Hb G-Philadelphia Trait/α-Thalassemia-2 trait
	HG-03	Hb Lepore Trait
	HG-04	$\delta\beta$-Thalassemia Trait
	HG-05	Hb S/C Disease
	HG-06	Hb S/Hb E
	HG-07	Hb S/C/G-Philadelphia (neonate) (DL)
	HG-08	G-6-PD Deficiency
	HG-09	Hb S Trait
	HG-10	Hb S/G-Philadelphia
	HG-11	Hb S Trait
	HG-12	Hb G-Coushatta Trait
	HG-13	Hb D-Los Angeles Trait
	HG-14	Hb E Trait/α-Thalassemia Trait (neonate) (DL)
1992	HG-01	Hb S Trait
	HG-02	Hb O-Arab Trait
	HG-03	Pyruvate Kinase Deficiency
	HG-04	Normal
	HG-05	Homozygous Hb E
	HG-06	Hb S/Hb N-Baltimore
	HG-07	Hb S/O-Arab (neonate) (DL)
	HG-08	Hb S Trait Transfused
	HG-09	Hb S/C Transfused
	HG-10	Hb Lepore Trait
	HG-11	Hb S Trait
	HG-12	Hb Köln Trait
	HG-13	Homozygous Hb S
	HG-14	Hb S/C-Harlem (DL)

Year	Survey Number	Result
1993	HG-01	Hb S Trait
	HG-02	Hb E Trait
	HG-03	Hb Kempsey Trait
	HG-04	Hb Q-Thailand/H Disease (DL)
	HG-05	Iron Deficiency in SE Asian
	HG-06	Hb S/Korle Bu
	HG-07	β-Thalassemia Trait
	HG-08	HPFH/β$^+$-Thalassemia Trait
	HG-09	HPFH/Hb C Trait
	HG-10	Hb S Trait
	HG-11	Sickle Cell Anemia with High F (DL)
1994	HG-01	Hb S Trait
	HG-02	Hb I Trait
	HG-03	Hb Zürich Trait
	HG-04	Normal Adult
	HG-05	Hb D-Los Angeles Trait
	HG-06	Hb C Trait
	HG-07	Hb H/Hb Constant Spring (DL)
	HG-08	Hb S Trait
	HG-09	Normal Adult
	HG-10	Hb Lepore Trait
	HG-11	Homozygous Hb S with Hb G-Philadelphia (DL)
1995	HG-01	Hb S Trait
	HG-02	Hb G-Philadelphia Trait
	HG-03	Hb A$_2$' Trait
	HG-04	Normal Adult
	HG-05	Hb Andrew Minneapolis Trait
	HG-06	Hb C Trait
	HG-07	Artifacts (DL)
	HG-08	HPFH
	HG-09	Hb C Trait
	HG-10	Hb S Trait
	HG-11	Hb S/Hb J-Baltimore (DL)
1996	HG-01	Hb S Trait
	HG-02	Hb E Trait
	HG-03	Hb O-Arab Trait
	HG-04	Hb C Trait
	HG-05	Hb S Trait
	HG-06	Hb Köln Trait
	HG-07	Hb C/G-Philadelphia (DL)
	HG-08	Hb S Trait
	HG-09	Normal
	HG-10	Hb D-Los Angeles Trait
	HG-11	Bart's Hydrops Fetalis (DL)

Year	Survey Number	Result
1997	HG-01	HPFH (diluted)
	HG-02	Hb S Trait
	HG-03	Hb Malmö Trait
	HG-04	Hb E/β°-Thalassemia (DL)
	HG-05	β-Thalassemia Trait
	HG-06	Hb M-Saskatoon Trait
	HG-07	Hb S Trait
	HG-08	Hb S/Hb E (DL)
	HG-09	Hb S Trait
	HG-10	Hb S/C Post-transfusion
	HG-11	Hb H/Hb Constant Spring
	HG-12	Homozygous S/Hb G-Philadelphia (DL)
1998	HG-01	Hb S Trait
	HG-02	Hb S/Hb Hope
	HG-03	Hb I Trait
	HG-04	Hb Hasharon Trait (DL)
	HG-05	Hb C Trait
	HG-06	Hb S Trait
	HG-07	Hb Russ/Hb Raleigh
	HG-08	β-Thalassemia Trait (Severe) (DL)
	HG-09	Normal Adult
	HG-10	Hb D-Los Angeles Trait
	HG-11	Hb S Trait
	HG-12	Hb S/Hb A_2' (DL)
1999	HG-01	Normal Adult
	HG-02	Hb S Trait
	HG-03	Hb E Trait
	HG-04	Normal
	HG-05	β-Thalassemia Trait
	HG-06	Hb S Trait
	HG-07	Hb S/Hb K-Woolwich (DL)
	HG-08	Increased Hb F
	HG-09	Normal Adult
	HG-10	Hb S Trait
	HG-11	Hb Q-Thailand/Hb E (DL)
2000	HG-01	Hb S Trait
	HG-02	Hb D-Los Angeles Trait
	HG-03	Hb S Trait/HPFH Trait
	HG-04	Hb S Trait
	HG-05	β-Thalassemia Trait
	HG-06	Normal
	HG-07	Homozygous β-Thalassemia vs. Homozygous HPFH (DL)
	HG-08	Increased Hb F
	HG-09	Hb C Trait
	HG-10	Hb S Trait
	HG-11	Hb H/Hb Constant Spring (DL)

Year	Survey Number	Result
2001	HG-01	Hb S Trait
	HG-02	Normal Adult
	HG-03	Hb E Trait
	HG-04	Hb C Trait
	HG-05	Normal Adult
	HG-06	Hb S Trait
	HG-07	Hb S/Hb D-Los Angeles (DL)
	HG-08	Increased Hb F
	HG-09	Hb S Trait
	HG-10	Normal Adult
	HG-11	Homozygous β^+-Thalassemia (DL)
2002	HG-01	Normal Adult
	HG-02	Hb S Trait
	HG-03	Normal Adult
	HG-04	Hb S Trait
	HG-05	Hb C Trait
	HG-06	Specimen with 8% Hb C
	HG-07	Hb E Trait/α-Thalassemia Trait (DL)
	HG-08	Elevated Hb F
	HG-09	Hb S Trait
	HG-10	β-Thalassemia Trait
	HG-11	Hb S/Hb G-Philadelphia/β-Thalassemia Trait (DL)

Index

A
Absorbance ratios, for M-hemoglobin, methemoglobin, and sulfhemoglobin, 203-204
Acanthocytes, 173, 305
Acid electrophoresis, 3
Alkaline electrophoresis, 3
α chain inclusion bodies, 170
α chain variants, associated with deletional forms of α-thalassemia, 67
α-thalassemia, 18-20, 170,
    α chain variants associated with deletional forms of, 67
    α-thalassemia-1, 18, 20, 217, 255, 263, 283, 294
    α-thalassemia-2, 18, 20, 133, 165, 217, 267, 283
        with Hb A2' and Hb S, 151-153
        with Hb Q-Thailand, 159-161
        homozygous, with Hb G-Philadelphia, 65-68
    α-thalassemia hydrops fetalis, 18-20
    α-thalassemia minor, 18, 19
    with Hb E, 51, 155-157, 241-243
    with Hb F-Texas, 223-227
    with Hb H and HbH disease, see separate headings
    with sickle cell disease, 259
Amino acid sequencing, 6-7
Ampholytes, 5
Artifacts, technical, in electrophoresis, 269-271
Aseptic necrosis, 81, 87, 257, 259
Asymmetrical hybrids
    in Hb British Columbia, 189
    in Hb Kempsey, 193
Autosomal traits, Mendelian inheritance of, 299
Autosplenectomy, 81, 87, 91

B
Basophilic stippling, 21, 23, 33, 37, 39, 65, 139, 147, 215, 233, 253, 281, 285, 289
β globin gene, anatomy of, 25
β-thalassemia, 24-27, 235
    β-thalassemia intermedia, 23, 37-40, 55
    β-thalassemia major, 23, 39, 55, 170, 305-308
    β-thalassemia minor, 18, 21-23, 39, 55, 137, 289-291
        β-thalassemia trait, see β-thalassemia minor
        β⁰-thalassemia, 24, 91
            with Hb C, 139-142
            with Hb E, 73, 285-288
            homozygous, 305-308
    β⁺-thalassemia, 24, 137
        with Hb C, 135-137
        homozygous, 37-40
    with Hb A2' trait, 147-149
    with hereditary persistence of fetal hemoglobin trait, 109-111
Bite cells, 169, 173
Buffy coat artifact, 271
Buffy coat band, 271

C
CAP Hemoglobinopathy Survey, samples used in, by year, 315-319
Capillary electrophoresis, 7
Capillary isoelectric focusing, 7
Capillary zone electrophoresis, 7
CAT box sequence, 24
Congenital heinz body hemolytic anemia, 170
Cooley's anemia, see β-thalassemia major
CO-Oximeter, principle of, 203
C-terminus, β chain variants near the, 180
Cyanosis, neonatal, 225

D
Dacrocytes, 263, 287
δβ-thalassemia, 33-35, 107
Diabetes mellitus, 121, 133, 165
Dithionate (sodium hydrosulfite), 3
DNA sequencing, 6-7
Drepanocytes, see Sickle cells

E
Electrophoresis
    acid, 3
    alkaline, 3, 6
    capillary, 7
    globin chain, 6
Embryonic hemoglobins, 283
Erythroblastosis, 39, 283
Erythrocytosis, 72, 133, 179
Extramedullary hematopoietic tumors, 73, 287, 308

F
FG corner, 179
    β chain variants in, 180
Flow cytometry for F cells, 31, 35, 107

G
Gallstones, 217
γ chain variants, 223-228
G helix, 189
    β chain variants near, 180
Globin chain electrophoresis, 6, 267
Globin gene loci, 25

Glucose 6-phosphate dehydrogenase deficiency, 170, 175
Glycerated hemoglobin, 5, 271
Glycosylated hemoglobin, see Hb A1c

H
Hand-foot syndrome, 247
Heinz bodies, 169, 170, 175, 291
Hematuria, 43
Hb A_2', 3, 5, 56, 63, 263
    with β-thalassemia, 147-149
    with Hb S and α-thalassemia-2, 151-153
    with Hb S, 153, 293-295
    homozygous, 143-145
Hb A_2-Babinga, 56
Hb A + E + Bart's Disease, 72, 157, 229-231
Hb A_{1C}, 5, 13, 111, 121, 133, 165
    Hb variants interfering with measurement of, 210
Hb Abruzzo, 180
Hb Alberta, 180, 189
Hb Andrew-Minneapolis, 133, 180, 183-185, 210
Hb Asabara, see Hb Q-Thailand
Hb B_2, see Hb A_2'
Hb Barcelona, 180
Hb Bart's, 5, 19, 255
    in alpha-thalassemia trait, 219-221, 223-228
Hb Bart's hydrops fetalis, see α-thalassemia hydrops fetalis
Hb Beth Israel, 180
Hb Bethesda, 180
Hb Brigham, 180
Hb British Columbia, 187-189, 193
Hb Buenos Aires, 175
Hb Bunbury, 180
Hb Bushwick, 175
Hb C, 3, 5, 26, 51, 62, 63, 103, 121, 129, 197, 243, 279
    with $β^0$-thalassemia, 139-142
    with $β^+$-thalassemia, 111, 135-137
    with Hb G-Philadelphia, 221, 277-280
    with Hb O-Arab, 133
    with Hb S, 85-88
        after transfusion, 195-197
        and Hb G-Philadelphia in a neonate, 237-240
    with hereditary persistence of fetal hemoglobin, 109-111
    homozygous, 75-78
    trait (heterozygous), 45-48, 52, 83
Hb Camden, 133, 299
Hb C-Georgetown, 62, 99
Hb C-Harlem, 3, 51, 63, 81, 99, 266
    with Hb S, 249-252
Hb Chemilly, 180

Hb Cochin-Port Royal, 180
Hb Constant Spring, 18, 217, 231
    with Hb H, 261-264
Hb Cowtown, 180
Hb D-Los Angeles (D-Punjab), 5, 43, 57-60, 63, 98, 99, 114, 115, 247
    with Hb S, 309-312
Hb Deer Lodge, 210
Hb Detroit, 180
Hb Djelfa, 180
Hb Duan, 67
Hb E, 3, 6, 26, 72-74, 121, 169, 284
    with α-thalassemia, 155-157, 241-243
        and Hb Constant Spring, 72
    with $β^0$-thalassemia, 73, 285-288
    with Hb H disease, 72
    with Hb Q-Thailand, 301-304
    with Hb S, 101-104
    homozygous, 69-71, 72
    with iron deficiency, 72-73
    trait (heterozygous), 44, 48, 49-52, 83
Hb E-associated disorders, 72-74
Hb Evanston, 67
Hb F, 6, 31, 35, 38, 105-107, 141, 307
Hb F-M Fort Rippley, 225
Hb F-M Osaka, 225
Hb F-Poole, 225
Hb F-Texas I, 223-228
Hb F variants, 226, 227
Hb Fannin-Lubbock, 210
Hb Fukuyama, 210
Hb G_2, 67, 95, 115, 239, 267, 295
Hb G-Accra, see Hb Korle-Bu
Hb G-Coushatta, 113-118
Hb G-Hsin-Chu, 115
Hb Gower-1, 283
Hb G-Philadelphia, 5, 43, 96, 115, 121, 161, 175, 219-221, 295, 302, 303, 311
    with Hb C, 221, 277-280
    with Hb S, 91, 93-96, 98, 311
        and Hb C, 237-240
        homozygous, 265-268
    with homozygous α-thalassemia-2, 65-68
Hb Graz, 210
Hb G-San Jose, 175
Hb G-Saskatoon, 115
Hb G-Taegu, 115
Hb G-Taichung, see Hb Q-Thailand
Hb H, 5, 18, 121, 125, 169, 175,
Hb Hasharon, 67, 115, 161-166, 169, 175
Hb H disease, 19, 20, 170, 215-218, 263, 269-271
    with Hb Constant Spring, 20, 261-264
    with Hb Q-Thailand, 253-255
Hb Heathrow, 180

Appendix

Hb Hifiyama, 210
Hb Hiroshima, 180
Hb Hokusetsu, 210
Hb Hope, 210, 299
    with Hb S, 131-134
Hb Hotel Dieu, 180
Hb I, 5, 63, 121, 123-125, 129, 217
Hb I-Burlington, see Hb I
Hb I-Philadelphia, see Hb I
Hb I-Skamania, see Hb I
Hb I-Texas, see Hb I
Hb I-Toulouse, 217
Hb J, 121, 129, 217
Hb J-Baltimore, 161, 119-122
    with Hb S, 273-275
Hb J-Capetown, 67
Hb J-Oxford, 275
Hb J-Tongariki, 67
Hb K, 133, 299
Hb Kansas, 180
Hb Kempsey, 180, 189, 191-193
Hb Kodaira, 180
Hb Köln, 167-171, 171, 180, 193
Hb Korle-Bu, 59, 60, 251, 311
    with Hb S, 97-99
Hb Kurashiki, see Hb Q-Thailand
Hb K-Woolwich, with Hb S, 297-300
Hb Le Lamentin, 210
Hb Lepore, 3, 53-56, 115, 311
Hb L-Ferrara, 165
Hb Lisbon, 210
Hb Little Rock, 180
Hb Mahidol, see Hb Q-Thailand
Hb Malmö, 5, 177-181, 193, 210
Hb Marseille/Long Island, 210
Hb McKees Rocks, 180
Hb Mequon, 175
Hb M Hyde Park, 225
Hb Mito, 180
Hb M Saskatoon, 199-205, 225
Hb N, 121
Hb N-Baltimore, 175
    with Hb S, 127-130
Hb Nigeria, 67
Hb Nottingham, 180
Hb N Seattle, 129
Hb O-Arab, 3, 51, 61-64
    with Hb C, 133
    with Hb S in a neonate, 245-248
Hb Okayama, 210
Hb Old Dominion, 180
Hb Olomouc, 210
Hb Osler, 133, 180, 210
Hb Peterborough, 175

Hb Portland, 19, 283
Hb Potomac, 180
Hb Q-Chinese, see Hb Q-Thailand
Hb Q-Iran, 175
Hb Q-San Jose, 175
Hb Q-Thailand, 67, 115, 121, 133
    with Hb H disease, 253-255
    with Hb E, 301-304
    with α-thalassemia-2, 159-161
Hb Radcliffe, 180
Hb Rainier, 180
Hb Raleigh, 210
    with Hb Russ, 207-211
Hb Rancho Mirage, 180
Hb Richmond, 180, 189, 279
Hb Rush, 180, 189
Hb Russ, with Hb Raleigh, 207-211
Hb S, 3, 5, 51, 121
    associated haplotypes, 258-259
    with β^0-thalassemia, 91, 233-235
    with β^+-thalassemia, 89-91
    with Hb A_2', 153, 293-295
        and α-thalassemia-2, 151-153
    with Hb C, 3, 85-88, 129, 247
        after transfusion, 195-197
        and Hb G-Philadelphia, 237-240
    with Hb C-Harlem, 103, 249-252
    with Hb D-Los Angeles, 309-312
    with Hb E, 101-104
    with Hb G-Philadelphia, 91, 93-96, 98, 311
    with Hb Hope, 131-134
    with Hb J-Baltimore, 273-275
    with Hb Korle-Bu, 97-99
    with Hb K-Woolwich, 297-300
    with Hb N-Baltimore, 127-130
    with Hb O-Arab, 103, 245-248
    with hereditary persistence of fetal hemoglobin, 105-108, 307
    hemoglobin variants resembling, 115-117
    homozygous, 44, 48, 52, 77, 79-83
        with Hb G-Philadelphia, 265-268
        with high Hb F levels, 257-260
        pathophysiology of, 82
    trait (heterozygous), 41-44, 48, 52, 83
        with α-thalassemia and Hb Bart's in a neonate, 133
Hb Saint Mande, 180
Hb S Antilles, 81
Hb Sealy, 165
Hb Shepherd's Bush, 175
Hb Sherwood Forest, 210
Hb Sinai, 165
Hb Sogn, 115
Hb South Florida, 210

Hb Stanleyville, 63
Hb Syracuse, 180
Hb Tacoma, 210
Hb Tarrant, 115
Hb Tatras, 210
Hb Torino, 175
Hb Wood, 180
Hb Yakima, 180, 189, 193
Hb York, 180
Hb Ypsilanti, 180, 189, 193
Hb Zürich, 173-176
Heinz bodies, 169, 170, 173, 175, 217, 291
Hemolysis/Hemolytic anemia, 18, 24, 77, 81, 87, 137, 141, 165, 169, 170, 175, 216, 217, 263, 311
Hereditary persistence of fetal hemoglobin (HPFH)
    with β-thalassemia trait, 109-111
    with Hb C, 109-111
    with Hb S, 105-108, 307
    heterozygous (trait), 30-32
    homozygous, 31, 305-308
    Swiss type, 259
High performance liquid chromatography (HPLC), 6
Howell-Jolly bodies, 37, 39, 79, 81, 173, 249, 305, 308
HPFH. see Hereditary persistence of fetal hemoglobin (HPFH)
Hydrops fetalis, see α-thalassemia hydrops fetalis
Hypochromia/Hypochromic red cells, 15, 21, 23, 37, 39, 53, 65, 69, 91, 101, 133, 137, 139, 141, 143, 147, 155, 167, 215, 217, 229, 253, 281, 283, 289
Hyposplenism, 81, 87, 103,

I
Inclusion body β-thalassemia, 291
Ingram, Vernon, 43
Ion-exchange chromatography
    In the measurement of Hb A_{1C}, 111, 121
Iron deficiency anemia, 15-17
    in Hb E trait, 157
    with beta-thalassemia trait, 26
Isoelectric focusing, 5

K
Kleihauer-Betke acid elution test
    in hereditary persistence of fetal hemoglobin, 31, 107
    in δβ-thalassemia, 33, 35

L
Leftward deletion, in α-thalassemia-2, 18, 255, 259
Leg ulcers, 81, 82, 87, 217

M
Mendelian inheritance of autosomal traits, 299
Methemoglobin, 5, 269-271
M-hemoglobins, 6, 199-205
Microcolumn chromatography, in the measurement of Hb A_2, 23, 26, 137
Microcytosis/Microcytic anemia, 15, 17, 18, 21, 23, 35, 37, 39, 45, 47, 49, 51, 53, 55, 65, 69, 71, 72, 89, 101, 103, 133, 135, 137, 139, 141, 143, 145, 147, 155, 159, 229, 233, 241, 253, 255, 257, 261, 263, 269, 281, 283, 285, 287, 289, 291, 301, 303, 305
Microvascular occlusion, 81
Monoclonal paraprotein, 269-271

N
Neonatal cyanosis, 225
Normal adult, electrophoretic patterns in, 12-13

O
Oxidant stress, 170, 175
Oxygen affinity, hemoglobin variants with altered, 177-193

P
Pappenheimer bodies, 37, 81, 305
Pauling, Linus, 43
Peroxidase, due to high WBC or PLT count, 269-271
Pigment gallstones, 81
Polychromasia, 75, 81, 141, 167, 173, 217, 229, 241, 253, 261, 265, 269, 281, 289, 305
Polymerase chain reaction (PCR) amplification, 7
Precipitated hemoglobin, disorders associated with, 170
Pulmonary artery occlusion, 73

R
Renal papillary necrosis, 87
Retinopathy, proliferative, 87
Rightward deletion, in α-thalassemia-2, 18, 259

S
Scleral icterus, 37, 79, 167, 169, 249, 253, 265
Sickle(d) cells, 79, 81, 233, 247, 249, 265, 309, 311
Sodium metabisulfite test, 83
Solubility test for sickling hemoglobulins, 3, 43, 83, 161, 247, 251
Spherocytes, 33, 75, 287, 135, 141, 169, 287
Splenic infarction, 81, 87
Splenic sequestration crisis, acute, 87, 91, 247
Splenomegaly, 71, 75, 87, 91, 103, 137, 139, 143, 169, 215, 217, 255, 261, 263, 265, 287, 291, 311
Spontaneous abortions, 87

Sulfonamides, 175
Sulfones, 175

T
Target cells, 21, 23, 37, 39, 45, 47, 49, 51, 53, 55, 65, 69, 71, 75, 77, 79, 81, 89, 101, 135, 137, 139, 141, 147, 155, 173, 195, 215, 217, 229, 233, 241, 247, 249, 253, 261, 269, 277, 279, 281, 285, 287, 289, 301, 305, 308, 309, 311
TATA box, 24
Thalassemia intermedia, 35, 255
Thromboembolic complications, 87
Tryptic peptides, 7
Typsin digestion, 7

U
Unstable hemoglobin variants, 163-176

V
Vaso-occlusive crises, 87
Vaso-occlusive phenomena, 81